Nurses After War

Mary Ellen Doherty, PhD, RN, CNM, is a professor at Western Connecticut State University, Danbury, Connecticut, teaching nursing students at the undergraduate, master's, and doctoral levels. Dr. Doherty is also an active researcher specializing in women's health and midwifery, although her most recent work focuses on nurses' experiences in the Iraq and Afghanistan wars and their reintegration. She has been a certified nurse-midwife for more than 30 years, working in both the public and private sectors. Dr. Doherty was the founder and president of Concord Nurse-Midwifery Associates, a private midwifery practice with delivery privileges at Emerson Hospital in Concord, Massachusetts. Her research articles have been published in the *Journal of Midwifery and Women's Health*, the *Journal of Nursing Scholarship*, *The Journal of Perinatal Education*, *The International Journal of Childbirth Education*, *MCN: The American Journal of Maternal–Child Nursing*, and the *Journal of Psychosocial Nursing*. She is an active member of the American College of Nurse-Midwives, three chapters of Sigma Theta Tau, the Association of Women's Health, Obstetric, and Neonatal Nurses (AWHONN), Lamaze Inc., and the International Childbirth Education Association. In 2013, Dr. Doherty received the Norton Mezvinsky Award for Excellence in Research from the Connecticut State University System Board of Regents. This was the first time the award was given to a nurse. Dr. Doherty is a reviewer for two maternal–child nursing journals and is an expert witness on maternal–newborn cases for the legal system. She has presented her research throughout the United States and in Ireland, England, Austria, and Denmark.

Elizabeth Scannell-Desch, PhD, RN, OCNS, is associate dean for undergraduate studies and a professor at the Rutgers University School of Nursing, Camden, New Jersey. Her research focuses on women's health and military nursing. She is a retired colonel in the U.S. Air Force Nurse Corps, having served 25 years on active duty, including 8 years overseas. Her last military assignment was at the Pentagon as the chief nurse executive for the entire Air Force Reserve. She was also chairperson of the nursing division at Mount Saint Mary College, Newburgh, New York, coordinator for graduate and undergraduate studies at Adelphi University, College of Nursing, Hudson Valley Center, New York, and a faculty member at Rutgers University, College of Nursing, Newark, and New Brunswick, New Jersey. Dr. Scannell-Desch has many data-based publications in national and international peer-reviewed nursing journals, including *The Western Journal of Nursing Research*, *The Journal of Nursing Scholarship*, *The Journal of Psychosocial Nursing*, *MCN: The American Journal of Maternal–Child Nursing*, *The Journal of Transcultural Nursing*, and *The Journal of Advanced Nursing*. Much of her published research has focused on nurses serving in the Vietnam War and the Iraq and Afghanistan wars. Dr. Scannell-Desch served as visiting faculty in the summer of 2001 at the University of Medicine and Pharmacy, Cluj-Napoka, Romania, and as a military consultant to the surgeon general for nursing research and oncology nursing. She received the Rita C. Kopf Memorial Research Award from the Foundation of New York State Nurses in 2010 and the Sustained Professional Performance Award from the Foundation of New York State Nurses in 2012. Dr. Scannell-Desch is a reviewer for *Military Medicine*, and has presented her research nationally and internationally.

Nurses After War

The Reintegration Experience of Nurses Returning From Iraq and Afghanistan

Mary Ellen Doherty, PhD, RN, CNM
Elizabeth Scannell-Desch, PhD, RN, OCNS

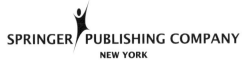

SPRINGER PUBLISHING COMPANY
NEW YORK

Springer Publishing Company, LLC
11 West 42nd Street
New York, NY 10036
www.springerpub.com

Acquisitions Editor: Joseph Morita
Senior Production Editor: Kris Parrish
Composition: Newgen KnowledgeWorks

ISBN: 978-0-8261-9413-8
e-book ISBN: 978-0-8261-9414-5

16 17 18 19 20 / 5 4 3 2 1

The author and the publisher of this Work have made every effort to use sources believed to be reliable to provide information that is accurate and compatible with the standards generally accepted at the time of publication. Because medical science is continually advancing, our knowledge base continues to expand. Therefore, as new information becomes available, changes in procedures become necessary. We recommend that the reader always consult current research and specific institutional policies before performing any clinical procedure. The author and publisher shall not be liable for any special, consequential, or exemplary damages resulting, in whole or in part, from the readers' use of, or reliance on, the information contained in this book. The publisher has no responsibility for the persistence or accuracy of URLs for external or third-party Internet websites referred to in this publication and does not guarantee that any content on such websites is, or will remain, accurate or appropriate.

Library of Congress Cataloging-in-Publication Data
Names: Doherty, Mary Ellen, author. | Scannell-Desch, Elizabeth, author.
Title: Nurses after war: the reintegration experience of nurses returning from Iraq and Afghanistan / Mary Ellen Doherty, Elizabeth Scannell-Desch.
Description: New York, NY: Springer Publishing Company, LLC, [2017] | Includes bibliographical references and index.
Identifiers: LCCN 2016012748 | ISBN 9780826194138 (alk. paper) | ISBN 9780826194145 (eBook)
Subjects: | MESH: Military Nursing | Nurses—psychology | Iraq War, 2003–2011 | Afghan Campaign 2001– | Stress Disorders, Post-Traumatic—rehabilitation | Social Support | United States | Personal Narratives
Classification: LCC RT86 | NLM WZ 112.5.N8 | DDC 610.73019–dc23
LC record available at http://lccn.loc.gov/2016012748

Special discounts on bulk quantities of our books are available to corporations, professional associations, pharmaceutical companies, health care organizations, and other qualifying groups. If you are interested in a custom book, including chapters from more than one of our titles, we can provide that service as well.

For details, please contact:
Special Sales Department, Springer Publishing Company, LLC
11 West 42nd Street, 15th Floor, New York, NY 10036–8002
Phone: 877-687-7476 or 212-431-4370; Fax: 212-941-7842
E-mail: sales@springerpub.com

Printed in the United States of America by McNaughton & Gunn.

This book is dedicated to all U.S. military nurses who have served our country. Military nurses truly exemplify the courage, dedication, commitment, leadership, and clinical expertise embodied in the nursing profession. It is also dedicated to our remaining family: Len, Chris, Meaghan, Jake, Sadie, Maxwell, and Maggie. You are the sun, the moon, and the stars to us. You motivate us to expand our horizons, seek truth, and continue our journey toward greater knowledge development. We could not do what we do without your support, understanding, and love.

Contents

Foreword   Melissa A. Rank, Major General (Ret.) USAF, NC   *ix*

Preface   *xiii*

Acronyms   *xxi*

1. Contemporary Historical Roots of the Wars in
   Iraq and Afghanistan   **1**

2. Military Medical Assets Deployed to the Iraq and
   Afghanistan Wars   **9**

3. Homecoming: A Positive Reception   **25**

4. Homecoming: A Disappointing Venture   **61**

5. Renegotiating Roles: A Family Affair   **83**

6. Painful Memories of Trauma   **91**

7. Sorting It Out: Getting Help   **115**

8. Needing a Clinical Change of Scenery   **155**

9. Petty Complaints and Trivial Whining: No Tolerance Here   **167**

10. Military Unit or Civilian Job: Support Versus Lack of Support   **175**

11. Family and Social Networks: Support Versus Lack of Support   **207**

12. Reintegration: Creating a New Normal   **227**

13. Discussion of Findings   **269**

14. Clinical Implications   **279**

15. Recommendations   **289**

Afterword   *297*

Index   *301*

Foreword

Sleepless nights consumed with images of wounded and dying soldiers and children. Enduring overwhelming guilt because a nurse lied to a patient when the patient asked, "Nurse, am I going to make it?" Vivid images of Balad trauma bays when a nurse took an art class post-deployment and the instructor splashed red, dripping watercolor across the canvas to provide more intense color. Preparing, cooking, and eating meat on the bone could no longer be tolerated. The images of the emergency department in Bagram when an uncut, large watermelon tumbled from a nurse's hand and crashed, spreading its pink juices and meaty contents across the floor. Still needing to have their helmets right beside their bedside to protect them in case of incoming attacks, long after their deployments have ended. Watching their child's baseball game for the first time after return from deployment and the crack of the ball against the bat triggered a memory and intense anxiety overwhelmed them. Vacations to sandy beaches were no longer possible after deploying to the sands of Iraq and Afghanistan. Intense frustration that they can't get over what happened in the war zone and why they cannot move on long after their combat assignments were ended. Still keeping the pictures of the wounded Iraqi and Afghani children on their cell phone and viewing them often, long after they had come home from war. A sense of great loss regarding their future direction because they were no longer serving a cause much greater than themselves. Upset, confused, and finding themselves angry in seconds over the smallest of things that never bothered them previously. Their angst that they were no longer loving, involved family members who enjoyed the presence of spouses, children, and relatives.

These are some of the stories still shared with me as nurses make their way back to the lives they led before deployment to a war zone. Stories like these unfold in this riveting book as you turn these pages.

As a hospital commander twice since September 11, 2001, and chief of the Air Force Nurse Corps, I believe the importance of the leadership team bidding farewell and welcoming home their deployers at the flight line or the airport, no matter what the hour, cannot be emphasized strongly enough. Time and again, officers and enlisted have shared how much it meant to them that, despite the fact that they left or returned in the wee hours of the night, their leaders were present on their return. Also key to their deployment was contact by e-mail, phone, and Skype, and "goodie" boxes sent from the hospital staff. It helped sustain them in knowing they were not forgotten during their time away, reminding them that their team was eagerly anticipating their return. Also, assigning a staff member from the deployers' squadron to stay in constant contact with family members and ensuring the leadership team touched base with the family throughout the deployment kept families in touch with the hospital. These families were comforted in knowing they were still anchored to us while their loved ones were away. These steps paid great dividends to the family when emergencies arose and when they were simply lonely and needed to talk. As a hospital commander and chief nurse, I felt it was my responsibility postreturn to personally see each troop, officer or enlisted, the following day to get "eyes on them" before they were released home for their recovery time with friends and family and to see them the first day they returned to duty.

What aided these deployers in beginning their personal journey toward reintegration? Alternative and complementary medicine assisted them to express their story. Composing a song about their combat experiences, creating a dance that portrayed their deployment, or painting a picture that expressed their thoughts, sights, and nightmares onto a canvas helped immensely in beginning their reintegration into society. Going back to school to further their education also helped. Throwing themselves fully into volunteer work on a local military base or in the community kick-started their recovery. Volunteering to train service animals that would eventually be assigned to a wounded warrior helped them serve a cause greater than their own. Efforts such as these were essential in assisting them to master their feelings and reset the refresh button.

Also critical in recovery were strategies that focused on relaxation and mindfulness, transporting them to a place of solace and peacefulness. Transcendental meditation proved very beneficial in quieting their minds and bodies. Exercises that included tai chi, progressive muscle relaxation, and yoga breathing, which lowered anxiety, reduced respiration, and lessened the number of posttraumatic stress symptoms, proved incredibly beneficial. Acupuncture helped make strides in restoring and rejuvenating energy. Guided imagery and horticultural therapy reduced stress. Finally, any pleasurable activities that promoted social interactions, such as horseback riding and learning new sports like surfing or skiing, had tremendous value.

"Veterans are the forward observers for the rest of us. They experienced life and death and moral anguish in which so many have been immersed" (Caplan, 2014, p. 24). "As an American, I take some responsibility for what you experienced in the military, and if you want to talk, I will listen as long as you wish to speak, and I will not judge" (p. 22).

Finally, the power of listening cannot be emphasized strongly enough. Allowing troops to share their stories of what they endured, appreciating what it means to serve in combat, and accepting without judgment the sights, feelings, smells, memories, and incidents in whatever way or order they wish to share their stories without prejudice by the listener is paramount. Listening is a higher order of communication than talking. Listening with 100% of your very fiber and intensely with your soul is critical to facilitating a recovery. No notes, no comments, and no questioning—just the fine art of listening. I have personally witnessed a nurse who told her story until she had exhausted all her anguish. She called me the next day to share that she slept through the night for the first time since she came home from the war 2 years ago. I have also listened to nurses over the phone who are now 5 years past their last deployment who are still experiencing vivid memories of combat. Yet, they tell me they are almost back to the person they were before they deployed.

The tincture of time heals the wounds of war to some degree. After experiencing the trauma of war, resilience for every officer and enlisted medic is an individual matter. The nurses in this book are on a journey of their own that is very personal, and so are many, many others who did not have this privilege of sitting around the kitchen table with Beth Scannell-Desch and Mary Ellen Doherty. To these two magnificent women and nurses, I give you my heartfelt thanks for allowing these 35 nurses to tell their stories for as long as it took them. This is the second of two books that catapults the reader vividly into the war zone and the heart-wrenching struggles endured emotionally, physically, personally, spiritually, and professionally during and after being assigned to a combat zone. Let us all hope that the tincture of time allows all to rediscover their resilience, rejuvenate holistically, and come to a place of restoration that returns our medics to the highly functioning individuals they are known to be in the workplace and at home.

Beth and Mary Ellen, thank you for inviting me to listen to the stories of these nurses and allowing me to be part of this account of their lives. You both made me feel like I was sitting at the kitchen table right beside you. It has been a journey of healing for me, as well, as I read the pages, and for that I am extremely grateful.

Melissa A. Rank, Major General (Ret.) USAF, NC
U.S. Air Force, Nurse Corps

REFERENCE

Caplan, P. J. (2014, June/July). Listening: A means to understanding war vets. *VFW Magazine, 4,* 22-24.

Preface

They hailed from the midwestern plains of Missouri and Nebraska, the oil field communities of Texas and Oklahoma, the historic cities of Baltimore and Philadelphia, and the shores of California. Some were recent college graduates, others were parents of young children, and still others were middle-aged professionals. A few were Latino Americans, whereas others were of Irish, African American, or Eastern European descent. Some were reared on farms; others grew up in suburbia or in urban centers. All were registered nurses serving the United States as members of the Army, Navy, or Air Force Nurse Corps. Many served in the active component, while others were Reserve or National Guard officers who were called to active duty for a specified period of time. Most of these nurses were women. All swore to protect and defend the United States in times of peace as well as war. Since 2003, these nurses have deployed to places such as Tikrit, Karbala, Ramadi, or Fallujah, Iraq; and Kabul, Kandahar, Mazar-e-Sharif, or Bagram, Afghanistan. As military officers, these nurses carried weapons to protect themselves and their patients. They were just as vulnerable to injury or death as anyone else in the war zones of Iraq and Afghanistan. As their medevac planes and helicopters were targeted by small-arms fire and their hospital compounds were subject to sporadic mortar attacks, these military nurses continued to provide care to wounded coalition troops, enemy prisoner patients, injured civilians, and children caught in the crossfire of war.

This book tells the nurses' reintegration stories once they returned to U.S. soil. The current study was born from finding previous studies examining the lived experiences of military nurses in the Iraq and Afghanistan wars (Scannell-Desch & Doherty, 2010), women nurses' health and hygiene experiences while deployed (Doherty & Scannell-Desch, 2012), and deployed nurse-parents' experiences (Scannell-Desch & Doherty, 2013). These aforementioned studies, using different sample cohorts from the current study, led the authors to wonder how military nurses would describe their homecoming and reintegration to the workplace, family, and community. Would these returning nurses use mental health services during their reintegration? What would they describe as challenges, triumphs, issues, and disappointments? What would they describe as helpful with homecoming and reintegration?

We identified a void in the current literature about nurse reintegration following wartime deployment to Iraq and Afghanistan. Review of the current research literature revealed only two studies that investigated characteristics of nurses' reintegration after returning from deployment to war. Rivers, Gordon, Speraw, and Reese (2013) examined the experiences of 22 active duty U.S. Army nurses transferred to two stateside army hospitals following an assignment in Iraq or Afghanistan. These investigators interviewed each nurse using one broad research question: "What stands out for you when you think about your experience of reintegration and coming home from deployment?" Data analysis produced five themes: (a) command support: no one cares; (b) check the blocks; (c) the stress of coming home; (d) they do not understand; and (e) it changes you.

Rivers and colleagues (2013) depicted the "command support" theme as the nurses believing that no one in their hospitals or in nursing administration knew or cared about their war experiences or appreciated that they had just returned from wartime deployment. Nurses portrayed a lack of acknowledgment or interest in their war zone service and a business-as-usual attitude toward getting them acclimated to the stateside practice milieu. The "check the blocks" theme described a succession of mandatory briefings administered at overseas transition centers in Germany or Kuwait, or at stateside bases once military personnel returned from war deployment. Nurses described these briefings as a rigid agenda of topics covered by trainers, most of whom had never deployed to war and were perceived as uncaring and in a hurry. The theme of "stress of coming home" focused on being overwhelmed with work and family responsibilities as the nurses struggled to keep abreast of all the changes in their environment. The theme of "they do not understand" centered on the perception that those who have not deployed to war, including family, friends, and even other military members, cannot truly comprehend and appreciate what these nurses experienced. Finally, the theme of "it changes you" emphasized that the nurses are not the same as they were before they deployed to war. Rivers and colleagues (2013) in their recommendations for the future called for enhanced reintegration support to be provided by the military services.

The second published study on nurse reintegration (Hopkins-Chadwick, 2012) investigated strategies to support nurses as they transitioned back to working in stateside U.S. Army hospitals. Hopkins-Chadwick conducted focus groups with 12 active duty U.S. Army nurses. These nurses were asked what actions would have enhanced their transition after returning from Iraq or Afghanistan. Five themes emerged from the focus groups:

- Recognize us and our families for our service and sacrifice with a "welcome home" event.
- Make an honest effort to give us assignments that move us forward in our careers.
- Treat all of us as though we plan to stay in the military.
- You make nursing work harder than it has to be.
- Periodically evaluate postdeployment health and well-being.

The nurses in this study (Hopkins-Chadwick, 2012) emphasized that homecoming recognition was very important and they were eager and excited about new career challenges after homecoming leave. Some nurses expressed frustration with peers and supervisors who appeared to not comprehend the level of work and new skills they mastered while deployed. Many of the nurses expressed indecision about remaining in the army, but stressed that all returnees should be mentored by superiors just as if they planned to make the army a career. This group of nurses agreed that their immediate supervisors should be crucial links to their successful reintegration. Based on the findings from this study, Hopkins-Chadwick constructed a list of tasks for peers and supervisors to use in supporting returning nurses.

This book originated from a qualitative research study examining the reintegration experiences of military nurses who served in the Iraq and Afghanistan wars from 2003 to 2013. In this study, 35 U.S. military nurses voluntarily told their stories of homecoming and reintegration with their families, stateside communities, and workplaces. All of the nurses had served at least one tour of duty in Iraq or Afghanistan, and included 11 army, 12 navy, and 12 air force nurses. Deployments for study participants ranged from 4 to 12 months. Thirteen nurses had served two tours of duty in Iraq or Afghanistan, and four nurses served three deployments to these wars. Of the 35 nurses, 32 were women and three were men (Doherty & Scannell-Desch, 2015). The nurses ranged in age from 25 to 57 years, with a mean age of 37 years at the time of the study. Most had been home for 3 years since their last deployment. One-half of participants were married with children when they deployed.

Informants were willing to share their experiences, consented to having their interviews audio-recorded, and agreed to validate interview transcripts. We used Colaizzi's (1978) phenomenological method of data analysis to guide discernment of the lived experience of reintegration in our research study. This method includes facets of both descriptive and interpretive phenomenology, seeks to describe the experience in terms of essential structures, and focuses on the subjective accounts of individuals telling their stories. Phenomenologists study human experience from the viewpoint of those living through or encountering a particular human phenomenon. For example, the phenomenon could be witnessing the death of a soldier, taking care of enemy prisoner patients, or working in a triage tent. Phenomenology as a method seeks to describe and construct the meaning of a human experience through intense interviewing and dialogue with persons who are living, or have lived, the particular experience (LoBiondo-Wood & Haber, 2014). Phenomenology is grounded in the assumption that there is a structure and there are common components to shared human experiences (Marshall & Rossman, 2011).

Our study participants included military registered nurses assigned to combat support hospitals, aeromedical evacuation aircraft and helicopters, mobile surgical teams, detainee prison hospitals, and local Iraqi and Afghan hospitals. Sampling criteria for inclusion in this study included study participants who were (a) registered nurses; (b) able to read, write, and speak English; (c) current or former members of the Army, Navy, or Air Force Nurse Corps; (d) able to recall their experiences of homecoming and reintegration as military nurses returning from a deployment to Iraq and/or Afghanistan; and (e) willing to discuss their war and homecoming experiences. This group included active duty component nurses as well as those from the Reserves and National Guard. Contact information for this population of nurses was not readily available, so a purposive sample was drawn employing "snowball sampling" (Polit & Beck, 2011).

To gain access to this population of interest we contacted two national veteran organizations and one nursing organization. All three organizations advertised a short description of our study purpose and contact information for any interested nurses. We received nine inquiries from nurses who met our study criteria. We began snowball sampling with these nurses. We mailed all potential participants who contacted us a letter describing the purpose and aim of the study along with a self-addressed, stamped return form indicating interest and demographics, e-mail address, telephone contact information, and an informed consent form to voluntarily agree to participate in this study. After we received the returned forms, an e-mail was sent to schedule an interview. The nine nurses who expressed interest in participating in the study contacted other nurses who met our study inclusion criteria. As a result, more nurses agreed to participate in the study. Sequential participants were selected for participation as data collection and data analysis proceeded. These practices served to expand the scope, range, and depth of information (Denzin & Lincoln, 2011).

Interview locations were selected by study participants. These included cafés, restaurants, offices, and residences. Most interviews were conducted face to face; however, due to geographical constraints, several were conducted via speaker-phone. Face-to-face interviews were conducted in the northeastern and southeastern United States. Most telephone interviews included nurses in the western continental United States and Hawaii. Interviews ranged from 40 to 90 minutes. All interviews were audio-recorded. Approval from the university institutional review boards where the investigators were employed was obtained before commencing data collection, as was approval from the funding agencies. Participants were told that the research question and the follow-up probing could trigger upsetting memories of their war or reintegration experiences. Although the plan was to refer anyone having difficulties to a mental health practitioner who agreed to provide counseling if needed, none of the participants needed to be referred. Before each interview, the investigator conducting the interview discussed the purpose of the study, informed consent, and study withdrawal procedures with participants. Participation was explained as a voluntary action that could be withdrawn at any time. Procedures about how interview and demographic data would be collected, stored, analyzed, and used were explained. Data collection took place over a 4-month period in late 2013.

The single research question was: What can you tell me about your reintegration experience? Probing was employed to enrich data and to clarify responses to the research question. Probing also helped to ensure that study participants would address the multiple facets of reintegration, such as family, workplace, and community. The researchers took notes to document emotional reactions such as crying or laughing during interviews. Interviews were transcribed verbatim. Approximately 8 weeks later, participants were sent their transcripts to validate content, provide feedback to the researchers, and to check for accuracy of description and meaning in their verbatim statements.

Study data were analyzed using Colaizzi's (1978) procedure for analyzing phenomenological data. Audio-tapes were listened to several times by the researchers to achieve familiarity with content, feeling, and tone. Following finalization of verbatim transcriptions, participant interview narratives were reviewed. Significant statements were extracted and grouped into thematic clusters. As analysis of data proceeded, study findings were integrated into an exhaustive description of the lived experience of military nurses' reintegration following wartime deployment in the Iraq and Afghanistan wars. Although all experiences and all interview content were respected and valued, within the margins of this book it was not feasible to include all interview statements. Since there was redundancy within answers to the research question, statements that best represented the substance and spirit of an experience in our judgment were those we included in this book.

The reader will meet each of the 35 military nurses in the first half of this book. These nurses' stories powerfully portray the emotional, visceral, and highly personal experiences of homecoming and reintegration after serving their country and caring for their patients in the war zones of Iraq and Afghanistan. Although the main focus of our research study was homecoming and reintegration, some nurses' stories also reflected back to their war experiences and the stresses of combat casualty care. In discussing the troubles some faced in reintegration, they also provided a vivid "snapshot" of the sights, sounds, vibrations, hardships, and fears they experienced in the war zone. These nurses' stories form a rich mosaic of the path to homecoming and reintegration they walked singly as well as collectively with their returning comrades. For every nurse who served in these wars, there is a story. Their paths to reintegration are individual and of varying chronological lengths. Their stories will now provide a piece of the fabric called "U.S. military nursing history." This book gives these nurses a voice.

We believe that nurse reintegration is an important and timely topic for the nursing profession as a whole. Nurses, nursing students, families of nurses, other health care professionals, and anyone interested in military nursing or military history would benefit from knowledge development in this area. We can all learn from reading the nurses' narratives; the positive, the negative, and the neutral. Our book attempts to paint a realistic picture of the reintegration experience and emphasizes that reintegration is very individual and has no set timetable. The knowledge gleaned from our research will benefit future generations of nurses in better preparing them for wartime deployments, humanitarian missions, and natural and man-made disasters. In addition, they will be better prepared to navigate homecoming and reintegration.

Although the reintegration experience may be essentially the same or similar regardless of career field and/or branch of military service, to date nurses reintegrating have lower rates of posttraumatic stress disorder (PTSD), suicide, and major mental health problems than other returning service members. It is hoped that a better reintegration experience will positively impact the morbidity and mortality rates for returning veterans.

We are exceedingly grateful to the 35 nurses who shared their stories with us. We recognize and value their openness and honesty. We salute and celebrate their courage, commitment, valor, and dedication as they exposed themselves to the risks inherent in serving in a war zone. They represent the best that the profession of nursing has to offer.

At Springer Publishing Company, we thank Joseph Morita, our senior editor, for his advice, encouragement, and support. We are indebted to Brigadier General Linda Stierle, USAF, NC (Ret.), and Major General Melissa Rank, USAF, NC (Ret.), for review of our manuscript and thoughtful advice. We want to thank veteran organizations and professional nursing associations for their help in advertising our research study to potential participants. We acknowledge support of the granting agency, Connecticut State Universities/American Association of University Professors in funding the research study that was the basis of this book.

The nurses who participated in the research study that led to this book were candid, generous, and articulate in describing their reintegration experiences. This sharing provides very helpful anticipatory guidance for returning nurses. It is our hope that knowledge development in this area will continue and that more programs will be developed to aid returning veterans and their families. We believe that the nurses' narratives contained in this book will inspire and guide future generations of nurses.

REFERENCES

Colaizzi, P. (1978). Psychological research as the phenomenologist reviews it. In R. Valle & M. King (Eds.), *Existential-phenomenological alternatives for psychology* (pp. 48–71). New York: NY: Oxford University Press.

Denzin, N., & Lincoln, Y. (2011). *The SAGE handbook of qualitative research.* Thousand Oaks, CA: Sage.

Doherty M. E., & Scannell-Desch, E. A. (2012). Women's health and hygiene experiences during deployment to the Iraq and Afghanistan wars, 2003 through 2010. *Journal of Midwifery and Women's Health, 57,* 172–177.

Doherty, M. E., & Scannell-Desch, E. A. (2015). After the parade: Military nurses' reintegration experiences from the Iraq and Afghanistan wars. *Journal of Psychosocial Nursing and Mental Health Services, 53*(5), 28–35.

Hopkins-Chadwick, D. L. (2012). Strategies to support nurse work reintegration after deployment: Constructed from an analysis of Army nurses' redeployment experiences. *U.S. Army Medical Department Journal, 3,* 59–63.

LoBiondo-Wood, G., & Haber, J. (2014). *Nursing research: Methods and critical appraisal for evidence-based practice.* St. Louis, MO: Elsevier-Mosby.

Marshall, C., & Rossman, G. B. (2011). *Designing qualitative research* (5th ed.). Los Angeles, CA: Sage.

Polit, D. F., & Beck, C. T. (2011). *Nursing research: Generating and assessing evidence for nursing practice* (9th ed.). Philadelphia, PA: Lippincott Williams & Wilkins.

Rivers, F. M., Gordon, S., Speraw, S., & Reese, S. (2013). U.S. Army nurses' reintegration and homecoming experiences. *Military Medicine, 178,* 162–166.

Scannell-Desch, E. A., & Doherty, M. E. (2010). Experiences of nurses in the Iraq and Afghanistan wars, 2003–2009. *Journal of Nursing Scholarship, 42*, 3–12.

Scannell-Desch, E. A., & Doherty, M. E. (2013). Nurse parents: Parental separation during deployment to Iraq and Afghanistan, 2003–2010. *American Journal of Maternal-Child Nursing, 38*, 3–8.

Acronyms

AE	Aeromedical evacuation
AEF	Air expeditionary force
AEW	Air Expeditionary Wing
Air evac	To move patients by air using fixed or rotary wing aircraft
AMBUS	Ambulance bus
AMC	Air Mobility Command
ANA	Afghan National Army
Army JAG	U.S. Army Judge Advocate General Corps
ART	Air Reserve technician
ASTS	Aeromedical Staging Transportation Squadron
Battle Rattle	Military personal protective gear consisting of Kevlar helmet, Kevlar protective flak vest (also referred to as "body armor"), pistol belt, pistol or semi-automatic rifle, goggles, and sometimes Mission Oriented Protective Posture (MOPP) gear, etc.
BCT	Behavioral couples therapy
BRAC	Base Realignment and Closure Commission
BSN	Bachelor of science degree in nursing
CASH	Combat army support hospital
CCATT	Critical Care Air Transport Team
CIA	Central Intelligence Agency
CNM	Certified nurse-midwife
CNS	Clinical nurse specialist
COPD	Chronic obstructive pulmonary disease
CRNA	Certified registered nurse anesthetist
CSH	Combat support hospital

DKA	Diabetic keto acidosis
DNP	Doctor of nursing practice
DOA	Dead on arrival
Drill	Reserve weekend duty
Dustoff	A medevac helicopter
EFT-C	Emotion-focused couples therapy
EFT	Emotion-focused therapy
EMDR	Eye movement desensitization and reprocessing
EO	Equal opportunity
EOO	Equal opportunity officer
ER	Emergency room
FNP	Family nurse practitioner
FOB	Forward operating base
Freedom Bird	Flight home to the United States
FRSS	Forward resuscitative surgery system—a mobile forward surgical system used by the U.S. Navy to perform life and limb-saving surgery in the field on casualties who will not survive without immediate surgery
FST and FFST	Forward surgical team, fast-forward surgical team—mobile surgical teams used in the field to perform surgery before medevac to a combat support hospital
GWOT	Global war on terrorism
IA	Individual augmentee
ICU	Intensive care unit
IED	Improvised explosive device
IG	Inspector general
IRR	Individual Ready Reserve is an inactive reserve status, which includes retired U.S. military personnel and former honorably discharged veterans
ISAF	International Security Assistance Forces
ISIS	Islamic State of Iraq and Syria is a Jihadist radical terrorist group occupying territory in the Middle East to include Iraq and Syria
LPN	Licensed practical nurse
MASH	Mobile army surgical hospital
MBSR	Mindfulness-based stress reduction
MOPP Gear	Mission-oriented protective posture gear—protects against chemical, biological, and contact with very low-level radioactive material. Suit is rubberized, moisture-proof, and puncture resistant. Includes gas mask with hood, heavy-duty rubberized boot covers and gloves.

MRAP	Mine-resistant ambush protected personnel vehicle is a heavily armored vehicle designed specifically to counter the land mine and roadside bomb threat in the Iraq and Afghanistan wars.
MSC	Medical Service Corps
MUST	Medical Unit Self-Contained Transportable is a package of tentage and medical gear used by the U.S. Army from the end of the Vietnam War until after Operation Desert Storm.
NATO	North Atlantic Treaty Organization
NKC	New Kabul Compound
NP	Nurse practitioner
NROTC	Navy Reserve Officer Training Corps
OEF	Operation Enduring Freedom
OIC	Officer-in-charge
OIF	Operation Iraqi Freedom
OR	Operating room
PA	Physician's assistant
PCA	Patient-controlled analgesia
PCS	Permanent change of station is when a military member has orders to report to a new assignment
PMS	Premenstrual syndrome
PRN position	Temporary position whenever necessary
PRT	Provisional reconstruction team
PT	Physical training
PTSD	Posttraumatic stress disorder
R & R	Rest and relaxation
Regs	Regulations, military regulations
RPG	Rocket-propelled grenade
SSRI	Selective serotonin reuptake inhibitor
SRP	Soldier reprocessing center
STP	Shock trauma platoon
TBI	Traumatic brain injury
USAID	United States Agency for International Development
USCENTCOM	United States Central Command
UTA	Unit training assembly
VA	U.S. Veterans Administration
Vents	Ventilators
VFW	Veterans of Foreign Wars
WMD	Weapons of mass destruction
WRNMMC	Walter Reed National Military Medical Center—located in Bethesda, Maryland.

Nurses After War

1

Contemporary Historical Roots
of the Wars in Iraq and Afghanistan

THE FIRST PERSIAN GULF WAR (1990–1991)

The bloody 8-year Iran–Iraq war ended in a stalemate in 1988. After the end of the war, Iraq was in considerable debt to Kuwait and Saudi Arabia. Iraq also accused Kuwait of exceeding its Organization of the Petroleum Exporting Countries (OPEC) quotas for oil production and for driving oil prices down. The resulting lower Iraqi oil revenues could barely support the government's basic costs, let alone repair Iraq's damaged infrastructure from the Iran–Iraq war (Finlan, 1994).

In early July 1990, Iraq complained about Kuwait's behavior, such as not respecting their oil-production quota, and openly threatened to take military action. Various meetings among Iraq, Kuwait, and other interested nations failed to remedy the situation or to reduce tensions (Cordesman & Wagner, 1996). Saddam Hussein, the fifth president of Iraq, ordered the Iraqi Army's occupation of Kuwait. On August 2, 1990, Iraq launched a surprise invasion with about 100,000 Iraqi ground troops against Kuwait and quickly overran the country, initiating the Gulf War. This action was met with international condemnation. The United Nations (UN) Security Council passed Resolution 661, imposing a trade embargo on Iraq (Blair, 1992).

The president of the United States, George H. W. Bush, deployed U.S. military forces to Saudi Arabia and urged other countries to send their own forces to the region. The first U.S. ground troops arrived in Saudi Arabia on August 7, 1990. An array of nations joined the coalition, the largest military alliance to configure since World War II. The greater bulk of coalition forces came from the United States, the United Kingdom, and Egypt (Hutchison, 1995).

On August 8, 1990, Saddam Hussein proclaimed the annexation of Kuwait, designating Kuwait as Iraqi territory. Coalition forces initiated a naval blockade of Iraq that same day (Brune, 1993). Iraq declared Kuwait as its 19th province and renamed Kuwait City as al-Kadhima (Head & Tilford, 1996). As the fall of 1990 passed, the multinational forces continued to assemble in Saudi Arabia to defend Saudi Arabia and to prepare for the liberation of Kuwait. This gathering of troops was labeled "Operation Desert Shield" by U.S. coalition forces. Iraq was sanctioned by the UN when the UN Security Council passed Resolution 678, setting a deadline for Iraq to withdraw from Kuwait before January 15, 1991, or face military action (Engel, 2013). On January 12, 1991, the U.S. Congress passed a joint resolution authorizing the use of military force to drive Iraq out of Kuwait. The votes were 52–47 in the U.S. Senate and 250–183 in the U.S. House of Representatives. These were the closest margins in authorizing force by Congress since the War of 1812 (Hutchison, 1995).

Iraqi-occupying forces failed to withdraw from Kuwait by the deadline (Long, 2004). The initial conflict to expel Iraqi troops from Kuwait began in the middle of the night with an intense aerial and naval bombardment on January 17, 1991. Apache attack helicopters firing Hellfire missiles led the way to neutralize radar sites, weapons batteries, command and control infrastructure, and troop concentrations. U.S.-led air force and navy warplanes attacked sites in Baghdad, Kuwait, and other military targets in Iraq (Cipkowski, 1992). A few days into the air war, Iraq began to launch Scud missiles into Israel, whereas the United States quickly deployed Patriot missile batteries to Israel and Saudi Arabia. In addition, Iraqi forces began to blow up and set fire to Kuwaiti oil wells and refineries, and dumped millions of gallons of crude oil into the Persian Gulf waters (Hutchison, 1995).

The coalition forces' aerial campaign continued for 5 weeks, considerably damaging Iraqi ground fortifications and killing many Iraqi troops. The first Gulf War was the formal combat debut of the U.S. Air Force's F-117 Nighthawk aircraft. This was the first operational aircraft to be designed around stealth technology. It was commonly referred to as the "stealth-fighter," but was a truly ground-attack aircraft, used in the war to attack ground-based radar sites, missile batteries, and troop concentrations (Dunnigan & Bay, 1992).

The Boeing AH-64 Apache is an attack helicopter used by the U.S. Army. It is armed with a 30-mm gun and has four firing pylons, which usually carry a mixed configuration of Hellfire air-to-ground missiles and Hydra rocket pods. The Apache was designed to perform in frontline combat environments, including operating at night and during adverse weather situations. The redundant electronic sensors and avionics configurations allow this helicopter to perform safely and accurately in much less than optimal weather. On January 17, 1991, eight Apaches destroyed part of Iraq's radar network in the operation's first attack (Dunnigan & Bay, 1992).

On February 22, 1991, U.S. President George H. W. Bush issued a 24-hour ultimatum that either Iraqi forces withdraw from Kuwait or the coalition would commence the ground war. Iraq did not withdraw its forces, and the U.S.-led coalition forces invaded Iraq under the cover of night on February 24, 1991. British forces were the first to enter Iraqi territory (Bin, Hill, & Jones, 1998).

During the 100-hour ground war, Apache helicopters destroyed 278 tanks, numerous armored personnel carriers, and many other Iraqi vehicles. One AH-64 was lost in the war to a rocket-propelled grenade (RPG) hit at close range. Although the Apache crashed, the crew survived (Hutchison, 1995). The Iraqi armored forces and infantry were overwhelmed by the coalition forces' air- and land-based power. On February 26, 1991, Saddam Hussein ordered Iraqi-troop withdrawal from Kuwait. Approximately 10,000 retreating Iraqi troops were killed when coalition aircraft bombed their civilian and military vehicles. In the retreat, abandoned and incapacitated Iraqi tanks, armored personnel carriers, and civilian trucks littered the main highway. This was labeled the "Highway of Death" by coalition journalists covering the war (David, 1991).

On February 27, 1991, U.S. Marines and Saudi Arabian ground forces entered Kuwait City. Later in the day, U.S. Army ground assets fought the Iraqi Republican Guard forces in several tank battles on Iraqi territory. This was known as the "Battle of Medina Ridge" (Blackwell, 1991). On February 28, 1991, U.S. President George H. W. Bush announced a cease-fire and that Kuwait had been liberated from Iraqi occupation. On March 1, 1991, a cease-fire plan was negotiated in Safwan, Iraq. On March 3, 1991, Saddam Hussein and his Iraqi general accepted the terms of a cease-fire from the UN Security Council. The first of thousands of deployed U.S. forces arrived back on U.S. soil on March 17, 1991 (Friedman, 1991).

THE WAR IN IRAQ (MARCH 2003–DECEMBER 2011)

Following the defeat of Saddam Hussein's forces in the Gulf War of 1991, the Iraqi government agreed to surrender or destroy several types of armaments, including chemical and biological weapons caches. In early 2003, U.S. President George W. Bush and British Prime Minister Tony Blair accused the Saddam regime of continuing to hide weapons of mass destruction (WMD) and having ties to the Islamic al-Qaeda terrorist organization headed by Osama bin Laden. The United States gave Saddam a deadline to relinquish the presidency or face a U.S.-led attack on Iraq. Saddam refused to step down (Ballard, Lamm, & Wood, 2012).

President Bush ordered the start of a war against Iraq on March 19, 2003, and U.S. forces poised on Iraq's southern border and at sea began strikes to disarm the country. President Bush told the people of the United States in a late evening newscast that coalition forces were beginning to strike selected targets of military importance to destroy Saddam Hussein's ability to wage war. In his newscast, President Bush cautioned that this war could be of longer duration than most people expected, and that casualty counts could be considerably higher than in the first Persian Gulf War. On March 20, 2003, U.S., British, Australian, Danish, and Polish ground forces invaded Iraq. Most troops met minimal resistance (Haass, 2009). Coalition forces moved into Baghdad, toppled the large statue of Saddam, and quickly ended the 24-year reign of Iraqi President Saddam Hussein on April 10, 2003 (Shimko, 2010).

When the U.S. forces invaded Iraq, they promised to destroy Iraqi WMD as well as end the rule of Saddam. However, the Central Intelligence Agency (CIA) and other intelligence-gathering agencies failed to recognize that Iraq had abandoned its efforts to produce large quantities of chemical and biological weapons after the end of the first Persian Gulf War in 1991. After this failure to find WMD current production capability or hidden WMD stockpiles, sentiment in both Iraq and some coalition countries changed. The insurgency against the occupation of Iraq by coalition forces escalated and support for the continued war waned to a degree in most of the coalition countries (Hoeffel, 2014).

After the collapse of Baghdad in 2003, the second phase of the Iraq war began. This phase was characterized by ground operations, house-to-house urban combat in the cities, and troop and equipment convoys being blown up as they rolled over hidden roadside bombs and improvised explosive devices (IEDs). Coalition forces' civil engineering and provisional reconstruction teams worked to improve Iraqi urban and village infrastructure; however, it was a dangerous duty because of the increased level of insurgency. This second phase of the war was fraught with increased coalition and civilian casualties. The third stage of the Iraq war began on September 1, 2010, when the drawdown of U.S. and coalition forces commenced. This stage was characterized by a reduction in forces as well as a redistribution of coalition forces remaining in Iraq. The third stage ended in December of 2011, when the last of the U.S. combat forces left Iraq by order of U.S. President Barack Obama (Gordon & Trainor, 2012). It is important to note that the characteristic injuries of this war were blast and traumatic brain injuries (TBI).

The years 2012 through 2015 saw variations in the number of residual U.S. troop trainers working with Iraqi Army and police forces in the urban centers of Iraq. During this time, the terrorist group Islamic State of Iraq and Syria (ISIS) gained momentum in taking control of some major cities, such as Mosul. To date, the Iraqi Army and police have failed to hold ISIS back (Devins, 2015).

THE WAR IN AFGHANISTAN (2001–PRESENT)

The Soviet Union deployed occupying ground forces, including Soviet-led Afghan forces, to Afghanistan in December 1979. Soon after this invasion, thousands of Muslims from all over the globe traveled to Afghanistan to become part of the Afghan resistance. This resistance was composed of multinational insurgents, known as the "Mujahedeen." The Mujahedeen received training as well as weapons from the United States, the United Kingdom, and Saudi Arabia (Williams, 2012). A wealthy man from a prominent Saudi Arabian family, Osama Bin Laden, traveled to Afghanistan and joined the fight. He also created a terrorist organization, al-Qaeda (translated as "the base"), on August 11, 1988. He helped finance and lead a force of about 20,000 Muslim freedom fighters in Afghanistan. The fight lasted until February 1989, when the Soviet forces were withdrawn. The election of Mikhail Gorbachev as Soviet general secretary in 1985 and his fresh perspective on foreign and domestic policy were probably the driving force in the Soviets' decision to retreat from Afghanistan. Bin Laden also left Afghanistan after the fighting had ceased in 2009, and subsequently he stepped up fund-raising for al-Qaeda while working for the family construction group firm, the Bin Laden Group. Over subsequent years, Osama bin Laden became more and more militant toward the West, especially the United States (Coll, 2004; Feifer, 2009).

The United States went to war in Afghanistan after the terrorist attacks of September 11, 2001, in New York at the World Trade Center Twin Towers; in Virginia at the Pentagon; and in Shanksville, Pennsylvania, where the fourth plane, which had targeted the U.S. Capitol Building, crashed. Global intelligence resources determined that Osama bin Laden and his radical terrorist network, al-Qaeda, were responsible for these devastating attacks. At the time, Bin Laden was thought to be hiding in a remote mountainous region of Afghanistan with his key protectors and advisers. After several failed attempts to broker the surrender of Bin Laden to U.S. Special Forces personnel, the United States initiated bombing and mortar attacks on Afghanistan, most specifically on Taliban fortifications and the mountains of Tora Bora, where Bin Laden was thought to be hiding. Years later, the U.S. Naval Special Forces killed Osama bin Laden in a surprise attack on his residential compound in Abbottabad, Pakistan, on May 2, 2011 (Owen & Mauer, 2014).

The U.S. drawdown in Afghanistan began in July 2011, when the first U.S. troops left Afghanistan as part of President Obama's planned drawdown. Later, in April 2012, the United States and its coalition and North Atlantic Treaty Organization (NATO) allies finalized agreements to wind down the war in Afghanistan by formalizing three commitments: to gradually shift the Afghans into a lead-combat role; to keep some international troops in Afghanistan beyond 2014; and to pay billions of dollars to help support the Afghan security forces. In May 2012, Afghan President Hamid Karzai and President Barack Obama signed a partnership agreement in Kabul between the two countries. The agreement provides the long-term framework for the relationship between Afghanistan and the United States after the drawdown of U.S. forces in the Afghanistan war. The agreement went into effect in July 2012 (Gunaratna & Woodall, 2015).

After the signing of the aforementioned partnership agreement, President Obama laid out his plans to end the war in Afghanistan responsibly. The plans called for removal of 23,000 U.S. troops by September 30, 2012; Afghan security forces to then take the lead in combat operations by the end of 2013 while International Security Assistance Forces (ISAF) trained, advised, and helped Afghans and fought alongside them when and if needed; and the complete removal of all U.S. troops by the end of 2014, except for trainers who will assist Afghan forces and a small contingent of special forces troops to combat al-Qaeda through counterterrorism operations. To date, this plan is currently in place and about 9,000 to 11,000 ISAF forces remain in Afghanistan in a training and advisement role (Gunaratna & Woodall, 2015).

REFERENCES

Ballard, J. R., Lamm, D. W., & Wood, J. K. (2012). *From Kabul to Baghdad and back: The U.S. at war in Afghanistan and Iraq.* Annapolis, MD: Naval Institute Press.

Bin, A., Hill, R., & Jones, A. (1998). *Desert Storm: A forgotten war.* Westport, CT: Praeger.

Blackwell, J. (1991). *Thunder in the desert: The strategy and tactics of the Persian Gulf War.* New York, NY: Bantam.

Blair, A. H. (1992). *At war in the Gulf: A chronology.* College Station, TX: Texas A & M University Press.

Brune, L. H. (1993). *America and the Iraqi crisis, 1990–1992: Origins and aftermath.* Claremont, CA: Regina Books.

Cipkowski, P. (1992). *Understanding the crisis in the Persian Gulf.* New York, NY: Wiley.

Coll, S. (2004). *Ghost wars: The secret history of the CIA, Afghanistan, and Bin Laden, from the Soviet invasion to September 10, 2001.* New York, NY: Penguin.

Cordesman, A. H., & Wagner, A. R. (1996). *The Gulf War.* Boulder, CO: Westview Press.

David, P. (1991). *Triumph in the desert: The challenge, the fighting, the legacy.* New York, NY: Random House.

Devins, R. (2015). *ISIS: Terrorists on the rise: Origins of the new war on terror.* New York, NY: Tisdale.

Dunnigan, J. F., & Bay, A. (1992). *From shield to storm: High-tech weapons, military strategy, and coalition warfare in the Persian Gulf.* New York, NY: Morrow.

Engel, J. A. (2013). *Into the desert: Reflections on the Gulf War.* Oxford, UK: Oxford University Press.

Feifer, G. (2009). *The great gamble: The Soviet war in Afghanistan.* New York, NY: Harper.

Finlan, A. (1994). *The 1991 Gulf War: Historic essentials.* Oxford, UK: Osprey.

Friedman, N. (1991). *Desert victory: The war for Kuwait.* Annapolis, MD: Naval Institute Press.

Gordon, M. R., & Trainor, B. E. (2012). *The endgame: The inside story of the struggle for Iraq from George W. Bush to Barack Obama.* New York, NY: Pantheon.

Gunaratna, R., & Woodall, D. (2015). *Afghanistan after the Western drawdown.* Lanham, MD: Rowman & Littlefield.

Haass, R. N. (2009). *War of necessity, war of choice: A memoir of two Iraq wars.* New York, NY: Simon & Schuster.

Head, W., & Tilford, E. H. (1996). *The eagle in the desert: Looking back on U.S. involvement in the Persian Gulf War.* Westport, CT: Praeger.

Hoeffel, J. M. (2014). *The Iraq lie: How the White House sold the war.* San Diego, CA: Progressive Press.

Hutchison, K. D. (1995). *Operation Desert Shield/Desert Storm: Chronology and fact book.* Westport, CT: Greenwood.

Long, J. M. (2004). *Saddam's war of words: Politics, religion, and the Iraqi invasion of Kuwait.* Austin, TX: University of Texas Press.

Owen, M., & Mauer, K. (2014). *No easy day: The firsthand account of the mission that killed Osama Bin Laden.* New York, NY: Penguin.

Williams, B. G. (2012). *Afghanistan declassified: A guide to America's longest war.* Philadelphia, PA: University of Pennsylvania Press.

2

Military Medical Assets Deployed to the Iraq and Afghanistan Wars

The United States and coalition partners sent thousands of nurses, physicians, and support medical personnel to Operation Desert Shield/ Operation Desert Storm in 1991. Because of the ground war's limitation of 4 days of combat, the coalition medical resources cared for a very limited number of casualties. At the end of the first Gulf War on February 28, 1991, 2,215 Army Nurse Corps officers were deployed to the Gulf region (Sarnecky, 2010.) The U.S. Army, Navy, and Air Force deployment of medical personnel in support of Operation Desert Shield and Operation Desert Storm was massive, expensive, multifaceted, and very challenging.

In the early 1990s, the Army Medical Service was in the process of converting from its Vietnam-era Medical Unit Self-Contained Transportable (MUST) hospital structure to a more current and mobile deployable system of medical equipment and modern environmentally controlled tentage. A significant number of medical units deployed to the Gulf were deployed with the older MUST equipment and tentage. The deployed medical personnel found the desert environment very tough on their outdated MUST systems. As a result, the Army Medical Department was compelled to rapidly replace the old MUST systems with the much newer deployable systems (Sarnecky, 2010). In addition, the beginning of Operation Iraqi Freedom marked the last wartime use of an active Mobile Army Surgical Hospital (MASH). During this operation, the army officially replaced its last active MASH with the new combat surgical hospital and fast-forward surgical teams (e.g., King & Jatoi, 2005).

In addition to modernizing deployable medical facilities, the Army Medical Service also implemented a new doctrine and concept of operations, called "Medical Force 2000." The two most significant changes in doctrine included employing far forward surgical assets and an increased breadth and depth of psychiatric support (Sarnecky, 2010). To understand how care was delivered by U.S. military personnel in a war zone, one has to appreciate the structure of military medical care. Military medical doctrine supports a system of triage, treatment, evacuation, and then return of military troops to duty in the most efficient and effective manner. Troops not fit for duty are returned for further evaluation, treatment, and rehabilitation in the United States. This current paradigm dictates an "evacuate and replace" philosophy, which places considerable demand on the transport and en route care abilities of all the military services (Joint Publication 4–02, 2012, p. I-6).

The wars in Iraq and Afghanistan commenced the extensive use of the U.S. Army's forward surgical teams (FSTs) to support military operations in Operation Enduring Freedom and Operation Iraqi Freedom (Counihan & Danielson, 2012). For example, the army's 102nd FST was deployed to Kandahar, Afghanistan, to provide trauma and surgical services in support of the army's 101st and 82nd Airborne Divisions during the beginning of Operation Enduring Freedom. Later, the unit's medical tasking was expanded to include local humanitarian assistance (Beekley & Watts, 2004).

The U.S. Air Force was considerably downsized after the end of the Cold War and the first Persian Gulf War. The Base Realignment and Closure (BRAC) commission proceedings resulted in the closure of several stateside and overseas air bases. With the closure of overseas bases and potential involvement in areas with little, if any, U.S. military facilities, it became crucial to reexamine, update, and alter U.S. air power doctrine to deal with future threats (Looney, 1996). In addition, to enforce the no-fly zone over Iraq in the mid-1990s, Operation Northern Watch and Operation Southern Watch placed additional burdens on airframe, logistical, and personnel assets (Air Force Doctrine Document 2, 2007).

Air force leadership crafted a new doctrine to demonstrate how it planned to meet its future global commitments. The Air Expeditionary Force (AEF) concept was designed, developed, and implemented to meet these worldwide demands. Under this concept of operations, the air force leadership mixed active duty; reserve forces; and Air National Guard airframe, logistical, equipment, medical, and other assets into a combined force (Nowak, 1999). Instead of deploying an entire active duty unit, such as a fighter aircraft squadron or a deployable hospital unit with all of its equipment and personnel for a year or longer, now specially sized "aviation packages," "logistical packages," or "medical packages" from several active duty, reserve, and Air National Guard wings would deploy together as a single AEF to carry out the deployment mission. These package sizes are flexible and tailored to meet specific mission requirements and capabilities (Nowak, 1999). Usually after a 4- to 6-month deployment, another AEF package would replace them in the operational theater. The air force "relies on the AEF as a force management tool to establish a predictable, standardized battle rhythm ensuring rotational forces are properly organized, trained, equipped and ready to sustain capabilities while rapidly responding to emerging crises" (Air Force Pamphlet 36–2241, 2013, p. 82).

Recent history has demonstrated that, over time, the U.S. experience in war increasingly demands cooperation, coordination, and integration of all U.S. military services. Today, joint operations are routine. It is not uncommon for air force personnel to augment army soldiers on convoy operations, or for army and navy medics to be assigned to an Air Force Theater Hospital in the Iraq and Afghanistan wars (Air Force Doctrine Document 2, 2007). On the battlefield, effectively integrated joint forces are able to rapidly and efficiently identify and engage enemy vulnerabilities, without exposing their own weaknesses to ensure mission accomplishment. In today's combat environment, U.S. armed forces must always be ready to operate in smoothly functioning joint teams (Air Force Pamphlet 36–2241, 2013).

In summary, the air force has taken its combat and mobility wings (active duty, reserve, and Air National Guard), and assigned them to one of 10 AEFs. Several of these 10 wings have contributed to the force mix in the Iraq and Afghanistan wars. The AEF is one that can conduct military missions on short notice in response to operational requirements or sudden crises with specific force packages tailored to achieve limited and clearly stated objectives. Several AEF organizations are defined as provisional in nature, organized to meet a specific mission or national commitment. As such, they are activated and inactivated as necessary (Air Force Doctrine Document 2, 2007).

In terms of AEF medical assets, they are a total force endeavor with staffing coming from the active duty, air reserve, and Air National Guard components. At times when medical specialists, such as neurosurgeons or otolaryngologists, are needed, it is not uncommon to have a few U.S. Army and/or U.S. Navy medical personnel attached to a predominantly air force unit. The USCENTCOM (United States Central Command) area of responsibility (AOR) covers the "central" area of the globe and consists of 20 countries: Afghanistan, Bahrain, Egypt, Iran, Iraq, Jordan, Kazakhstan, Kuwait, Kyrgyzstan, Lebanon, Oman, Pakistan, Qatar, Saudi Arabia, Syria, Tajikistan, Turkmenistan, United Arab Emirates, Uzbekistan, and Yemen (U.S. Centcom, 2015).

The U.S. Navy had historically relied on fleet surgical teams to provide surgical and critical care onboard large deck ships and hospital ships, both having helicopter landing pads to receive casualties. However, because of the geographical distances involved in the Afghan and Iraqi war theaters, this aforementioned strategy was deemed impractical. As a result, the U.S. Navy designed, developed, and implemented a new type of surgical unit, the Forward Resuscitative Surgery System (FRSS) to provide a light weight, mobile, forward surgical and stabilization capability (Bohman, Stevens, Baker, & Chambers, 2005).

The goal of the FRSS is to "save life and limb" of those casualties who would die, mostly from blood loss, caused by delayed access to surgical and resuscitative care by minimizing transport time between point of injury and surgical intervention. In order to meet this goal, the FRSS staff perform what they call "damage control" surgery. The aim of this surgery is to restore normal life-saving physiology rather than providing anatomical repair. Anatomical repair would be accomplished later at a higher echelon of surgical care. An FRSS is usually staffed by one or two general surgeons, an orthopedic surgeon, a critical care nurse, an anesthesia provider, two operating room (OR) technicians, two hospital corpsmen, and a transport nurse. During Operation Iraqi Freedom, each deployed FRSS was matched with a navy shock–trauma platoon (STP). The STP is a mobile expanded emergency care facility staffed by two emergency room (ER) physicians, a physician's assistant (PA), an ER nurse, 14 corpsmen, and seven marines. When matched with an FRSS, the STP provides care to patients not needing FRSS services, but also supplements the preoperative and postoperative care provided by the FRSS (Bohman et al., 2005).

More than 2.5 million military veterans have been deployed for service in Iraq and Afghanistan since 2003 (Conard, Allen, & Armstrong, 2015). The austerity and danger of the war zone intensifies the complexity of providing critical care in the airborne and ground environments. Medical facilities and medevac aircraft have to operate with limited resources, medical and nursing personnel may be asked to assume unexpected roles out of necessity, and combat injuries can involve multiple areas of the body and organ systems (Venticinque & Grathwohl, 2008).

Current military medical doctrine directs five echelons of care. The first echelon commences in the combat zone when a military member is injured. Immediate first aid is delivered by the injured soldier (self-aid), by a fellow soldier (buddy-care), or by a military medic. First echelon care includes such activities as assessing the patency of the airway, breathing, circulation, controlling bleeding, and requesting evacuation to a FST facility or combat support hospital (CSH). FSTs and CSHs have been developed and used extensively only during the wars in Afghanistan and Iraq (Schoenfeld, 2012).

The second echelon of care is the FST, sometimes called the "Army Battalion Aid Station," which is located in the wider combat zone. Staffing for FSTs or aid stations usually includes physicians' assistants or nurse practitioners, one or two nurse anesthetists, and two or three physicians (one usually being a general surgeon). Third echelon care takes place once the injured soldier is evacuated by ground or air to the CSH. Here, more definitive surgery and care is provided by surgeons and other specialists (Joint Publication 4–02, 2012; Schoenfeld, 2012).

The CSH has larger inpatient medical–surgical care units as well as an intensive care unit (ICU) and several ORs. Most CSHs usually operate at 44 to 50 beds, but can be expanded. CSHs need to be located close to an airbase with runways capable of handling the air force's large aeromedical transport aircraft, the C-17 Globemaster III, C-130 Hercules, and the C-135 Stratolifter. The fourth echelon of care is provided at a large medical center that has specialty care capabilities such as a burn care unit, neurosurgery, special hand surgery, and cardiac surgery outside the combat zone. The Joint Services Military Medical Center (formerly the 2nd Army Regional Medical Center) in Landsthul, Germany, next to Ramstein Air Base, is an example of a fourth echelon medical facility. Fifth echelon care is provided in large medical centers in the United States, such as Walter Reed National Military Medical Center in Bethesda, Maryland (Kenny & Hull, 2008; Korzeniewski & Bochniak, 2011). The war in Afghanistan and the second Iraq war became a long-term test of current military medical doctrine.

In the Iraq war, the air force medical assets were formed around the new AEF doctrine as noted earlier. One of the key air force medical assets deployed in the Iraq war included the 332nd Expeditionary Medical Group (Joint Base Balad Air Force Theater Hospital). This hospital was located at Joint Base Balad, Iraq, in the Sunni Triangle about 40 miles north of Baghdad. It was staffed by more than 350 medical, nursing, and support personnel. It was the biggest U.S. hospital in Iraq and had a survivability rate of 97%. Over the course of the Iraq conflict, about 30,000 wounded military personnel and civilians passed through Balad for treatment and/or aeromedical evacuation (AE). At the height of the Iraq war, the hospital housed many medical specialties, including anesthesia, general surgery, vascular surgery, neurosurgery, nutritional medicine, ophthalmology, orthopedics, physical and occupational therapy, radiology, clinical psychology, urology, ear, nose, throat, oral-maxillofacial surgery, pediatrics, emergency medicine, and trauma and critical care. The hospital was the referral hospital for any head injury in Iraq, and it was also the place everyone went through before going to the United States for further treatment (Maureen, York, Hirshon, Jenkins, & Scalea, 2011).

In the war in Afghanistan, several key medical assets provide much needed trauma, illness, and surgical care. The 455th Expeditionary Medical Group is located at Bagram Air Base, Afghanistan, under command of the 455th Air Expeditionary Wing (AEW). The group is the air force component for Task Force Med, which provides combat medical and medical support services to U.S. and coalition forces throughout Afghanistan. The hospital, called the Heathe N. Craig Joint Theater Hospital, is a 50-bed military hospital named after SSG Heathe N. Craig, a U.S. Army medic who died while trying to save a wounded comrade in Afghanistan. This hospital has modern clinical facilities that rival modern hospitals in the United States (Dierkes, 2011).

The hospital at Kandahar Air Base, Afghanistan, is a 50-bed expandable state-of-the art hospital. It was completed in mid-2010 replacing a semipermanent plywood structure in disrepair. The U.S. Navy makes up about 70% of the 200 to 300 personnel assigned to the hospital, with others from Canada, the United Kingdom, Australia, the Netherlands, Denmark, and Romania. Many badly injured troops are treated and transported within hours to Bagram Air Base, north of Kabul, and then on to the U.S. Joint Military Medical Center in Landstuhl, Germany (Brisebois et al., 2011).

Camp Bastion was a British Ministry of Defense airbase located northwest of the city of Lashkar Gah in Helmand Province, Afghanistan. Between 2005 and October 2014, it was the logistics hub for ISAF operations in Helmand Province. Camp Bastion's Hospital was operated by regular and reserve personnel of the British Army, Royal Navy, and Royal Air Force as well as medical assets from the U.S. Navy and Canada. The medical staff included orthopedic surgeons, general surgeons, anesthetists, nurses, and medics. Wounded military personnel from the British, U.S., and other ISAF forces in Helmand Province were evacuated from the battlefield for treatment at Bastion Hospital and then were medevaced to the Theater Hospital in Bagram or directly to the U.S. Joint Military Medical Center at Landsthul, Germany (Vassallo, 2015).

The Joint Military NATO Hospital—Kabul was located at the Kabul International Airport in the ISAF compound. The hospital is staffed by NATO medical personnel, including French, Spanish, Danish, and U.S. Navy personnel. The hospital provides comprehensive care to NATO forces, Afghan National Security Forces, and local Afghans. Patients are quickly surgically and medically stabilized for AE to the Theater Hospital in Bagram, Afghanistan, or directly to the U.S. Joint Military Medical Center at Landsthul, Germany (Brondex, Viant, Trendel, & Puidupin, 2014).

The U.S. military medical forces also performed a mentoring role at several of the largest Afghan military hospitals. Navy nurses were assigned to mentoring teams, for example, at the regional Afghan National Army (ANA) Hospitals in Kandahar and Mazar-e-Sharif. Other teams were assigned to the mentoring role at ANA Regional Military Hospital—Gardez, ANA Regional Military Hospital—Herat, and Afghan National Police Hospital—Kabul, and the ANA National Military Hospital—Kabul. Here, several senior U.S. Navy nurses were on 12-person imbedded training teams to mentor senior

Afghan nurses. In addition, several senior U.S. Army, Navy, and Air Force certified registered nurse anesthetists (CRNAs) were sent to mentor and teach modern anesthesia care and procedures as well as pain management therapies at these Afghan hospitals (Scannell-Desch & Doherty, 2012).

During combat actions in the Iraq and Afghanistan Wars, U.S. Army nurses have served in a new role—providing en route care in military helicopters for patients being transported to a higher tier of care. From battalion aid stations and FSTs, medical personnel have provided life- and limb-saving resuscitative care along with coordinated movement to the next higher echelon of care at CSHs. Helicopter and fixed-wing medevac missions required military nurses with specialized critical care skills to safely care for these critically wounded or burned patients en route to the CSH (Nagra, 2011).

More than 6,200 Americans have been killed and more than 37,000 wounded in the Iraq and Afghanistan wars to date. Military medical personnel are among those who died. A total of 262 military medical personnel were killed in the conflicts in Iraq and Afghanistan from October 2001 through the present time, according to the Military Health System. Our service in Afghanistan continues to this day.

U.S. AIR FORCE CRITICAL CARE AIR TRANSPORT TEAMS

The Critical Care Air Transport Team (CCATT) is a unique, highly specialized medical resource that can establish and run a mobile ICU on board U.S. Air Force transport aircraft during flight. It is a valuable component of the air force's AE system. The CCATT is a three-person team consisting of a physician, a critical care nurse, and a respiratory therapist (Beninati, Meyer, & Carter, 2008). The physician is usually one specializing in critical care or pulmonology. The team has advanced training in the medical aspects of flight including the effects of flight on the physiology of medical conditions, oxygen limitations at altitude, and medication administration requirements while airborne (Hurd et al., 2006). The team is experienced in caring for critically injured or ill patients with severe multisystem trauma (Brewer & Ryan-Wenger, 2009), shock (Mora, Ervin, Ganem, & Bebarta, 2014), burns (Hamilton, Mora, Chung & Bebarta, 2015), respiratory failure (Fang et al., 2011; Kashani & Farmer, 2006), multiple organ failure, TBI (Dukes, Bridges, & Johantgen, 2013), and other life-threatening conditions. The criticality and instability of these types of patients warrant continuous monitoring, ongoing stabilization measures, and may involve life-saving invasive interventions during the flight.

In the Iraq and Afghanistan wars, current military medical doctrine has emphasized an "evacuate and replace" (Joint Publication 4-02, 2012, p. I-6) philosophy regarding the care and transport of injured and ill soldiers. This strategy has led to a significant reduction in the air force's forward, in-theater medical posture, requiring the development of a strong and flexible medevac capability. The AE system is now directed to rapidly evacuate casualties from many forward locations that are supported by small medical units, such as FSTs or battalion aid stations (Galvagno et al., 2014; Ingalls et al., 2014). This has produced the need to shift from evacuating only "stable" patients to evacuating "stabilized" patients, and thus developing the expertise and right mix of medical personnel to care for these "stabilized" patients during air transport.

The idea for developing the CCATT was introduced and developed in the early 1990s in an effort to expand the air force's aeromedical capabilities. The airborne critical care team would facilitate the early transfer of stabilized seriously injured or ill patients by providing an ICU capability on any available transport aircraft. The CCATT pilot-program commenced in 1994. In mid-1996, CCATT was formally approved as part of the AE system, and has been established throughout the active duty forces, the Air National Guard, and the Air Force Reserve (Ingalls et al., 2014). CCATT expertise was implemented to support quickly mobile FSTs on the ground with elevated capability for emergency resuscitation and limited capacity for postresuscitation casualty care. The CCATT permits rapid evacuation of stabilized casualties to a higher echelon of care. Recognizing that the aeromedical environment presents complex challenges for the delivery of care, all equipment used in this environment must be tested for safety and effectiveness before use in flight. The team members must incorporate current standards of practice and standards of care with the limitations levied by the stresses of flight on their patients (Beninati et al., 2008).

Since the onset of U.S. fighting in the Iraq and Afghanistan wars, explosive blasts have been the top mechanism of injury for patients requiring CCATT. IEDs became the primary ordinance causing blast injuries, and TBI became the signature injury caused by IEDs. Other frequent injuries caused by IEDs and roadside bombs included traumatic limb amputations and severe burns. The distribution of injuries requiring CCATT appears to have changed compared with previous conventional conflicts. Understanding the epidemiology of casualties evacuated by CCATT during modern warfare is a prerequisite for the development of effective predeployment training to ensure optimal outcomes for critically ill and injured troops (Galvagno et al., 2014).

CCATTs have participated in numerous missions since inception. Such missions have included Operation Joint Endeavor in Bosnia, the evacuation of U.S. soldiers from Somalia, the *USS Cole* bombing, several hurricane evacuations, and numerous humanitarian missions (Alkins & Reynolds, 2002).

Within days of the onset of Operation Enduring Freedom and Operation Iraqi Freedom, CCATTs were present in the theater of operations (Collins, 2008; Galvagno et al., 2014; Ingalls et al., 2014), and were saving lives by transporting the wounded and burned from austere airfields after receiving stabilizing treatment by FSTs (Bridges & Evers, 2009; Lairet, King, Vojta, & Beninati, 2013).

Aeromedical capability has grown and matured over the last decade of war. The addition of CCATT has significantly enriched the flexibility and medical expertise that can be delivered to the battle zone, giving our combat troops and their commanders the confidence that we can deliver a timely evacuation platform and emergent medical care should they need it. CCATT has the capability of providing care over a long duration and distance, such as the Middle East or Africa to Germany and Germany to the United States (Alkins & Reynolds, 2002).

Critical care air transport nurses improvise and provide nursing care based on past experiences using a broad and deep critical care knowledge base (Topley, Schmelz, Henkenius-Kirschbaum, & Horvath, 2003). Flight nursing, whether as a traditional flight nurse or as a CCATT member, is a physically tough and mentally demanding profession that calls for tremendous energy, stamina, flexibility, leadership, organizational abilities, and expert clinical skills. However, most of these nurses claim it is the most rewarding experience in their professional lives (Pierce & Evers, 2003).

PROVINCIAL RECONSTRUCTION TEAMS

A few nurses introduced in this book have served on what is called a "Provincial Reconstruction Team" (PRT). As PRTs are mentioned by these nurses, we believe a brief description of a PRT is warranted. A PRT is a small unit of personnel initiated by the U.S. government composed of military officers, diplomats, and reconstruction subject matter experts, functioning to support reconstruction work in unstable states (Roe, 2012).

The first PRTs were created in Afghanistan in 2003, and later operated in Iraq before U.S. forces left Iraq. The purpose of these teams in Iraq and Afghanistan was to empower local governments to govern their people more effectively (Maley & Schmeidl, 2015). Most teams are generally led by a senior official representing the U.S. State Department or USAID (United States Agency for International Development), a senior U.S. military officer of the rank of lieutenant colonel or commander, and representatives from the Department of Agriculture and sometimes the Department of Justice. Other NATO countries also staff PRTs in Afghanistan (George & Rishiko, 2010).

The PRT experience combines civil action and security to enable regional development and affords a crucial interface of information sharing

and problem solving among the local people and governmental, nongovern-
mental, and international aid agencies. The PRT programs in various regions
of Iraq and Afghanistan have varied significantly in their compositions, roles,
operational environments, and resourcing (Roe, 2012). In Afghanistan, time
will chronicle the success, or failure, of the PRTs over the long run.

One might ask: "Why would Nurse Corps Lieutenant Colonels or Naval
Commanders be chosen to be the senior military member on a Provisional
Reconstruction Team." Nurse Corps officers are officers first and nurses second. Most Nurse Corps officers of this rank are graduates of their intermediate
service school, such as Army General Command and Staff College or the Air
Force Command and Staff College. Furthermore, many may have already graduated from the Army, Navy, or Air Force War College, which are the respective
services' senior service schools. As senior officers with advanced formal military education, Nurse Corps officers are as well prepared as their nonmedical
counterparts of the same rank to perform PRT duties. Also, Nurse Corps officers possess and demonstrate the "people" skills to work successfully on a
team, the listening skills to astutely hear what people are saying and needing,
the public health acumen to assess the needs of poor and vulnerable populations, and the leadership abilities to make a positive difference in people's lives.

REFERENCES

Air Force Doctrine Document 2. (2007). *Airpower doctrine: The Air Expeditionary
Wing*. Washington, DC: Office of the Secretary of the Air Force.
Air Force Pamphlet 36-2241. (2013). *Professional development guide*. Washington,
DC: Department of the Air Force.
Alkins, S. A., & Reynolds, A. J. (2002). Long-distance air evacuation of blast-injured
sailors from the *USS Cole*. *Aviation, Space, & Environmental Medicine, 73*(7),
677–680.
Beekley, A. C., & Watts, D. M. (2004). Combat trauma experience with the United
States Army 102nd Forward Surgical Team in Afghanistan. *American Journal
of Surgery, 187*(5), 652–654.
Beninati, W., Meyer, M. T., & Carter, T. E. (2008). The critical care air transport
program. *Critical Care Medicine, 36*(7), S370–S376.
Bohman, H. R., Stevens, R. A., Baker, B. C., & Chambers, L. W. (2005). The U.S.
Navy's forward resuscitative surgery system during Operation Iraqi Freedom.
Military Medicine, 170, 294–297.
Brewer, T. L., & Ryan-Wenger, N. A. (2009). Critical care air transport team (CCATT)
nurses' deployed experience. *Military Medicine, 174*(5), 508–514.
Bridges, E., & Evers, K. (2009). Wartime critical care air transport. *Military
Medicine, 174*(4), 370–375.
Brisebois, R., Hennecke, P., Kao, R., McAlister, V., Po, J., Stiegelmar, R., & Tien, H.
(2011). The Role 3 Multinational Medical Unit at Kandahar Airfield 2005-2010.
Canadian Journal of Surgery, 54(6 Suppl.), S124–S129.

Brondex, A., Viant, E., Trendel, D., & Puidupin, M. (2014). Medical activity in the conventional hospitalization unit in Kabul NATO Role 3 Hospital: A three month long experience. *Military Medicine, 179*(2), 197–202.

Collins, S. T. (2008). Emergency medical support units to critical care transport teams in Iraq. *Critical Care Nursing Clinics of North America, 20*(1), 1–11.

Conard, P. L., Allen, P. E., & Armstrong, M. L. (2015). Preparing staff to care for veterans in a way they need and deserve. *Journal of Continuing Education Nursing, 46*(3), 109–118.

Counihan, T. C., & Danielson, P. D. (2012). The 912th Forward Surgical Team in Operation New Dawn: Employment of the forward surgical team during troop withdrawal under combat conditions. *Military Medicine, 177*(11), 1267–1271.

Dierkes, D. (2011). Deployment to Afghanistan: Perioperative nursing outside the comfort zone. *Association of Operating Room Nursing Journal, 94*(3), 271–278.

Dukes, S. F., Bridges, E., & Johantgen, M. (2013). Occurrence of secondary insults of traumatic brain injury in patients transported by critical care air transport teams from Iraq/Afghanistan: 2003–2006. *Military Medicine, 178*(1), 11–17.

Fang, R., Allan, P. F., Womble, S. G., Porter, M. T., Sierra-Nunez, J., Russ, R. S.,…Dorlac, W. C. (2011). Closing the "care in the air" capability gap for severe lung injury: The Landstuhl Acute Lung Rescue Team and extracorporeal lung support. *Journal of Trauma, 71*(7-1), S91–S97.

Galvagno, S. M., Dubose, J. J., Grissom, T. E., Fang, R., Smith, R., Bebarta, V. S.,…Scalea, T. M. (2014). The epidemiology of Critical Care Air Transport Team operations in contemporary warfare. *Military Medicine, 79*(6), 612–618.

George, R. Z., & Rishiko, H. (Eds.). (2010). *The national security enterprise: Navigating the labyrinth.* Washington, DC: Georgetown University Press.

Hamilton, J. A., Mora, A. G., Chung, K. K., & Bebarta, V. S. (2015). Impact of anemia in critically ill burned casualties evacuated from combat theater via US military critical care air transport teams. *Shock, 44*(1), 50–54.

Hurd, W. W., Montminy, R. J., De Lorenzo, R. A., Burd, L. T., Goldman, B. S., & Loftus, T. J. (2006). Physician roles in aeromedical evacuation: Current practices in USAF operations. *Aviation, Space, and Environmental Medicine, 77*(6), 631–638.

Ingalls, N., Zonies, D., Bailey, J. A., Martin, K. D., Iddins, B. O., Carlton, P. K.,…Johannigman, J. (2014). A review of the first 10 years of critical care aeromedical transport during Operation Iraqi Freedom and Operation Enduring Freedom: The importance of evacuation timing. *Journal of the American Medical Association Surgery, 149*(8), 807–813.

Joint Publication 4-02. (2012). *Health service support.* Washington, DC: Office of the Joint Chiefs of Staff, Medical Department.

Kashani, K. B., & Farmer, J. C. (2006). The support of severe respiratory failure beyond the hospital and during transportation. *Current Opinion in Critical Care, 12*(1), 43–49.

Kenny, D. J., & Hull, M. S. (2008). Critical care nurses' experiences caring for casualties of war evacuated from the front line: Lessons learned and needs identified. *Critical Care Nursing Clinics of North America, 20*(1), 41–49.

King, B., & Jatoi, I. (2005). The Mobile Army Surgical Hospital (MASH): A military and surgical legacy. *Journal of the National Medical Association, 97*(5), 648–656.

Korzeniewski, K., & Bochniak, A. (2011). Medical support of military operations in Iraq and Afghanistan. *Journal of International Maritime Health, 62*(2), 71–76.

Lairet, J., King, J., Vojta, L., & Beninati, W. (2013). Short-term outcomes of US Air Force critical care air transport team (CCATT) patients evacuated from a combat setting. *Prehospital Emergency Care, 17*(4), 486–490.

Looney, W. R. (1996). The Air Expeditionary Force: Taking the air force into the twenty-first century. Maxwell Air Force Base, AL. *Air and Space Power Journal, 2*, 1–6.

Maley, W., & Schmeidl, S. (Eds.). (2015). *Reconstructing Afghanistan: Civil-military experiences in comparative perspective.* New York, NY: Routledge.

Maureen, M., York, G. B., Hirshon, J. M., Jenkins, D. H., & Scalea, T. M. (2011). Trauma readiness training for military deployment: A comparison between a U.S. trauma center and an Air Force Theater Hospital in Balad, Iraq. *Military Medicine, 176*(7), 769–776.

Mora, A. G., Ervin, A. T., Ganem, V. J., & Bebarta, V. S. (2014). Aeromedical evacuation of combat patients by military critical care air transport teams with a lower hemoglobin threshold approach is safe. *Journal of Trauma and Acute Care Surgery, 77*(5), 724–728.

Nagra, M. (2011). Optimizing wartime en route nursing care in Operation Iraqi Freedom. *Journal of the U.S. Army Medical Department*, Oct-Dec, 51–58.

Nowak, M. J. (1999). *The Air Expeditionary Force: Strategy for an uncertain future?* Maxwell Air Force Base, AL: Air War College/Air University.

Pierce, P. F., & Evers, K. G. (2003). Global presence: USAF aeromedical evacuation and critical care air transport. *Critical Care Nursing Clinics of North America, 15*(2), 221–231.

Roe, A. M. (2012). *A Contemporary "blueprint" for North Atlantic Treaty Organization provisional reconstruction teams in Afghanistan.* Fort Leavenworth, KS: School of Advanced Military Studies.

Sarnecky, M. T. (2010). *A contemporary history of the U.S. Army Nurse Corps.* Washington, DC: The Borden Institute.

Scannell-Desch, E. A., & Doherty, M. E. (2012). *Nurses in war: Voices from Iraq and Afghanistan.* New York, NY: Springer Publishing Company.

Schoenfeld, A. (2012). The combat experience of military surgical assets in Iraq and Afghanistan: A historical review. *American Journal of Surgery, 204*(3), 377–383.

Topley, D. K., Schmelz, J., Henkenius-Kirschbaum, J., & Horvath, K. J. (2003). Critical care nursing expertise during air transport. *Military Medicine, 168*(10), 822–826.

U.S. Centcom. (2015). About U.S. Central Command: Fact sheet. Retrieved from http://www.centcom.mil

Vassallo, D. (2015). A short history of Camp Bastion Hospital: Preparing for war, national recognition and Bastion's legacy. *Journal of the Royal Army Medical Corps, 465*, ii.

Venticinque, S. G., & Grathwohl, K. W. (2008). Critical care in the austere environment: Providing exceptional care in unusual places. *Critical Care Medicine, 36*(7), 284–292.

Photo courtesy of U.S. Navy.

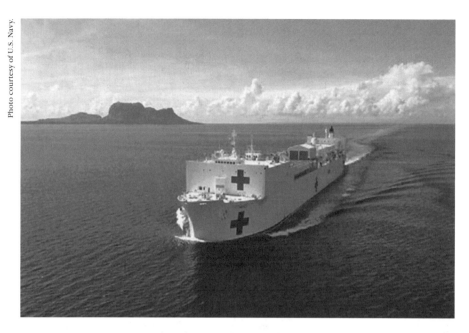

U.S. Navy hospital ship, *USN Mercy*, at sea.

Photo courtesy of U.S. Air Force.

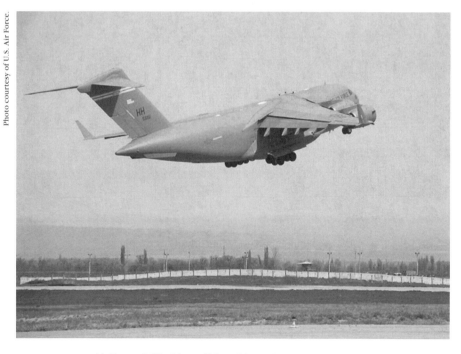

Air Force C-17 taking off from Manas Air Base, Kyrgyzstan.

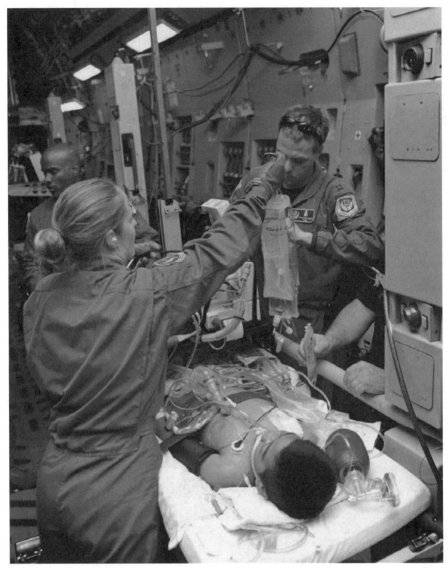

Air force flight nurses providing critical care inflight.

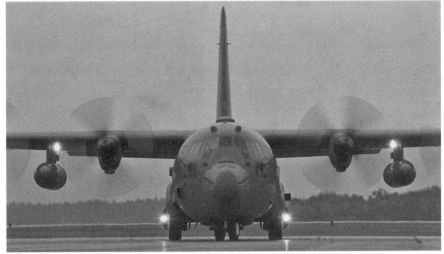

Air Force C-130 aircraft frequently used for in-theater aeromedical evacuation between bases in Afghanistan.

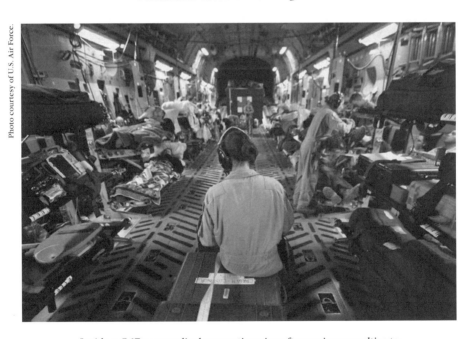

Inside a C-17 aeromedical evacuation aircraft carrying casualties to Ramstein Air Base, Germany.

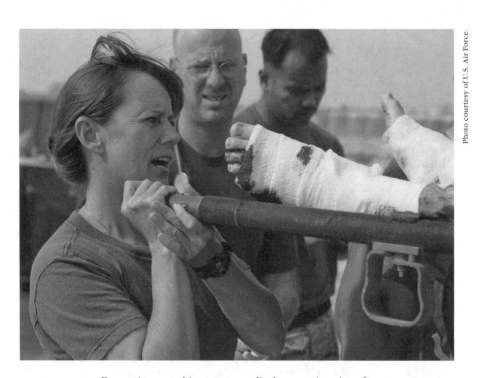

Photo courtesy of U.S. Air Force.

Evacuating casualties to aeromedical evacuation aircraft.

3

Homecoming: A Positive Reception

Homecoming was usually anticipated as a positive experience for most of the military nurses. However, communication between deployed personnel and their family and military unit back home was often compromised because of myriad connectivity problems. During the early years of the Iraq and Afghanistan wars, communication infrastructure for personal communication was poor to nonexistent. Sometimes, the only method of communication with family and friends back home was through slow regular mail service. Because of the austerity of some remote assignments on forward operating bases (FOBs) in Iraq and Afghanistan, a fair number of nurses reported great frustration with poor Internet connections and intermittent telephone service even in later years of these wars. Nurses assigned in population centers, such as Baghdad, Mosul, Balad, Kabul, Kandahar, and Bagram, fared much better in using Internet and telephone services. As a result, loved ones and even military colleagues often did not know the specifics regarding the date, time, and location of the nurses' arrival in the United States. For example, some nurses arrived at an airport or an air base on the east coast when their family or military unit was on the west coast. Others arrived in the middle of the night without any prior notification of their family or military unit. Occasionally, veteran or retired military organizations, located near aerial ports of entry, met returning flights. Some nurses recalled a joyful homecoming that left a lasting memory; they felt welcomed and appreciated.

LIEUTENANT COLONEL REGINA

Regina was raised in Buffalo, New York, one of six children in a middle-class family. She attended nursing school and college in upstate New York. She and her husband both joined the Army Reserve several years after they were married and their children were in school. They joined because they wanted to give something back to their country, it was a time of relative peace, and they wanted to earn extra income. Regina was an Army Nurse Corps Reserve lieutenant colonel when she was deployed to Iraq in April 2007 for 11 months.

Regina described her deployment and her homecoming:

I was assigned in Ramadi, Iraq, on an embedded provincial reconstruction team. We were part of President Bush's surge strategy into Iraq. Even though I was a registered nurse, I was cross-trained in civil affairs. We were to use our professional expertise, in my case as a nurse, to help the civil affairs team to rebuild Iraq and its necessary infrastructure. The embedded provincial reconstruction teams were originally set up with three members. The lead member was from the U.S. Department of State, the second team member was from U.S. Agency for International Development (USAID), and the third member was a senior military officer.

When the U.S. invaded Iraq, most of the wealthy and professional people left the country. So, about 90% of Iraq's physicians left. Many of the nurses in Iraq left, too. The directorate general for health was an industrial engineer. The cities were left with mostly working class and poor people. When I first got there and got a tour of the city it looked like post–World War II Berlin. Most buildings were damaged, and there was raw sewage in the streets. The hospital had no electricity or running water. They used emergency generators at the hospital when they had to. I learned a lot while I was in Iraq. I think it changed me by giving me a whole different perspective about the challenges of rebuilding after a locality is devastated by war and what war does to a population center and its people.

I came back in late February 2008, to Fort Benning, Georgia. I was lucky that my husband was also an Army Reserve officer who was on active duty at the time. He was my greatest support. I could not have done this without his support. I came back, again I was very blessed, that the army gave my husband the time off to drive from Florida to Fort Benning, and my husband was in the reception area when I got off the plane. It took me like five days to travel in Iraq to get on the Freedom Bird [flight] for the trip home. You are almost kind of "shell shocked" to finally be back on U.S. soil. When I got off the plane they had a band playing, they had big banners saying "Welcome Home." I had never experienced anything quite like this in my life. When I walked in the hangar, I saw the band playing, the banners flying, and my husband standing off to the side. I got to give him a hug right away and then we were ushered to the bleachers and got some type of briefing. That was my initial welcome home. I did my out-processing at Fort Benning, filled out lots of forms, turned in my weapon and all my other gear. It was kind of a blur, I want to say I was there for five to seven days. My husband actually left me a vehicle to get around. Then, he came back to Benning and we drove together to where he was assigned in Florida. I came off active duty to be in the reserves again. My homecoming could not have been better and I was thankful to be home safe and sound with my husband.

LIEUTENANT COMMANDER CATHERINE

Catherine hailed from a small town in north Texas. She grew up riding horses, driving farm equipment, and raising calves and pigs with her local 4-H Club. She describes herself as adventurous with a passion for travel and trying new things. After college, and a year of working in a local community hospital, Catherine joined the Navy Nurse Corps. Catherine is a family nurse practitioner in the navy with two deployments under her belt. Her first deployment was to Fallujah, Iraq, for 6 months, which she described as a "blood bath." Then she was at a remote site called Camp Korean Village for 2 months. Camp Korean Village was located near the Jordanian and Syrian borders. Her second deployment was in Afghanistan from 2009 to 2010. Catherine had 4 months of training away from home before going to Afghanistan for 9 months—a total absence of 13 months. She was in Khost province, which is in the eastern part of Afghanistan near the Pakistan border. Catherine was with a provincial reconstruction team. To prepare for this role, she spent time at Camp Attaberry, Indiana, with the army, and also in San Antonio, Texas.

Catherine described her homecoming:

My initial homecoming was great. My family had done all kinds of nice things. My husband had gotten a big Welcome Home poster and they put lots of flags all around the sidewalk. [*She starts crying as she tells me this and her voice is all choked up.*] Now he knows that I cared about all the things they did [because he's listening to this phone interview] and now he's gonna make fun of me all night long for crying and getting choked up as I tell you this [*she starts laughing*]. They really made a nice homecoming for me with decorating the house and all that stuff.

And this is true of both of my deployments. Your command wants to know when you are coming home. I felt strongly that I didn't want them to know when I was coming home. I didn't want the command at the airport. You don't want to be anything other than the mom or the wife. I didn't want to be the family nurse practitioner or the lieutenant commander. I didn't want to do that or be in that role. I just wanted to go home. I think I just told my husband not to tell them.

LIEUTENANT COLONEL TAMMY

Tammy was the daughter of an army officer, who grew up in Germany, Kansas, Georgia, and Texas. After college, she joined the Army Nurse Corps and had assignments the states of Washington and Virginia. After several years, she left the army and worked as a recovery room nurse for 2 years. She then joined the Air National Guard. After more than a decade in the Air National Guard, she volunteered for deployment.

Tammy stated:

I was deployed in 2011 to Kabul, Afghanistan. I was assigned as an IA (individual augmentee) to an imbedded mentoring team. I was deployed for 6 months. I mentored the director for the Afghan National Army Nurse Training Program. I mentored the director as well as a cadre of instructors.

I had a very good reunion with my family. The kids had missed me a lot and they welcomed me with open arms. I had really good support from home, and I was able to communicate almost every day with my husband while I was gone. So I was pretty well informed about how everyone was doing and what activities the kids were engaged in. It was a pretty easy transition back into our family. I had quite a bit of notice that I was going to deploy, so we had time to put the necessary supports in place so that my husband wouldn't be overwhelmed with his job plus being a single parent with kids. I would say that I had almost a year's notice to get myself and my family ready for me being gone. Our youngest kids were 6 and 8 when I deployed and we had a 14-year-old at home and a 21-year-old in college.

MAJOR ANITA

Anita is a "southern belle" from the heart of Charleston, South Carolina. She joined the air force after college to gain valuable nursing experience and see the world. She is married to another air force officer and she describes their life together as an adventure because they love to travel, they are gourmet foodies, and they are into having lots of fun. She reports that at this point in life they are not interested in having children, although they enjoy other people's children in limited doses.

She described her deployment experiences and homecoming:

I am in the air force and have had two deployments, the first one to Pakistan and the second one to Bagram Air Base, Afghanistan. My first deployment was right at the beginning of the war in early 2003 to Pakistan. We were at Jacobabad Air Base in Pakistan near the Afghanistan border. Our mission there was to take care of the army guys who were on the front lines. They would come to Jacobabad to rest up, get hydrated, and then go back to the fighting. We provided health care as needed. It was pretty basic, the bare minimum to take care of their health care needs. If we had a critical patient, we'd have to ship them out. We would have a C-130 air evac flight come in to get any patients that were beyond our capability.

I went to Bagram, Afghanistan, in July 2012 and I got back to the States in February 2013. I was at Bagram Air Base the whole time working in the ICU as a nurse. I was solely dedicated to the ICU for 6 months. When I first got there in the summer, it was peak season, every single bed was full every single day. My orientation to the unit was like, "Here you go," so I just had to jump in and start working. We were all replacing somebody, so you kind of just "high five it" and wish them well as they leave for home. It was super, super busy. We had 14 beds total, we could expand to 20, but we hardly ever did that, and if we did that would only be for a few hours. I would say that 98% of our patients were trauma. We did occasionally have a few medical patients, meaning someone with cardiac issues or a pediatric patient with congenital issues.

Anita went on to talk about her homecoming stating:

My homecoming was great. I was able to talk to my husband every
day I was gone. I was able to call him on the regular phone. We
couldn't rely on Skype all the time because it was inconsistent. My
husband didn't like Skype because it tended to be in and out, not
a good connection. I would call him on the regular phone and we
had a set time. It would be a 2-minute phone call because if you
talk every day, there's not a whole lot to talk about [*laughing*].

My husband is military and he's deployed before so he understands the situation. He's in the air force, too, but we've never
been deployed at the same time. We don't have kids. The homecoming was good and I flew into Sacramento. We're stationed at
Travis AFB. My husband was there, some friends were there, and
some coworkers were there. They had a big "Welcome Home"
sign. It was wonderful. There's a funny story and it kind of
makes me a little teary-eyed when I think of it. When I was coming down the escalator, my favorite song is "Dancing Queen" by
Abba and everyone makes a little joke about it, it's even on my e-
mail. Well, my husband has this little tiny itty-bitty speaker thing,
I don't even know what it is really called, it is about 6 inches long
and you hook it up to your iPhone and it plays music. Well anyway, so when I was coming down the escalator, I see him with
this thing above his head because we're a product of the 80s
and we love 80s music and movies, so it was like John Cusack
holding up the boom box in the movie *Say Anything*, telling his
girl that he loved her. So, my husband is standing down there
holding up that thing playing "Dancing Queen." I was like "I love
it, it's great" [*laughing*]. It was precious, adorable, and when I
think of it, I get a little teary-eyed. It was sweet.

LIEUTENANT COMMANDER ZOE

Zoe grew up as a navy brat because her father was a career naval officer.
Her family had lived in Rota, Spain; Kenitra, Morocco; Jacksonville, Florida;
Norfolk, Virginia; and San Diego, California. Zoe was an active duty navy
family nurse practitioner. She had deployed to Kuwait from 2006 to 2007
and to Afghanistan from 2009 to 2010. The Afghanistan mission was with
a provincial reconstruction team, which was a tri-service augmented role.
It was an army mission but it involved the army, navy, and air force. They
were all on the same team.

She found out about her first deployment to Kuwait while her husband was out on a submarine. They were both on active duty navy. He had been away for 3 months when she found out that she would be deployed, but, thankfully, they never got deployed at the same time. At this time, their both daughters were quite young. They had only 1 week overlap between their two deployments, which was not good for them as a couple and as parents. It was very stressful for both of them.

With the second deployment to Afghanistan, they were much more prepared as a couple and as parents. The timing and communication were better. They had time to prepare. They had learned a lot from Zoe's first deployment. Even on returning from Afghanistan, Zoe reported, "We didn't have the marital strain of the first deployment."

Zoe recounted:

My husband was in Hawaii with our kids. It was planned that they would not come to San Diego. I wanted to be able to come back to our home and have them be there. I think I was in San Diego for about 2-1/2 days. Then, in preparation for coming back to Hawaii, I told them that I didn't want a big homecoming. I just wanted to see my family and have it be low key. I'm not someone who likes to be the center of attention. It makes me feel uncomfortable and embarrassed. So, I traveled in uniform and during the flights some people made positive comments like, "Thank you for your service." It was nice and it was helpful to be recognized in that way.

I arrived at the airport in Hawaii, I got through security, and then [*laughing*] there was a huge group of people to greet me. It was my husband and my daughters and one of our best friends and her family and ten of my coworkers. We're in Hawaii, so there were leis. My initial reaction was "Oh, no" [*laughing*]. I wanted a small group. I was tearful; I was hot; I was tired; I was emotional. But, it was interesting because as we walked down to the baggage claim together, this huge gaggle, and then other people were there, and they saw that I was being welcomed home. More people said, "Thank you for your service" [*laughing*], and then I realized, I really did need this. I needed it to be a celebration and a welcoming full of excitement. It was mostly people I knew. It was my coworkers and my immediate boss. It wasn't the whole town. No one was a stranger. I was OK that I was crying [*laughing as she told me this*]. Everyone just wanted to be helpful. My boss said, "Your job now is to spend time with your family and take time." It was actually a really good experience. We lingered after the bags were gathered.

We took pictures. They brought Martinelli's sparkling cider and we're toasting. It was such a funny random thing, toasting at the airport [*laughing*]. It was joyful!

Later, my husband said, "I didn't tell them to come." [*Laughing*] I said, "It's OK, it really is" [*laughing*]. Ahead of time, I wouldn't have known this would be OK with me, but it was [*laughing*]. Maybe if it had just been my husband and daughters, it might have been less celebratory. We still talk about it to this day. So, my immediate homecoming was celebratory and joyful. I got home in November, just a couple of weeks before Thanksgiving and the whole Christmas season. I was excited about that but was also worried. It can be such a "false" time for people—being stressed, but at the same time you are supposed to enjoy and be thankful.

LIEUTENANT LAUREN

Lauren was raised in the suburbs of Philadelphia, Pennsylvania, and attended a local university on a Naval Reserve Officer Training Corps (NROTC) Scholarship. Once she graduated, she attended medical officer basic training. Her first duty station was in San Diego, California, at the large Balboa Naval Medical Center.

Lauren stated:

I was deployed to Kuwait in 2007. In 2008, I was sent to the naval hospital in Japan. Then in 2010, I was deployed to Afghanistan right next to Camp Leatherneck. First, before I deployed, I did some trauma training at the University of Southern California— Los Angeles County Level 1 trauma center for 3 weeks. Then, I was sent to York, England, because I was joining a unit that was British. So, it was a collaboration between the U.S. and the British in Helmand Province, Afghanistan, at Camp Bastion. I trained in York, England, for almost a month and then went to Afghanistan for 6 months. We hit the ground running when I got to Afghanistan. It was a pretty intense and bloody time. It was the busiest trauma hospital in the world.

When I got back from my Kuwait deployment, I was up in Maine and it was the most phenomenal experience. All these old people and veterans were there to greet us when we landed in Bangor. It was really kind of cool.

When I returned from Afghanistan, it was me coming off the plane solo. I think it was Dulles airport and that place is sort of a ghost town. There was my boyfriend who I had not seen in ages because he was in Sicily and then he also got deployed. He was in Iraq when I was in Afghanistan. It was the closest time zone on the phone that we had in years for him to be in Iraq and me to be in Afghanistan. I was just so thrilled to see him and we literally had about 2 hours at Dulles airport before I had to jump on another plane and go down and do that decompression thing in Norfolk, that deployment evaluation. I remember that he picked me up in the dark. He picked me up in DC. He had gone and checked out an apartment for us. He had already moved his stuff in and my stuff was not there yet from Japan. I hadn't gone back to Japan yet. I spent a few nights in DC with him at this new apartment. It was just him who got me at the airport, no family. I was exhausted and then the next day I had to do the return from deployment interviews. At least I had a home. He had gotten the apartment. I remember being upset that I had to go to Norfolk so soon. So, I saw him for 2 hours at the airport. We waited together and then I flew to Norfolk. Then, I got a flight back that night. I remember that he picked me up in the dark.

CAPTAIN SCHUYLER

Schuyler joined the army shortly after graduating from college. She considers the state of Washington her home, having lived there with her parents since she was 10 years old. She considered herself an "outdoors adventurer" and somewhat of a tomboy growing up. She liked to camp and hike, play sports, and stay physically fit.

Schuyler related:

I was in the Army Nurse Corps. I was active duty and now I'm in the inactive reserves (individual readiness reserves). I had 4 years of active duty. I deployed to Iraq in April 2006 to April 2007. I was assigned to a combat support hospital in the beginning of the deployment at Abu Ghraib, but then we shut down and moved all the detainees to a new location near the airport and that was Camp Cropper. My whole deployment was the detainee care mission.

My homecoming was very successful. I feel like I coped and transitioned very well. One of the biggest reasons was because I was well-supported by my family. I kept in contact with them a lot through e-mail. I wrote them letters, particularly my parents.

I also had two of my close friends at the time from my duty station in Germany deploy with me at the same time. I had a good network of people—men and women who I either went to college with or went to officer's basic with or were stationed with. When I was done with my deployment I flew back to Texas and went on leave. I then went home to my family in Washington state. I think the first few days back in the States were the hardest. It was hard to realize that I was not going back to Iraq; to realize that I wasn't there anymore. It was hard, too, because I was in a relationship with someone who was still in Iraq. The realization that we were no longer close was hard. Flying home from Texas to Washington, I was really weepy. Once I got there it was better. They were very welcoming. My dad had been in the military in Vietnam and that helped. My mom had siblings who had gone to Vietnam. So, I think they had prepared how to handle me. I think they put a lot of thought into things. I spent probably about 15 leave days with my family and then I left to go back to Europe because I had been stationed in Germany. Then, I went to Iraq to see my fiancé at the time. We ended up spending time in Turkey. Then, I went back to work in Germany. I went back to work taking care of soldiers who had just gotten injured in Iraq or Afghanistan. I was around a lot of people who had been deployed and they understood where I had been and what I had been doing. My work was similar except for the fact that I wasn't taking care of detainees anymore. However, it was very much the same type of injuries we had been seeing.

I spent another year in Germany before I got off of active duty. During that time my fiancé and I got married. We were in Germany together and it was just him and I. We were able to deal with any stress that might have been left over from Iraq and our war experiences. We came back and reintegrated into my family and community here in Washington state.

FIRST LIEUTENANT ALLISON

Allison was raised in the suburbs of Hartford, Connecticut, and attended college in the Boston, Massachusetts, area. After working as a civilian nurse for 2 years, she joined the air force because she wanted to travel, meet new people, and experience life overseas. She was assigned to a large Air Force Medical Center in California as a Coronary Care ICU nurse for only 2 years before being deployed to Gazi Province, Afghanistan. She volunteered for deployment because she "wanted to be where the action was."

Allison remarked:

I'm a first lieutenant on active duty in the air force, and I deployed to Afghanistan in December 2012 and returned to my California base in late July 2013. Everything we did in Afghanistan was quite different than what we were used to. It was a really awesome experience. Over there we kind of worked at everything. I was an ER Triage nurse. I was actually the blood bank officer. I stabilized patients in the emergency room. Once we stabilized patients we would bring them to our operating room. In the operating room, they had a permanent staff assigned, so that was about the only place that I never worked in. I recovered patients in a recovery room ICU setting as well. So, my role over there was ER, triage, trauma stabilization, recovery room, and ICU. I would say about a quarter of the patients we treated were American soldiers and the remaining three quarters were local civilian Afghan men, women, and children. Our hospital was on a FOB, which was quite small. I think the perimeter of our FOB was only about 2 miles. The hospital was fairly small and made of plywood. It was not the most secure location because we did have rocket attacks some nights. Even though I'm air force, I was assigned as an individual augmentee to an army unit. We went for training with the army prior to deployment. There were 28 of us air force personnel coming from different bases and different specialty occupations going for training on an army post. Only one other air force officer coming from my base in California was in my group. Once we got to Afghanistan, all 28 of us were dispersed to other FOBs. We never saw each other again until we were reunited at the end of our deployment when we were leaving Afghanistan.

When I got to my hospital they were set up as a Forward Surgical Team [FST] and I was replacing one person on that team. That way you don't have 28 new people coming to a unit at the same time. They incrementally add new people and take out the old people so as to control the flow of experienced versus inexperienced personnel. I walked in with one medical technician, so we were the "newbies" for this unit. It was a pretty easy transition because the team that was already there was still intact. They gave us very good guidance. The first day we got there had a mass casualty event about 4 hours after we arrived. This is when we have more patients than we can handle at once and we need all staff to come in, even if they are off duty. They just threw me in the mix of everything. They said, "Here's the chart, fill out what you can, and do a head-to-toe assessment." I said, "OK." I guess that is the best way, just kind of jump right in and get your hands wet with the job. I think this was a good way to get oriented to the facility and how the patient flow works. I was an ICU nurse and used to ICU care, but not trauma ICU. I was used to critical situations with patients that could crash at any moment. I was used to ventilators and blood pressure medications and various IV drips. Of course the deployed environment can be very chaotic and overwhelming because you know you are in a war environment and you can be attacked while you are taking care of patients with critical raw trauma injuries.

When we left Afghanistan we stopped in Germany for about 4 days. We attended a 3-day reintegration program just to kind of decompress and go over things we might have seen, and get emotions expressed. The program described helpful ways to deal with things when we get back, like driving a car, or taking public transportation, and having more freedom since we had been confined to such a small space for almost 7 months. This program in Germany was at Ramstein Air Base, Germany, where all the air evac flights from Afghanistan come in and where most troops redeploy to the U.S. from. This is where I met up with the 28 air force people I had done the army training with before deploying. It was nice and very comforting to meet up with those 28 air force people again. Everyone made it through the deployment safely, and we all shared stories and experiences. I kept in touch with five or six of them through our deployments to various FOBs in Afghanistan to see how folks were doing and to see what kind of patients they were seeing. It was nice to sort of "compare notes" over the 7 months. It was so comforting to recognize familiar faces again that you had been with prior to deployment and I have to admit those 7 months went by really fast. We all took commercial flights out of Germany to the U.S. commercial hubs near the bases we were assigned to in the U.S. We all went our separate ways out of Germany. For me, I took a commercial flight to Los Angeles, and then connected to a flight into Sacramento. Other folks were stationed in Texas, or Florida, or Washington, DC.

When I landed in Sacramento, one of the OR techs, that I had met while deployed, was also stationed at my base in California. She came home 3 months before I did, and she agreed to come to Sacramento and pick me up when I came home. She picked me up at the airport and we went out for a nice dinner before she dropped me off at my apartment. I had kept my apartment while I was gone and let someone from the base live in it till the week before I came home. It was nice to be back in my place in familiar surroundings and not have to start all over finding a place to live.

I didn't want a crazy, over-the-top homecoming party. For me, I was deployed to do my job, which is what I trained for. Deploying is part of what military nurses and other military people do. So when I got back to Travis AFB, I had to inprocess through the base to just make sure my medical clearance and personnel records are up-to-date. Since I came back alone, the next day I did the inprocessing and met with my supervisor. We also did computer-based training where we did several question-naires asking about our experiences and how we were doing mentally and physically. It was kind of a self-assessment to see how we were doing. My supervisor also met with me to assess how I was doing and to see what I needed. I didn't have to go to a psychiatric evaluation, it was a computer-assisted program where I answered a bunch of questions about my temperament, such as "was I angry, depressed, wanting to hurt myself, wanting to hurt others, etc." Another computer questionnaire asked about nightmares, flashbacks, intrusive thoughts, etc. I didn't have any issues. I enjoyed my deployment. It was a truly awesome experi-ence. I'd go back in a heartbeat, it was that good. I guess if people answered the questions that they were having issues, they would be seen by the mental health folks before they were allowed to go on R & R [rest and relaxation]. We got 2 weeks of R & R. It was nice, but you can't leave the local area. Since I kept my apartment while I deployed, I didn't have to go house hunting or do any-thing stressful like that. I was able to sleep in my own bed, and my surroundings were the same as what I had left. It's not like I had to worry about finding a new apartment or buying a car, or any of that stressful stuff. So for my 2 weeks I had my mom and my stepdad come out and visit me. We did stuff in the area and visited San Francisco and Napa Valley and got reacquainted. It was a nice visit. It was good but we weren't allowed to fly home to Connecticut to visit family or anything like that.

After my 2 weeks of R & R I went back to work at my hos-pital in California. I wanted to go home to Connecticut, but peo-ple's schedules and vacations were already programmed. So, I decided to work for a month and then go on leave to Connecticut to visit family. My unit gave me 3 days of orientation even though I was returning to the coronary ICU that I have left 7 months

before. The orientation was good and it was totally more than
adequate to get back in the groove. I quickly got refamiliarized
with the charting and routine, and then went back working the
usual 12-hour shifts. We had some new people on my unit, but
many people I had worked with before. That is just the way it is
in the military and I was used to that. I think my transition back
was pretty smooth and uneventful.

LIEUTENANT COLONEL TONI

Toni grew up in the suburbs of Charlotte, North Carolina. Toni was one of
five children. After working as an ICU nurse for several years, she joined
the Air Force Reserve forces with a work colleague. At the time they were
both single and wanted to broaden their horizons as military nurses, see
more of the world, but wanted to keep their civilian jobs in the ICU near
Richmond, Virginia.
Toni recalled:

I'm in the Air Force Reserve. I've been in the Air Force Reserve for
18 1/2 years. I've had three deployments overseas. My first deployment was to Kuwait in 2003, and we were in a hospital at Camp
Wolverine where we provided care to some of the first casualties.
I was there for 102 days. Coming home wasn't too bad. My family
missed me and my kids missed me, and they were teenagers then.
I got good support from my employer, which is still my employer.

My second deployment was at Balad Air Base, Iraq. It was
in 2006 into 2007. I was there for 10 months. I was the charge
nurse in the Combat Aeromedical Staging Facility (CASF). There
we cared for all the patients after surgery awaiting aeromedical
evacuation, usually to Germany on their way home. My additional duty on my day off was in the ICU since I'm a trauma critical care nurse with lots of experience. Also, if the hospital got
overwhelmed with casualties, I'd get pulled to work in the ICU.
I'm also trained as a CCATT (Critical Care Air Transport Team)
nurse, but I didn't fly much on the air evac planes, I was generally on the medevac helicopters with very critical patients.

Flying medevac on helicopters was an interesting experience. I had never been shot at before. At first I didn't notice it
until we were on our way back after we had dropped off our
patients in Baghdad. At night you could really see the tracers
and fire in the area of our helicopter. I was by myself on these

missions, because there was no physician or medic to help me. A lot of my patients were amputees or patients that had had general surgery and now were being transported to Baghdad for specialty surgery. Some of these patients were locals, so it wasn't just our soldiers that we transported to Baghdad. We also cared for the enemy insurgents who were wounded at our hospital in Balad. You might be caring for the insurgent in the evening in the ICU who had shot up the village earlier in the day and we had saved his life in the operating room. Caring for the enemy never crossed my mind until the first day I worked in the ICU and an insurgent was my critical care patient.

Toni found her third deployment to be her most difficult deployment. She recalled:

My third deployment was Kandahar, Afghanistan. I was there from 2009 to 2010. I was on a CCATT team the whole 7 months that I was there. We flew patients to Bagram Air Base, Afghanistan, or to Ramstein Air Base, Germany, and we went downrange in Afghanistan to some of the smaller bases and took those patients to Kandahar, Bagram, or Germany. I did not fly any missions to the States, I stayed in theater except for missions to Germany. This deployment was devastating for me. I had not seen raw trauma like that before. It was so fresh and so raw. I was prepared clinically, but I don't think I was prepared mentally. When you see it day after day after day, it has a cumulative effect on you. Your CCATT team is the extra trauma team onboard the aircraft, and many times we didn't just care for the one or two most critical and unstable patients, we frequently had four very critical patients. And the CCATT team is just four people usually, the critical care physician, nurse, respiratory therapist, and medic. Most of our patients are on ventilators, monitors, getting blood, and on various IV drips. In 49 missions our team cared for 74 patients and we were the team with the most flying hours and critical patients. They finally added a second CCATT team at Kandahar because we were simply exhausted. We had been "quick-turned" too much. We primarily used the KC-135 aircraft, and sometimes the C-17.

Toni recalled her difficult reintegration:

It was great to come back to my family, but they didn't understand sometimes when I was depressed, or when loud noises startled me. We had had IED explosions in Kandahar frequently so loud noises bothered me when I came home. Sometimes I couldn't sleep at night because I was thinking about some of the patients I took care of, and wondering how they fared once they got home.

CAPTAIN AMANDA

Amanda was born and bred in Boston, Massachusetts. She has the accent to prove it, and cheers for the Boston Red Sox, Boston Celtics, and the Boston Bruins.

She was happy to tell her story:

I am in the U.S. Air Force Reserve. I am currently on full-time orders down here at Robins AFB, Georgia, as part of the Yellow Ribbon Program. But, usually I'm a traditional reservist, or as some folks call us "weekend warrior" before I deployed. I was a civilian ER nurse in Boston. I was a traditional reservist until June of this year. I think I'm gonna be at Robins AFB for 3 to 4 years. I'm on active duty orders but I'm still a reservist. I may not be active duty the whole time I am here, I don't know yet. My husband is an ART [Air Reserve Technician], which is a full-time reservist and we came to Georgia because of his job. He looks like an active duty officer in uniform, but he's actually a GS [Government Service] employee.

I've been deployed twice. My first deployment was in 2010, May through December, to Ramstein Air Base in Germany and I worked at the aeromedical staging unit there. My job was a nurse on a bus pretty much. We would go on the big ambulance bus (AMBUS) that you put litters on and receive a bunch of patients off an air evac plane that just came back from Iraq or Afghanistan. We'd bring the patients to the hospital at Landstuhl. It was the largest military medical center in Europe. On the way to the hospital, we'd medicate them, check their vital signs, monitor their IV fluids, and make sure they were doing OK. Then, a few days later we'd pick up patients at the hospital and transport them to the large aeromedical evacuation transport plane, usually a C-17 Globemaster III, that would be going to Andrews AFB in Maryland, near Washington, DC.

My second deployment was last year from June 2012 till January 2013. I went to FOB Wagman in Qalat in southeast Afghanistan. For about 5 weeks in the middle of the deployment, I was temporarily assigned to the big combat support hospital at Bagram Air Base, Afghanistan. When more replacements arrived at Bagram, I went back to my FOB in Qalat.

Amanda shared some of the positive memories of her first deployment:

With my first deployment, I had just met my husband in January and I deployed in May. He was a new boyfriend back then. So, he came to visit me in the middle of the deployment in Germany. We drank Riesling every night in my room out of my little Boston mug. Great food, we traveled and had fun. The biggest positive was that I got to take care of the greatest patients on earth; 99.9% of my patients were American. They were fantastic. They didn't want for anything. They didn't ask for anything. They were the opposite of entitled. They appreciated anything that I ever did for them. A constant, constant thing with them was that they wanted their buddies taken care of first. They wanted their "brothers" to be medicated first. "Can you help out my buddy, I think he's in more pain, I don't need this." They were just the best patients on earth and I couldn't be more thankful that I had that opportunity to take care of them.

She went on to mention the flip side of the coin relating some of her negative deployment memories of that same deployment:

Some people, when they deploy, they lose their minds. I deployed with a friend and she got a little racy over there. She forgot where her morals and ethics were. We ended up not really being friends towards the middle of the deployment. She cheated on her boyfriend, she completely slept with a lot of people over there. People that you would never, ever want to sleep with when you are a lieutenant. We had joined the military within a month of each other. We were in the same reserve unit, we were very close. I made captain before we deployed. We deployed together. I stuck to the rules and she completely did not. So, that was a negative thing. She disappointed me greatly and I think she disappointed herself by her behavior, but sometimes that happens. She was one in a million who did that. It might have been the first time she was away. I know she went to an all-girls college. We just grew apart during the deployment and it was largely due to her behavior.

Amanda told what touched her deeply during the deployment:

I was affected by the men. I was affected by every single American I spoke with and touched and took care of. That wasn't like me. I am an old ICU and ER nurse from Boston. I really don't get affected by anything, I am almost numb. They affected me, they did, I'll admit that. It's a mixed bag, positive and negative. I wasn't numb. I took care of them with every morsel of love and gratefulness. I was just so appreciative of their service. Our country really did appreciate their service and I did appreciate them. It was a good deployment all in all.

She talked about her homecoming:

My homecoming was great. I look back on all of this from the eyes of the Yellow Ribbon Program. I'm on full-time orders with the Yellow Ribbon, it's the Reintegration Program. So now, I look at this and say that it is so textbook. I didn't realize that at the time. The first night, you are full of excitement and it's great. Then, I woke up in the morning the next day with a great, great sense of guilt. I had left those guys over there. I had so many nightmares. I had left the men at Landstuhl with no nurse, there was no nurse in sight. They were all lined up moaning. I really thought I left them without a nurse. I was replaced by two nurses. We were so busy that summer. All of us were replaced by double the staff. It was insane to think that I left them without help. I recovered fairly quickly from those sleepless nights. It's like when I was a waitress and you'd wake up with waitress nightmares [*laughing*].

LIEUTENANT COLONEL VIOLA

Viola comes from a military family and has lived all over the United States. She considers San Antonio, Texas, her home because that is where her father was assigned the longest, that is where she graduated from high school, and that is where she has had two assignments.
    She stated:

I am in the army and I am currently stationed in Landstuhl, Germany. I was deployed to Iraq. I was in Bagdad in the Green zone. I was with the 86th Combat Support Hospital, so we were providing Level 2 trauma care and I was one of the nursing supervisors. We got there in November 2007 and we returned to the States on December 31, 2008. When I first came back, it was just me and my husband in our household because our kids are grown and gone away. We have three each so it's a total of six young adults.

Homecoming was good and reintegration was OK. My husband was in the Navy Reserve at the time. He's retired now. He was pretty understanding. The extended family, which is out in New Mexico, who we just visited, were all pretty good. My father is a Korean war and Vietnam veteran. My brother is retired army. I also have another brother in the air force. So, I have a very understanding family. I guess you could say my family "gets it."

COMMANDER ROBIN

Robin reported that she has lived all over the world with the military. She joined the navy while in college and met her husband in the navy, although they are currently getting divorced. She was deployed to Afghanistan from April 2010 to October 2010.

She recalled:

I was on ground for 6 months at Camp Bastion, Helmand Province, next to Camp Leatherneck. Camp Bastion is British and Camp Leatherneck is the Marine Corps base. I worked primarily as an ER nurse. I have been in the navy for a long time, let me put it this way, I can retire in 18 months. I've always been active duty.

My sister and her family drove from New York to meet me during my layover at Baltimore–Washington International (BWI) airport. It was great to see them and we had a nice visit. There was also a large group of USO volunteers and retired military there to greet us as we came down the ramp from the jet way. It made us feel very special and appreciated. It meant the world to us to be received this way.

She commented on her family situation:

You have to understand, I took deployment orders so I could come back here because my kids are here [Portsmouth, New Hampshire]. We were already in the process of separating [marriage] before I went and I wanted the orders so I could come back and be stationed here again. So, I came back here. I didn't tell my kids when I would be coming back exactly because I didn't want to disappoint them again because I had first told them when I was gonna deploy in October 2009 and then I didn't really deploy until February 2010 because it got changed. When I left in 2010, the kids were 7, 10, and 13. My youngest is high-functioning autistic, so that's what was really hard when my dates got changed. So, I let their dad know approximately "around the dates" so that way I could surprise them, that's what we had planned. I told them I'd come back in November at the latest and I ended up coming back in late October. My soon to be ex-husband and I met in the military, but he had been out of the military long before I deployed. He had been out for about 15 years or so. He understood and was supportive. He had never deployed, but he had been out on ships. So, with my homecoming, I was very glad to get back to my kids.

LIEUTENANT COLONEL CHRISTA

Christa hailed from a small rural New England town but now calls upstate New York her home. Her two older brothers had served in the Air Force Reserve, so Christa joined the Air Force Reserve a few years after graduating from college. She grew up hearing about the travels of her brothers, so she wanted to get in on the action, too. Her family was very patriotic with her father and uncles serving in World War II. She was the first female member of her family to join the military.

Christa recalled:

I was a lieutenant colonel in the Air Force Reserve when I deployed to Iraq. I served in the Air Force Reserve for 22 years retiring in March 2013. I first deployed to Al Salem Air Base in Kuwait in 2004 and my second deployment was in 2007 to Balad Air Base, Iraq. We performed the ASTS (Aeromedical Staging Transportation Squadron) mission. I came home from Iraq in May 2008 after being in Iraq for a year.

An ASTS is the ground-based unit of people involved in aeromedical evacuation. We meet the air evac aircraft and move the patients off the planes. We decide which patients need to go to the hospital and which patients are stable enough to go to our aeromedical staging facility to be cared for there and wait for their flight to Germany. We then evaluate the patients medically and administratively to get them on a flight out of the theater of operations and up to Germany. We can hold patients up to 72 hours in the ASTS if they don't need to be further stabilized in the hospital.

Christa described her homecoming:

We flew from Germany to Baltimore, and then got a connecting flight to Hartford, Connecticut. Our base, Westover Air Reserve

Base, in Massachusetts sent a bus to pick us up and bring us back to the base. Once we arrived back at the base we were dispersed to return to our homes and did not have to report back to the base for another week. I did not have a car at Westover, so I got a ride with one of the guys from my unit that was heading back to the Albany, New York, area where I lived.

When I got home there was nobody there because I live alone. It was kind of weird walking around and looking at my house. I walked into the kitchen and looked out the window to my back yard and I saw a row of brand new planted tomato plants [*crying*]. My neighbors had cleaned up my garden and planted tomato plants for me as I had always done [*still crying*]. It was just so touching for me. It meant so much. It showed that people remembered and people cared. Then, I decided I needed to get some food. So I got in my car and drove off to the food co-op. I bought some really good salad fixings because I really missed my salads while I was deployed. The guys in the cheese section of the food co-op had been really good friends of mine. When I walked in they just came out from in back of the counter and gave me hugs. It meant so much to me to be hugged and recognized by people in my community. It was so heartwarming. Between these guys at the food co-op and my neighbors tending my garden, I felt remembered and cared about. I went home and enjoyed my first evening home from Iraq.

The day after I got home from Iraq was Memorial Day. Now, I had always carried the American flag for my church in our town's Memorial Day parade. I called them up when I got home from the food co-op and they were so excited that I was home and that I agreed to carry the flag in the parade again. I walked in the parade with my church and I carried the flag. Afterwards, they have this ceremony down in the cemetery. Someone had mentioned to the master of ceremonies that I had just come home from Iraq the day before and it was my birthday. I was sitting in the audience with another woman who had been assigned in Iraq with the 42nd Aeromedical Evacuation Squadron. All of a sudden they made this announcement about my return from Iraq and a little bit about my work and my unit. They had me stand up and I got a substantial and enthusiastic ovation from the audience. It was a little embarrassing, but it also felt good. People don't always think of the contributions women military members and nurses make, but we are in harm's way just as any military member is since in these wars there are no front lines or safe places. At the ceremony, they also did a roll call of our VFW [Veterans of Foreign Wars] post and as they finished calling the names it dawned on me that there was not one female member.

Christa described the simple pleasures she enjoyed on coming home:

I was so happy to sleep in my own bed that I didn't feel alone or lonely at all. I had gone to my friend's house to pick up my two cats that afternoon so I was able to cuddle with my two cats in my own bed. When you have been sleeping in a really hot room with no air conditioning and a terribly flimsy mattress for 12 months, having the comforts of home makes a big difference. I was so happy to take a real shower in my own bathroom, sleep with real sheets on my bed, and make a hot cup of coffee in my kitchen. When I was in Iraq we frequently couldn't take showers because they were always running out of water. I was glad to be home and grateful for all that I had.

COLONEL SARAH

Sarah grew up on a farm in Wisconsin. After attending nursing school and getting a college degree she joined the air force. Her older brothers had all served in the military, as had her father and grandfather. She was not planning on a long-term commitment, just a few years to hone her nursing skills and to travel overseas. However, she enjoyed the military lifestyle and met her husband in the military. Both she and her husband gradually became more interested in making the military a career as the years passed by. Sarah was almost eligible for retirement and had never deployed to a war zone, so she volunteered for duty in Iraq in 2005.
    Sarah related:

I was an active duty air force nurse assigned to a large coalition forces hospital in Iraq for 6 months in 2006. At my hospital in Iraq, I supervised 128 nursing personnel. The majority were air force nurses and medical technicians, but I also had 15 army nurses and a handful of army medics. There were also some army physicians that provided our neurosurgical capability, but the majority of all medical occupations at our hospital were air force members.

    I would say that it was a very positive homecoming and reintegration. It was a different reintegration than I guess most people had returning from Iraq because within 3 weeks of getting home, I was moving my family from the Midwest to Florida. I didn't have to reintegrate to work life at my medical center because we were leaving and I had the 3 weeks essentially off before we left. The preparation for the move took my mind off all that I had experienced in Iraq. Our daughter had moved six times prior to our move to the Midwest, and she was lucky enough to have the general personality to make friends very quickly. The family of one of her friends helped her a lot during the time that I was gone. She speaks of them in loving terms and they sort of gave her a shoulder to cry on, if you will, while I was gone. My husband and I did kind of a role reversal. He stopped working outside our home and became the primary care giver. I guess in the reintegration he incorporated a lot of the routines that he was already following, but when I came home from Iraq we got into the PCS [permanent change of station] move routine which meant that all routines are kind of up in the air as the family prepares to move again.

CAPTAIN TENLEY

Tenley was raised in the Pacific Northwest. She grew up near a large sprawling army post in the state of Washington. As a nursing student she actually had several of her clinical rotations at the large army medical center there. She was impressed with the professionalism and clinical expertise of the army nurses she encountered during her student days. Shortly after graduation, Tenley applied to join the Army Nurse Corps. After receiving her registered nurse license and gaining 6 months of medical–surgical nursing experience, she was commissioned into the army.

Tenley commented on her reintegration:

I deployed twice. The second time was a whole lot easier, especially since I had been through it once before and I knew what to expect. I didn't question my sanity the second time. I thought "this is normal and I'll get over it." It was a lot easier to control my emotions.

My lesson learned from my first deployment: Family will be present when I return. They were there when I got home. After my second deployment, I flew into Fort Benning, Georgia. They made the trip from Washington State to Fort Benning, Georgia. I had 2 weeks off because it was only a 6-month deployment. But having family there to meet me was what I needed. I had no bad feelings.

I started nurse anesthesia (NA) school about a year after I came home from my second deployment. I was at my 3-year mark at Fort Bragg. It was my opportunity to do something new.

There were 35 nurses in my NA program. We probably lost about 10. There is a huge attrition rate. You have to be on your game— it's life and death. I got married during anesthesia school so I'm actually a newlywed [*laughing*]!

MAJOR FRED

Fred is a seasoned air force nurse, who has served in both the Air National Guard and Air Force Reserve. He and his wife and sons currently live near Orlando, Florida.

Fred stated:

I am in the Air National Guard in Florida. I have been in the military for 29 years. My first 10 years was in the army as a medic. Then that's when I decided to go to nursing school. Then, I took my commission with the air force. My first deployment was with the army as a medic during Desert Storm. My second deployment was in 2007, I went to Washington, DC, as a flight nurse and the wounded from Iraq and Afghanistan came into Germany and then would eventually be flown to Andrews AFB near Washington, DC. I would pick them up and fly them to home or a hospital at their duty station. In 2009, I went to Iraq as a critical care nurse and then in 2012 I went to Afghanistan as a critical care nurse. In Iraq, I was at Balad Air Base and in Afghanistan I was at a FOB, called Tarinkowt. It was northeast of Kandahar by helicopter.

Well, with my first two deployments with Desert Storm and being a flight nurse stateside, I really didn't have to reintegrate. When I went to Iraq, I really didn't notice any differences when I came home. I think I had a different outlook on life. Life became a lot more precious after seeing the war injuries. As far as reintegration, I don't remember any big deals. Coming back from Afghanistan, after being on a FOB, I had an 8-foot by 22-foot room. It was like living in the back of a semi-trailer. On my FOB, there were air force people with me and my two medics. We were attached to the army, but also with the navy. We were there to provide care and there were 33 people in our hospital pocket, our FST. There was turnover between the three services as well.

Fred summarized his homecoming and reintegration in two sentences:

I have a wife and two boys. Coming home to them was no problem, we have a strong family. The things that bothered me were crowds and dealing with the VA [Veteran's Administration].

LIEUTENANT COLONEL NATASHA

Natasha was raised in the suburbs near Worcester, Massachusetts. As a teenager, she had worked as a candy striper volunteer in a large community hospital. This experience sold her on becoming a registered nurse. She joined the air force a few years after gaining medical–surgical nursing experience in a Boston area hospital. Her older brother was also a career air force officer.
Natasha reported:

> I was in the air force and I deployed to Gardett, Afghanistan from August 2007 to January 2008. I was part of an embedded medical training team. We mentored Afghan National Army personnel in setting up their regional hospital. I was in the same place for 6 months. I was active duty with the air force for 20 years. I am now retired. I retired in June 2008.
>
> My homecoming itself was fine. I stopped first in Massachusetts to see my dad who was 90 years old. I came through Baltimore so it made more sense for me to see him first rather than go to Montana and then come back to the east coast. That was wonderful. Then, I came home to Montana. My son had had a hard year at school while I was gone. He may have been acting out and not turning in assignments and stuff like that. He had just turned 12 and was in sixth grade. I only have one child. My family was very happy to see me and I was happy to be home. I remember sleeping a lot at first. I had been looking forward to taking a shower without having to wear "shower shoes" [*laughing*]. It was nice to eat different things again.

CAPTAIN BRITTANY

Brittany is a California girl who grew up in close proximity to San Francisco. She joined the army as a nurse after college to "see the world" and to gain valuable nursing experience. Brittany described herself as an "adventurous free spirit" wrapped in an army uniform. She said she played by the rules as far as the army went, but she said she was always up for something new and different. She was deployed to both Iraq and Afghanistan.
She shared information about both deployment assignments:

> I was first deployed to Iraq in 2009–2010. I was with the 47th Combat Support Hospital based in Tikrit and I was a critical care nurse and did some flight missions when needed, both in helicopters and airplanes. I was there for 6 months. Then in

Afghanistan, I was assigned as a critical care nurse and spent 6 months with "dustoff" [medevac helicopters] in regional command east on FOB Schrada. My second 6 months I was with the Air Force Combat Search and Rescue doing medevac. I was there from June of 2011 to June of 2012. The original deployment was for 6 months, but before I left, my OIC [officer-in-charge] asked if I would consider staying for the full year for staffing purposes.

Homecoming was pretty easy. My cousin met me at the airport and I hung out with her for a little bit. My company commander was really welcoming when we all came home. She let us know in advance what to expect when we came home administratively and what our days would look like before we went on leave. She kept everything very low-key for us and without a lot of responsibilities. I came back with three or four other people. We were actually on loan to the 47th Combat Support Hospital. We went through 2 weeks of administrative leave, getting paperwork done. Then, we went on leave. I went back to California to see my family. I am from outside of San Francisco. Prior to Iraq, I was stationed at Walter Reed Army Medical Center in the Washington, DC, area. I was in their adult medical ICU and their pediatric ICU. With this deployment, I felt like administratively everything was lined up for us. There were a lot of communications before we got home. We knew what to expect. Everything was low key. For people who had a more difficult deployment, the leadership was very good. The support was there. People had time to catch their breath and get used to being home again.

MAJOR COLLEEN

Colleen is from the Midwest, having joined the army after college to gain nursing experience and travel. She met her husband in the army and was married for 2 years at the time of her deployment. She reports that she accepted her deployment thinking her marriage was strong only to find out at her R & R break that the relationship was in trouble. She is now divorced and has gone back to using her maiden name.

She shared the details of her deployment:

I have been deployed only once and that was to Herat, Afghanistan. It is in western Afghanistan and it is not a place that a lot of people have been to. The hospital is only on its third or fourth rotation. The hospital was started in 2006 but is Regional Command West, which is predominately NATO (North Atlantic Treaty Organization). The actual hospital is a Spanish hospital with some Bulgarian folks, too. When I went there this was the first iteration that we did, we were the first Americans to go into that area. There were some Americans north of us and south of us but they were in Role 2 (basic primary and resuscitative care). We were not quite a Role 3, but we were the highest level of care in western Afghanistan. It was an interesting one because diplomatically it was showing other countries that we could go into a foreign hospital and work under foreign government rules and get along. You know how Americans are seen as coming in and taking over [*laughs*], so that was the intent of us going there. There had been some Americans at a British Hospital who worked together and I think there were some at a French hospital but I think they were separated, they had separate wards. At our hospital, we were all working together.

Language could have been a problem at the Spanish hospital but my unit came from Fort Bliss, Texas, so most of the people from my CASH (Combat Army Support Hospital) who were enlisted were Spanish speakers. We actually did have a large number of people who could speak Spanish. Most of the officers did not speak Spanish, maybe a few of them knew some conversational words. We were not chosen to go because of language. We were chosen because we did not need a lot of oversight from our command. We were located on a post where there was open alcohol. It was very interesting. I was there for a year.

Colleen recalled the events leading up to her deployment:

When I arrived at the unit in July, I had deployed in December. When I arrived in July, I had initially thought I'd have a year in the States because I had previously been overseas. I was in Germany for 3 years. My unit told me that they were trying to move the deployment up. I was assigned to a medical–surgical ward at William Beaumont Hospital (Fort Bliss). I was organic to the 31st CASH, so the deployable unit went for a year as opposed to 6 months. I was loaned out to the hospital in Texas for about 6 weeks till they told me to mobilize. So I really didn't get a chance to integrate into the hospital there. Once I deployed, I was one of five American nurses and there were 10 nurses total in the hospital. I am a med–surg nurse and the other four nurses were ICU nurses. I had been given a choice of two missions, and I told them that I wanted to do the NATO mission. I reminded them that I was not an ICU nurse. They told me that I would basically be running my own medical hold ward. When we arrived there, the Spanish said that we all work together. So I would go out to the field and pick up the patients when they landed. I would take them back and work the trauma bay, and I would do sick call.

At night, we would only have one nurse on staff, and they would cover the ICU, med–surg ward, and medical hold unit. So, we covered everything. The one nurse at night would usually work with a Spanish medic. The most I usually had was nine or ten patients. One night I had four intubated patients and four or five med–surg ward patients. An LPN [licensed practical nurse] actually came in and worked with me. Those were busy nights. If we had high acuity because we were a small group of people, one of us would come in and help the other. Later, we started having people on call, if needed. Generally with trauma patients, once you stabilize them and get them settled in, especially if they are intubated, you could call someone in if you needed more help. My first night in the ICU was about 2 weeks after I got there. They left me there. I had trained for a couple of nights and then they said, "You're good." I think my first night on my own in the ICU, I had a two or three intubated patients. It was a little bit scary [*laughing*]. It was a good experience.

We were in a small facility. The difference with what we did was that we'd pick the patients up at the plane. I would be potentially bringing them off the plane, working on them in the trauma bay, sometimes going in the OR with them, and helping out in there, and then I'd go to the ICU with them. We get them out as soon as they were stable to fly to Germany.

We'd really work quite extensively with our patients and have a bit of continuity, too. In a lot of facilities, the ER nurses would stabilize them and then send them upstairs. Then, the med–surg nurses or ICU nurses take care of them and then someone comes to transfer them to go out on a flight. That was the difference. We did see some pretty severe injuries. As a mixed staff from other countries we worked well together. The staffing mix was actually very successful. A lot of other facilities did not do so well with this.

We were near the only FOB in western Afghanistan that was able to take six planes. We had two runways. We'd usually get the patients from a chopper, get them to the facility, treat them, and ship them out on an aeromedical aircraft flight if they were Americans. If they were other NATO troops, they'd stay a little bit longer depending on what their country wanted to do. We'd treat Afghans and then send them to a hospital in Herat. We also had some pretty high-level hospitals in the vicinity for Afghanistan. There was a pediatric hospital where they would ship kids from all over the country. So, we did a lot of moving people. About 75% of our patients were Afghans. We had very few Americans that came to us who were severely injured. More often than not, the Americans were killed, unless it was not a severe injury. The NATO troops, we would see some severely injured troops, but the majority of the severe injuries were Afghans because they were much easier targets. I saw a few bad injuries with NATO troops and Americans, but more so in the Afghans.

Colleen described her homecoming:

There were only 30 of us. We came home a month before the rest of our unit because we had deployed first. They did about 9 months, where we did a year. We ended up at Manus in Kurdistan. There were problems with the plane. We sat around there for a few days and ended up getting on the last plane out before Christmas. Flights stopped for Christmas. So we ended up in Fort Drum, Watertown, New York, and were supposed to catch a commercial plane back to Fort Bliss in El Paso, Texas. But, we were so delayed that we had missed our flights. We went down to Syracuse to get a commercial flight and we ended up arriving home on the 22nd of December, but we were all split up. My particular group was four of us and I was the top commander basically making sure that our soldiers didn't drink on the way back home [*laughing*]. When we arrived, it was 11 o'clock at night after stopping at three or four places across the country. There were only a couple people waiting for us. My husband came to pick me up. We were released for the evening and then we had to report the next morning for reintegration stuff. The next morning all 30 of us gathered, and we weren't allowed to drive for a couple of days. We started to do all of our stuff to demobilize. They initially told us that we were gonna have to be there for Christmas Day, but they ended up shortening it so we could get done by the 23rd. And so we were finished on December 23rd, so we did get Christmas Eve and Christmas Day off. I was married about 2 years when I deployed. I am divorced now and went back to using my maiden name.

LIEUTENANT DARLA

Darla is from a small hamlet outside of Philadelphia, Pennsylvania. She attended college in Pennsylvania and initially worked in Pittsburgh, Pennsylvania, after graduating from college. She joined the Navy Nurse

Corps about 3 years later. She was looking to serve her country, while at the same time to travel and see the world. Her first assignment was as an operating room nurse in San Diego, California. After several years there, she volunteered for deployment to Afghanistan.

Darla reported:

I am currently in the Navy Reserve, but I was active duty navy when I deployed to Kandahar, Afghanistan in December 2011 until June 2012. It is a Role 3 NATO hospital, where we had predominantly U.S. personnel working there, but also personnel from Belgium and Australia. Our patients were from several coalition countries including France, Germany, Spain, and local Afghans and even insurgents. I worked in the operating room, since I'm a navy OR [operating room] nurse. Our hospital was one of the largest hospitals in Afghanistan. We got a lot of "point of injury" patients, which means they were injured in the area close to our base. A lot of fighting was going on right outside of Kandahar. We got transfers in from Camp Bastion, too. We had three major case operating rooms and a minor procedures room. We had a 20-bed ICU and a large ward. We had a laboratory, pharmacy, radiology, and all the services you expect to find in a hospital that treats surgical and critical care patients. We had a neurosurgeon and an eye surgeon, which are two specialties a Role 3 NATO hospital has, plus many general and orthopedic surgeons. Air Evac flights would come in and transport patients out of theater to Ramstein Air Base, Germany.

I think our trip home was pretty much like what other military people experienced. We stayed in Kuwait for a couple of days to attend the warrior transition program. If you are trying to recover from a deployment, I suggest it not be Kuwait. We were in the desert there. I think they have now moved the transition program to Germany. It takes a while to acclimate in Kuwait. It was well over 100 degrees. We came from Afghanistan on a C-130, and you get off and run to the bathroom because there were no bathrooms on the plane, and you are sweating because it is over 100 degrees. From Kuwait we went to Germany, and we stayed at Ramstein Air Base for a couple of hours. After that we flew to San Diego. It was good, and there were people from work who greeted us and our friends were there. Almost our entire OR crew from San Diego had deployed, so I deployed with colleagues and we returned on the same flight. They had a nice reception for us when we got off the plane.

We landed at night. We had the next day off, and then the following day we all went to the processing station. It was used for people deploying and for people returning from deployment. I returned in June and then we had a week to in-process back into the hospital. In-processing only took 2 days, so I had the rest of the week off. That was pretty nice. I went back to work for 2 months before I separated from active duty in the navy in August. I'm in the Navy Reserves now.

My homecoming was good. I was single, so it was a little harder to take care of personal matters when you are gone. I had put all of my stuff in storage. I lived with a friend for a short time before deployment. I had put in my paperwork to get out of the military after I returned from deployment. I didn't want to move my stuff into an apartment because I wasn't sure where I was going to be heading to after I separated from the navy.

When I got back I was living with my boyfriend, and that ended up not working out. I was thinking about getting out of the military, and he pushed me over the edge to get out. Who knows if I would still be in the navy if it wasn't for him? I had already put my paperwork in to get out and he was transferred to Pensacola, Florida, in October. So I got off active duty in August. The plan was to move with him to Pensacola, and I would find a civilian nursing job there and join a Naval Reserve unit. However, that didn't work out because we did not get along very well after I came home from deployment. So I had some friends in Georgia, and I moved to Georgia close to my friends.

My boyfriend was being transferred from San Diego to Pensacola, Florida, so we drove across country. I stayed 2 days with him and then I came up to Georgia. When you join the reserves, you usually don't have to report to your gaining command for a month or so, so I didn't have to report till November. I took a whole month off to look for a place to live, interview for jobs, and learn my way around the area. I ended up taking a job in a city hospital and I no longer work in the OR, I now work in the ICU.

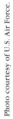

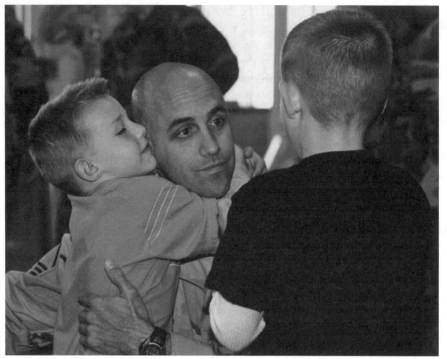

Air force dad reunited with his sons.

Photo courtesy of U.S. Air Force.

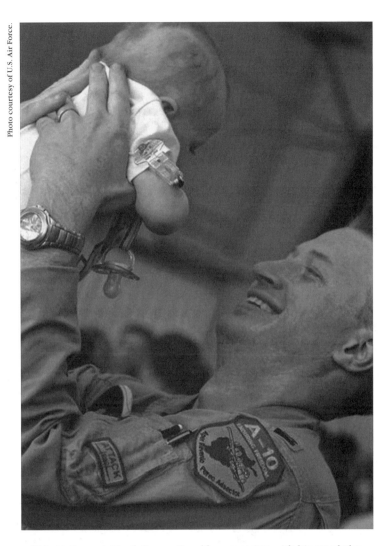

U.S. Air Force A-10 pilot's emotional homecoming with his new baby.

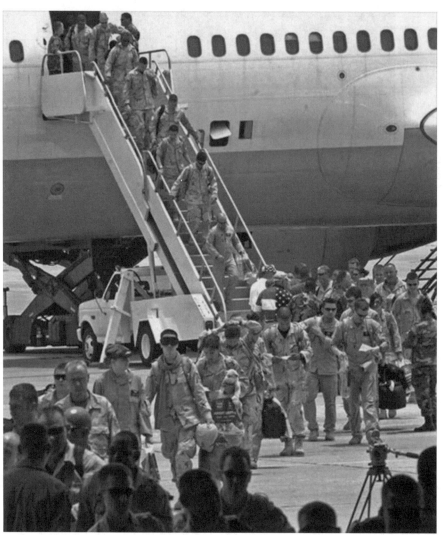

Welcome home, Hurlburt Air Force Base, Florida.

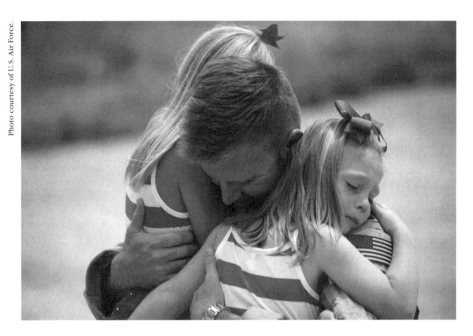

Air force dad is reunited with his daughters.

4

Homecoming: A Disappointing Venture

Some nurses expressed a personally disappointing homecoming experience that left a lasting negative memory. Thus, there was a dichotomy in the nurses' feelings related to their homecoming experience that were dependent on the responses of their families and military units to their return. Although family is impossible to mediate in terms of a response, military units could ensure that there was a familiar cadre of personnel to greet returnees. A reception with food and beverages is probably not too much to ask. A warm reception with expressed gratitude for their sacrifices and service would have been appreciated. Such actions could turn some negative, isolating, and disappointing memories into positive ones. How troops are treated on their return to U.S. soil can be critical in setting the tone for a successful reintegration.

It is important to note that the majority of nurses in this research study described more positive homecoming experiences than negative ones. It is quite possible that the military services learned over time that planning for an organized homecoming reception was expected and appreciated by returnees and their families. Likewise, as the years of wartime engagement passed, the services became more responsive to the needs and desires of returning personnel. Thus, over time, lessons were learned and priorities were established with sensitivity and respect.

LIEUTENANT COLONEL CHRISTA

Although Christa described an overall good homecoming with many thoughtful gestures from members of her neighborhood and community, one aspect that she related as negative was the lack of recognition by her reserve base when a large cadre of reservists returned home.

Christa recalled:

> There was no celebration at Westover Air Reserve Base when we finally returned: no band, no families, and no dignitaries. The bus just dropped us off in the parking lot near our unit. That was kind of odd that our unit and our base did not do anything for us. Previously, when I had deployed to Kuwait, it was the same way when we returned; no recognition ceremony and no celebration at all. It was kind of counter to what we had seen on television with other units from around the country when they returned home. It was kind of disappointing to not acknowledge our homecoming and mission accomplishment in some positive and visible way.

LIEUTENANT KATE

Kate was born in Japan while her father was assigned at the U.S. Naval Base in Yokosuka. She attended six schools before she finished high school in Rhode Island. Kate attended college in Rhode Island while her father was assigned to the Naval War College in Newport, Rhode Island. After working on a medical–surgical unit and then in the surgical intensive care unit (ICU) at a large Boston medical center for 4 years, Kate joined the Navy Nurse Corps.

Kate related:

> I was on active duty in the navy for 7 years when I was deployed to Afghanistan. I was a lieutenant in the Navy Nurse Corps. I was assigned to FOB Dwyer in Helmand province in Afghanistan, where there were mostly U.S. Marines. My hospital was a small combination shock–trauma and resuscitation unit. Once we stabilized patients we sent them to a Role 3 hospital at Camp Bastion or to Kandahar, or a local regional Afghan hospital, if the patients were locals.
>
> I was there from April 2010 until the end of November 2010, and this was my first deployment. Our job was to treat, resuscitate, and stabilize injured marines brought to us. We would resuscitate them using blood products, surgeries, and get them prepared for chopper medevac. I also served as a flight nurse, so I would fly on the chopper with them to Camp Bastion. They had more services at Camp Bastion, so more was clinically available there.

Kate reported the details of her return to the United States:

We flew into March Air Force Base in Riverside, California. It was not at all like you usually see on TV [*starts crying*]. We were not from there so there was no parade, no band, and no families to greet us. There were about five commanders from the base who had to be there to greet each returning plane. They thanked us for our time in Afghanistan, and told us what we needed to do to out process before we needed to make flight arrangements to return to our homes. We were then put on a bus to Camp Pendleton Marine Base. It was the middle of the night and most of us were from the East Coast. That is why there were no families to greet us. I was assigned to Portsmouth Naval Medical Center in Virginia, so all my friends were on the East Coast. For our deployment, they pulled medical people from all over the U.S, so many of us were not from California bases even though the plane landed in California.

This homecoming was really very difficult. We got our bags and had to pick up a rental car as there was no room to stay on base at Camp Pendleton. We got situated very late in our hotels and had to start our out-processing the next morning. Out-processing entailed handing in all our gear, filling out many forms, and going to various briefings, and all we wanted to do was to finish up and head home to our families. It was a week before Thanksgiving, so they were allowing people to take time off in the area, but most of us didn't want that, we just wanted to get home. I finished up at Pendleton after about 5 days, and took a commercial flight home. My husband and two nurses from work were there to greet me. That was pretty depressing also, knowing that I had been stationed there for 5 years. It was a big medical center and they had advertised ahead of time what flights people would be arriving on. I just expected more of my friends and co-workers to come out. Maybe it became routine for those left behind at the hospital, but it was not routine for me, and I just expected more, so I was very disappointed.

LIEUTENANT COMMANDER KATHLEEN

Kathleen hailed from the suburbs of Chicago, Illinois. She always wanted to be a nurse, and after graduating from college she joined the navy. She chose the navy because she liked the idea of travel and knew that, besides working in hospitals, navy nurses could be assigned to hospital ships as well. She had grown up sailing at her parent's summer cottage on Lake Michigan, so she chose the navy over the other military services.

Kathleen recalled:

I'm active duty navy. I've been active duty navy since 2003. I was deployed from September 2009 until May 2010 at Camp Bastion in Helmand Province, Afghanistan. That was my only deployment. I was an ER nurse by trade, so the ER at Camp Bastion was where I was assigned. Camp Bastion was run by the British Army, so we triaged patients and followed all the British protocols for caring for patients and resuscitations. We used their antibiotic protocol and their pain management protocol. We had a multinational medical team working there. It was pretty much U.K. and U.S. army and navy personnel, but we also had some Danish and Dutch military medical personnel, too.

We had eight beds in the ER. We also had an ICU. We had a multiservice unit that was always full. We had a pharmacy and a dental clinic, and our hospital was kind of a warehouse-type building. We had tile and linoleum floors, running water, air conditioning, and flush toilets in the hospital. We lived in a tent, but our tent had air conditioning. We had running water and flush toilets in an attached tent. We had eight women to a pod in the tent, and about eight pods came off like wings of this big tent. The attached bathroom tent had four showers and four toilets.

Kathleen described her trip home:

On our trip back to the U.S., we stopped in Kuwait for 4 days. I was left behind in Kuwait for 2 extra days by myself because my name was not on the flight manifest to fly home, so my entire unit left without me. Those 2 days were kind of lonely, but I survived. My flight landed in Dulles (Virginia) and then I was routed through Houston to my final stop in Chicago. I called my dad from Houston and told him my flight information. My dad met my flight in Chicago. I got home on Thursday and went back to work on Monday. I returned to my same navy job I had left as a clinical instructor at a navy school for young sailors learning medical skills.

I had to either take leave or come back to work. My best friend and I had booked a trip to Hawaii a month later, so I came back to work knowing that I had a month off coming later. Coming back was weird because I think people looked at me like I was different. Well, I was different because you grow in ways you don't expect.

People looked at me to see if I had become "nuts" from the trauma of war. I think some people were waiting to see if I broke down.

I taught a medical arts class right away about combat trauma, and it was hard for me to watch the video. I didn't think it would bother me. I never gave it a second thought, but I found it hard to watch. It was a lot of emotional stuff that came up for me watching war trauma videos having been in that setting so recently. I went into counseling right away. I'm a big proponent for mental health. It is like cleaning out the "junk drawers." So I didn't wait for my war trauma memories to become a problem, I was proactive about getting a professional to talk with. I went for about 16 sessions of counseling and just talked about it and it worked out fine for me. When I came back there was construction outside of my apartment, and when I was in Afghanistan we would hear the explosions in the distance, so the construction sounds took me back to Afghanistan. It was upsetting and unnerving to have to listen to the construction noise and have intrusive thoughts about the explosions in Afghanistan.

Kathleen discussed what helped her reintegration:

I found solace in talking to people at my base that had also deployed. We could share and there was a bond. But then there was survivors' guilt. I felt that I didn't do enough. I felt in some ways we had it too easy, the camp was pretty decent and we weren't out climbing rough terrain or being shot at regularly. Some of the navy corpsmen I worked with were deployed with the marines, so they were on the move a lot and in the thick of it in terms of danger. I found it difficult to have a conversation with people that hadn't deployed because they really didn't understand. My parents and my civilian friends looked at me as if I was going to be crazy when I came back, that was what they expected. I was 29 when I deployed and I turned 30 in Afghanistan.

Kathleen described visiting her parents:

When I went home to visit my parents as soon as I returned from Afghanistan, my dad had this postdeployment book sitting on the coffee table. He had chapters highlighted and paper clipped. I got mad and said, "Stop looking at me like I should be crazy, I'm fine, really I'm fine." I am just different now. It was a soul-awakening experience. I'm not different because I'm crazy, I'm different because

I grew up. War grows you up like no other life experience will. I like being by myself more now, but not because I'm crazy. When you live with someone 3 feet from you for 7 months, it is nice to have my space now. It was hard to be alone in Afghanistan because you lived and worked with so many other people. I don't need to go out all the time now. I'm good with only occasional social evenings. I don't like going out all the time and drinking like we used to do, because drinking just doesn't make me feel good. I got away from it, so it is not part of my life anymore. We used to be young and rowdy, but I've grown up and that isn't me anymore. Partying used to be a coping mechanism for me and my friends when we were in our mid-20s, but it is not who I am now, I've moved on.

I lost some friends when I came back. They wanted to go out and party like we used to do, and I had grown up and wasn't into partying anymore. So, I grew apart from some of my friends. Another thing that was weird was that in the States there are mirrors everywhere, and I never really noticed that until I came back from Afghanistan. There were virtually no mirrors in Afghanistan. Even in our tent bathroom, there was only one tiny brushed metal mirror that distorted your image. In the States, it seemed like you can't get away from your own image.

I had a lot of body image issues when I came home. It was like, "I'm not skinny enough, or I'm not working out enough." I talked to the counselor about it. She said I just have to do enough exercise that I'm comfortable with, and try to not overdo it. I was so used to working 12 hours at the hospital for 6 days a week. You were always at work and I only ate once a day. So, when I got home trying to eat three times a day made me sick. Eating real food was weird after eating all the processed food they served in the mess hall at Camp Bastion. I didn't feel good about myself physically after I came home. When I looked in the mirror after I came back I looked fat. When you deploy, people expect you to come back thin. A couple of people said to me, "I expected you to come back skinnier." People saying those kind of comments kinda bummed me out. It just kinda gets in your head. I also didn't get the awards that I was told to expect to get. I didn't expect anything, but people told me I'd get a Navy Commendation medal, but I only got a Navy Achievement medal. Well, people assume that when you come back from a deployment you'll get the Commendation medal. In reality, people got either one or the other. But there were just these little things that picked away at me, irritated me, and some of the comments were from people who had never deployed.

LIEUTENANT LORETTA

Loretta worked as an operating room (OR) nurse after graduating from college. Although she was from Maryland, she worked for several years in Los Angeles and San Francisco, California, before joining the navy. She decided to join the navy to experience a different way of life while still working as an OR nurse. She wanted to live abroad and to experience different cultures, while still being employed by a "stable" employer. She believed working for the U.S. government was about as stable an employer as anyone could possibly find.

Loretta described her homecoming:

> I saw my family for 2 hours at Baltimore airport when I got off the plane from Afghanistan. They had sat at the airport for 4 hours waiting for me to get off the plane. I went to dinner with them and that was that. Then, I had to fly back to San Diego. I didn't have very much time with my parents. My boyfriend actually flew out to San Diego to surprise me. He was there to meet me. That was very nice to have him waiting for me in San Diego. My boss picked us up at the airport. My boyfriend is military, too.
>
> I'm a navy nurse. I was deployed to Kandahar, Afghanistan. I worked in the operating room. I was deployed from August 2011 until March 2012. Our hospital was a NATO [North Atlantic Treaty Organization] facility, so we had a mix of British, Dutch, Canadian, and American military personnel. My home base was San Diego. Coming back was hard. I was the fourth and final person from my home base to deploy. One person who I was in Afghanistan with left for another assignment before I came back. The second nurse I was with was getting ready to go back to school on navy sponsorship. The third person I was deployed with did not want to talk about her experience in Afghanistan. So, it was kind of lonely when I went back to work in San Diego.
>
> When I came back, it was all new people. There was a lot of turnover and I did not know anybody. I had just spent 7 months over there. The person that I would really like to talk to about my experience and how I felt was already gone when I came back. We were individual augmentees, so we were picked from our respective clinical areas and sent over. Some of us were sent to one training site. A smaller group of us were sent to another site and then we combined in Afghanistan. There were a number of us from San Diego, but we came to Afghanistan at different times.

LIEUTENANT COMMANDER CATHERINE

Catherine was a navy family nurse practitioner who was deployed in 2004 to Iraq and again in 2009 to Afghanistan.

She described her first homecoming:

> As far as coming home, you knew that home was not going to look like Iraq [*laughing*]. That was a good thing! But not everyone shares the same experiences with you. So, as far as your family goes, my family knew that I was not in a safe place. They knew that there was a lot of risk inherent with that role. I think everyone was anxious. There was a lot of anxiety in terms of actually getting back home. There was worry about actually getting back home. When we did come back, we actually went to Camp Pendleton which was not where I was from. I had left out of Corpus Christi, Texas. When you come back there is a lot of military processing requirements that are not necessarily at your home. So that is a frustrating experience because mostly you don't care about un-loading your bags or getting on the next bus or waiting in a line or signing papers. I was pretty forceful and I was the most senior person in the group that was not from California. There were a lot of people who had deployed out of San Diego, so their first night home, their families were there and they put the unit on a "96," which is a 4-day leave period. Well, the people who weren't from California weren't home yet and we didn't want to be on a "96." We still needed support services to work for us so we could get on planes and go back to Texas where our families were. So this was very, very frustrating. It required a lot of independence and advocacy as the senior person. I felt responsible for other nurses and corpsmen who were from my hospital in Corpus Christi.
>
> So, I rented a vehicle, a passenger van because there was no transportation arranged for us to drop off all this gear. Camp Pendleton is a geographically vast base. There are a lot of miles. There were inadequate resources to expedite our actual home-coming. So, I rented a van on the base and helped people get their gear to warehouses so they could get through this as quick as possible. You are also on a completely different time zone. Your day is night and that takes a long time to get regulated. So when we got back, most of us stayed up all night. Then, when the morning came, we thought we could start processing our stuff. I remember going to some offices. I remember in one office we needed some signatures on a form and the poor guy at the

desk told me that the person who could sign the forms had gone to PT [physical training] and wouldn't be back till 9 a.m. and we were there at 7 a.m. when they were supposed to be open. So I said to him, "Well, I guess you are gonna sign these forms." I ordered him to sign them and gave him my cell phone number and said, if your lieutenant or whoever has any problems, he can call me directly but we're not waiting for him to get back from PT.

There was some frustration there. I probably was not the most patient person. I hope I didn't shoot the messenger or yell at people unnecessarily [*laughing*]. I'm sure that I was not at my very best in terms of my behavior. Anyway, we got through that and we did eventually get back to Corpus Christi. We were able to leave Camp Pendleton within a few days. There were commercial flights but you were not able to book those until you had done all the other things.

LIEUTENANT COLONEL NATASHA

Natasha is a retired air force nurse.
She remarked:

I retired in June 2008, so from the time I got back to the clinic I was sort of a "nonentity." I think that my experience was a bit different from the average person because while I was gone the entire leadership of the hospital had changed. The commander, chief nurse, and everybody I knew was gone. The hospital was now an Air Force Clinic. It was weird because the new people were not at all welcoming. One thing that my friend kiddingly had been saying to these new people was, "Wait until the colonel gets back, she's not going to like this." So, I stepped into a new situation where these new people already did not like me and they did not even know me. They had not even met me! [*laughing*] And so, I had a hellacious experience at the clinic for the remainder of my time there. I was dropped from every committee. I really was a "nonentity." I was the third highest ranking person in the clinic and it was awful.

So, when it came time for my retirement ceremony, I planned and executed my entire retirement ceremony myself. No one helped me. I don't know but this experience was a disaster. With that and the fact that I retired, we moved to a new city and I changed jobs. I scored really high on that depression scale. I tried to get through it but then I said to myself, "I really need to do something because I have a family history of depression." I felt like there was no joy in my life at all. So, I talked to the people at the VA [Veterans Administration] and I talked to a psychiatrist and started on some antidepressant medication. I'm convinced I did the right thing because I'm much better now. It was very hard. It was so hard [*voice gets very choked up*].

The turmoil in my workplace at the clinic was so hard because I felt like I had done a good job there. I came back to a group of strangers at work and they were already convinced that I was a "primadonna" without even meeting me or getting a chance to know me. I threw my own going-away party, but I still had one. All the junior staff came because I had had a really good relationship with them before deployment and after. I still see some of them. I just came home to my son and husband. A lot of my friends at the clinic had left while I was deployed. I had left in May to train with the army before going to Afghanistan. My husband took good care of our son while I was gone. He was supportive and did a good job with our son.

We lived on base until July and then we moved to a small town. My support system was actually stronger at the new place. I had friends there. It is just 30 miles down the road from the base where we had lived. It's a small community and they were very supportive. I didn't notice any problems at all getting back into my life. I have a wonderful husband who does an awful lot. He's been my son's primary care provider since he's been an infant.

LIEUTENANT COMMANDER JUSTIN

Justin was reared outside of Virginia Beach, Virginia. After college he worked for a few years as an ICU nurse before entering graduate school to become a certified registered nurse anesthetist (CRNA). He later joined the U.S. Naval Reserve after hearing about the travels, adventures, and benefits from two other CRNAs he worked with in a large civilian practice. When he deployed to Afghanistan, he had almost 10 years of naval reserve experience.

Justin stated:

I was deployed from 2010 till 2011 on a 15-month deployment in Kabul, Afghanistan. My role was as an embedded senior nurse mentor, even though by skill set I was a CRNA. I served in this mentoring role in a 450-bed, seven-story medical facility run by the Afghan National Army. When I got to this facility I found that we were terribly understaffed for this mentoring role. It was a difficult job for me because of a number of factors. The cultural differences between U.S. nurses and what Afghans believe are very great. This has direct bearing on the reintegration of us U.S. nurses once we come home. We put patient care ahead of personal needs and schedules. We work days, we work weekends, we work nights, and we work holidays, whatever it takes to provide the highest quality care. It is what we believe in and practice as RNs in America. This is completely different from what the Afghans believe. The Afghans will choose whatever they can find as a means to their end. Today they will be friends with you because it serves their purpose. Tomorrow, they may have to kill you. So this Afghan mindset is very difficult to stomach during a tour of duty working in an Afghan hospital. It is very stressful for U.S. nurses and medics because it "goes against the grain" of what we believe in and practice. It wears us down and adds to the futility we feel in trying to improve practice and outcomes in Afghan hospitals.

If you are a male patient and you are a Pashtun, I will not care for you because we have cultural differences. I had a patient tell me, "That's a bad guy." Being a U.S. military member, I perceived what he meant was that "This guy is an insurgent threat." So, when I questioned him more about what he meant by "a bad guy," he said his tribe killed 50 of my tribe's pigs 100 years ago. Some of the Afghan caregivers refused to feed some of the patients because of these types of old tales of tribal conflict. Some patients in the Afghan hospital in Kabul starved as a result.

I did not deploy with a unit. I was a naval individual augmentee. When I deployed, my assignment was not clear, and I was not sure what I was going to be doing. I'm a CRNA by education, but they put me in this nurse mentoring role. When I got to the hospital it reminded me of a New York City subway station because it was so dirty. It reeked of urine. There were flies flying around in the operating room landing on your surgical field. There was no air conditioning. You'd have a doctor come from one operating room to another, borrow an instrument to use on his patient, then come back in with the contaminated instrument and drop it right back on your patient's surgical field.

Justin described a rough homecoming readjustment:

My family really didn't have any idea what the heck to do with me once I came home. I got home and was quite a recluse, I didn't want to go out or do much of anything. I also got injured while I was in Afghanistan. I was involved with a bombing at the hospital. We were attacked and we were our own security at the hospital. I was getting out of a vehicle and I got kicked from behind and injured my right hip. I ended up having surgery on it, and I also have a disc herniation that I have to have surgery on as well. My wife and I were having problems before I left on deployment and this continued once I returned home. I needed some time to sleep, to rest, and to recover from my injuries, which I mostly ignored in Afghanistan and just "pushed forward." I really wanted time to connect with my son, as he was only 6 months old when I left for Afghanistan. I was gone for a long time during those important formative months. My wife and I had a rough time when I got home. She ended up changing the locks on the house so I had nowhere to sleep. She took money out of our joint bank account. Things were terrible and eventually led to our divorce.

CAPTAIN MARLEY

Marley grew up in Albuquerque, New Mexico, as the youngest of three children. She enlisted in the army after high school. The army trained her as a laboratory technician, but after 2 years she started taking nursing courses in a baccalaureate nursing program during her off-duty time. Later, she was selected for army sponsorship to finish the nursing program. Once Marley graduated, she was commissioned as an Army Nurse Corps officer.

Marley stated:

I have been in both Iraq and Afghanistan. I am actually a veteran now and out of the military. I was in the army for about 11 years. The first 4 years were enlisted and the rest were as an active duty officer. I'm a trauma nurse and emergency room nurse. When I first went to Iraq, I was a lieutenant. In Iraq, I went with the 21st Combat Support Hospital to Abu Ghraib prison hospital. I did the detainee health care mission in the emergency department. Later, I actually helped to close that place and we brought the detainees to Camp Cropper. It was all detainees and they were all men. We moved them from Abu Ghraib to Camp Cropper so I was in both places.

Occasionally, U.S. soldiers needed our care so it was probably 90% detainees and 10% U.S. soldiers. It was the highlight of our deployment when we got to take care of U.S. soldiers. This was my first wartime deployment from 2006 to 2007. My second deployment was to Afghanistan in 2009, and I was on a forward surgical team. We did surgery to stabilize wounded soldiers. I was in Ghasni and helped set up two forward surgical teams.

Marley described her homecoming after returning from Iraq:

When I came home from Iraq, we went back to Fort Hood, Texas, which was where we had mobilized from. We didn't like our unit and I didn't really want to be there. There were a lot of problems in the unit and not much support for us. When we got back to Fort Hood, we had to go on leave, which was a break as I dreaded going back to work there. I actually flew from Germany to Fort Hood. I went on leave and took 3 weeks off. I went back to Albuquerque, New Mexico, where I'm from.

MAJOR FRED

Fred, an Air National Guardsmen, who served in Iraq and Afghanistan, said that one of the most frustrating experiences in coming home was dealing with the Veterans Administration (VA).

He stated:

The VA seems to be stuck into thinking that everyone is retired and they call you up and give you an appointment saying that you need to show up on this day and at this time. Then, you have to call up and cancel because every appointment they give you is on a day you are scheduled to work. They seem to think everyone is retired and not working, which is not the case. The person I was assigned to see was a PA [physician assistant] and she only works Mondays, Tuesdays, and Wednesdays. So, as long as I call on one of those days, I might be in luck. She keeps an opening on each one of her days that she can put people in after four in the afternoon because now she knows that some of us work. In our community, we have healthy working people besides retired people. We have a big military reserve population, we have an Army Guard and an Army Reserve unit here, a Navy Reserve unit here, and up until last year there was a Marine Reserve unit here, and every one of these units has deployed. So, there are a lot of people who are still in the workforce. So she [my PA] finally adapted to that.

I've also had a dermatology issue. I've been home since January and I've tried to schedule an appointment six times. The one that was on a day that I could actually go was cancelled because the doctor broke his foot. It's frustrating. I live in the Tallahassee area. So,

after being home 9 months, I finally had my dermatology appointment yesterday. I work as a critical care nurse in a nearby hospital.
I train with the Air National Guard one weekend a month. In the
summer it's a little more than 2 weeks of Guard annual training. It
was more when I was a flight nurse, but right now I am not flying.

LIEUTENANT SANDRA

Sandra joined the navy after college wanting to expand her horizons, meet
people, and gain nursing experience. She says she was looking to find her
niche in the world. She was deployed from Guam to Afghanistan.
  She stated:

I was at Camp Bastion, Afghanistan. I was an ER trauma nurse. I
left Guam in February 2010 and went to England to train with the
Brits because they have a different approach to trauma training. So,
we went to England for a month and then off to Afghanistan. I was
at Camp Bastion for 6 months. Then, I returned to Guam where I
was stationed at the time. Now, I'm back in the U.S. in California.

  Camp Bastion was a British camp. I think the living conditions would have been different if it were a U.S. camp. We lived
in tents and slept on cots. The air conditioner worked sometimes
at best. It was usually over 100 degrees in any tent you lived in.
The camp in general was pretty run down and that killed morale.
I think the living conditions would have been considerably better if it were a U.S. camp. Absolutely, absolutely. We have a larger
military and we have more money to spend on the military. We
would be more willing to spend that money to elevate the morale
of our people. It wasn't that the British didn't care, they were used
to not having things as nice as we are. You know, that "stiff upper
lip" [*laughs*]. You know, make do with what you have. It was a
very, very busy hospital. There were U.S. personnel on the flight
line and in the hospital besides the British. We also had a Danish
camp on the same grounds. It was not primarily U.S. folks there,
but there were some of us. There were Australians there, too.

  I was really not wanting to come home. I mean I wanted to
and I didn't want to. I kind of lost touch with my family. I had my
husband and two boys. They shut down our Internet connection at
Bastion and we weren't able to Skype. So we couldn't really see our
loved ones on a screen at that time. They weren't willing to pay for
the extra bandwidth. I didn't really know what I was coming home

to, so there was a little bit of apprehension. I didn't know. I knew it was going to be awkward. Of course, I would be happy to see my kids. But I knew that getting back into a routine with them would be a challenge because I am more of the disciplinarian, Dad's not. I knew I'd be walking on eggshells for a little bit. My two boys were 8 and 6. I was gone in 2010. My husband is not military. He didn't have a job while I was gone. I am pretty much the one who mans the fort, I do everything. I am the one who works full-time, I take care of the money, and I take care of everything else. That's why I was stressed about leaving in the first place because I didn't know how he was gonna handle things. We had no family around because we were in Guam, and Guam is isolated. I knew I'd have to get acclimated there. Guam is hot all year round. Coming back, I had a lot of doubts about whether my relationship was gonna last with my husband cause it didn't go well while I was gone. We're almost at the peak of our divorce right now.

LIEUTENANT DOREEN

Doreen is a "Jersey girl," having grown up in northwestern New Jersey near the Pennsylvania border. She had been in the Naval Reserve for several years before her deployments. Her civilian nursing position is as an ER trauma nurse in a large inner-city medical center. Doreen described herself as "Jersey smart." When asked what she meant by that she said it was "the Jersey version of street smart."

Doreen stated:

I was deployed twice. I was in Iraq in 2008. I was in Afghanistan from 2010 to 2011. I was in Iraq for 6-½ months and I was in Afghanistan for 6-½ months. In Iraq, I was at Camp Korean Village in western Anbar province. I was a flight nurse. In Afghanistan, I was in Kandahar with the NATO Hospital and I was a full-time trauma nurse. I also did a mission out to a FOB Wilson for about 2-½ weeks.

Doreen described her homecoming from Iraq:

They flew us out of Iraq to Camp Lejeune and then to New Jersey. My homecoming was OK, the usual, meet all my friends at a bar [*laughing*]. I saw my dad, my cousin, and my aunt. My cousin was battling cancer at the time. They were all supportive. I am not married and never have been. I have no kids.

Coming back was not immediately problematic but down the road, I began to drink. I became extremely angry. I didn't know I could be such an angry person inside. I was angry with the military and eventually I lost my billet, my position with the Marine Corps as a "shock–trauma platoon nurse." I had to find myself a new billet. I got home in September of 2008 and I found a new billet by November 2009. I got a new billet with the hospital in Bethesda, Maryland. Upon returning, lots of people lose their billets. If you want it bad enough you can get it back. But, I was so disgusted with what had happened in Iraq that I didn't want it back. I was so upset about everything, to me it was "the good old boys' club." On top of that, I was the whistleblower because once the EOO [equal opportunity officer] came out to our unit, she couldn't believe my story and then when she interviewed everyone else, she realized that my story was exactly the same as everyone else's. The captain in charge demeaned most of us in front of junior enlisted folks. He found things, personal things, like your weight or the way you looked, and put you down in front of junior people. His behavior was just so inappropriate. First, she [the EOO] accused me of lying. I am not a liar, I served with my heart and soul. Lying just isn't my deal. Then, she found the truth.

I was not heartbroken about losing my position. It was fine with me. I work in a Level 1 Trauma Center in the ER in Newark, New Jersey. I haven't been at work for a year now, but I did go back after Iraq. After Iraq, it wasn't that bad. Of course, you have people ask you crazy questions like, "How many people did you kill?" People would come up behind me and make loud noises. One person continuously kept doing this. I think he was just trying to be funny and there was no malicious intent, but it was annoying. My anger did not come out at work. I did OK at work. What I saw in Iraq did not carry over to the ER at work. I didn't have mass casualties where I was in Iraq, I had people with seizures, finger amputations, a DOA [dead-on-arrival], fractures, heat exhaustion, and stuff like that.

It was OK getting back into my life. My anger was because of the command situation over there. "How could, how dare they," all the old man [captain] got was a slap on the hand and was asked to step down. He stayed with us, his position just changed, there was no place for him to go. The camp was small. He eventually became OK, almost an OK person. A physician's assistant became the OIC [officer-in-charge] and the captain kept his mouth shut and became an OK person. I mean nobody would sit with him and have a nice conversation with him, but he became OK, not a villain anymore because he wasn't in charge.

Doreen described her homecoming from Afghanistan in 2011:

My homecoming was horrible. As far as my family and friends, "Welcome home, you are great and we love you. Thank you for serving!" I did not have rocks thrown at me, nor was I spit on. I took my 3 months off from my job and from the reserves. I started very quickly to have nightmares. I came home to a new house, an extremely big empty house. I started to have horrific nightmares within a month of being home. Don't worry about this interview. I may cry, but I am not alone. I have a friend here with me.

I went out one night and managed to bring a man home and he sexually assaulted me. Fortunately, about 2 days later I went to where I graduated college from and I was with my friends for about a month. This was already planned. I went paragliding and had the time of my life. My sister was up there and I worked through it with her. It was a phenomenal trip. I did a lot of crying. I drank every day and didn't care about too much. I came home and continued drinking pretty much every day. It was really every day. I very quickly pushed my friends away. My cousin at that point was still battling cancer, so my aunt was really engulfed with that side of the family. I became very distant to them because I was embarrassed because of my issues. The last thing they needed was me around drunk, or whatever.

Doreen explained how things went when she returned to work:

I went back to work 3 months later. I could function pretty well at work. I was not drinking before work at all. I wouldn't drink at work at all. I was stupid, but not that stupid [*laughing*]. I realized that triaging just my own patient load was very difficult for me. I couldn't do med calculations in my head like I used to do. I know computers do it, but I was constantly questioning myself. Then management realized what I was doing in Afghanistan. Our ER is very separate, trauma ER, adult ER, peds ER [pediatrics]. So, anytime a bad trauma came in guess where they put me. They would put me in trauma a lot. Level 1 trauma. In the 6 months I worked there this time, I could take care of the patients. It was what happened to me afterwards. After the patient went off to the OR, or wherever, I would go into the bathroom and I would dry heave, not because it was grotesque, but because I simply could not do it again. My scrubs would be soaking wet, my heart rate would go up to like the 130s, I would cry and I just could not function after taking care of a bad trauma. It became habitual, and I would just request to go home. OK, go home. Of course, I would not go home. I would go to my hiding spots and drink at one or 2 o'clock in the afternoon. It became very habitual, my drinking. Nobody got it. People would say that they understand.

Long story short, I started to not eat, and I would vomit bile. I was not taking care of myself, period. I was not showering. I became one of my own patients. In 2012, I went to the VA and they sent me to the psych inpatient unit to "detox me," which I really didn't need. I didn't have the shakes or withdrawal. This was the VA in New Jersey. They did the Ativan thing, and, great, I got to sleep for 4 days. It was lovely. I agreed to do the outpatient program which allowed them to discharge me. I never went back to do the outpatient program. I came home and started drinking again. I finally went back and ended up in their inpatient drug and alcohol rehab unit. I was transferred to West Virginia, Martinsburg VA for 90 days in their PTSD [post-traumatic stress disorder] program. That lasted 45 days for me. I signed myself out. The entire time I was an inpatient in the drug and alcohol rehab unit, I was on a "line of duty" with the navy. So, the navy got involved and I was supposed to be getting paid. Long story short, I had a very belligerent conversation with my corpsmen when I was down in West Virginia and I told her that this was not working for me, this isn't the right place for me, blah, blah, blah. She said you need to get out of that program every time I talk with you about it, you seem to be getting worse. Also, I was not being paid by the navy. Nothing was working for me, so she was able to get me on med hold orders, active duty, and that happened in December of 2012.

I remain on active duty med hold. They have me down in Norfolk, Virginia, on med hold. They have had a physician assigned to me since December 2012 when I got there. He's a neuropsychiatrist and is very good. Of course, being a psychiatrist he orders all the medicine. When I got there, he almost blew his lid seeing the medicines that the VA had put me on. He said, "It's no wonder why you left the program, it's no wonder why you wanted to pull your hair out and poke everybody's eyeballs out." The VA had me on Wellbutrin and a bunch of other stuff. There was something for sleep, but I wasn't taking it. Now I'm getting something for migraines. It is helping. I can actually walk around and function. This has been the answer, I wish I had it when I got home from Iraq.

When I got down to Norfolk, and it actually just came up about 3 months ago, about a suspected TBI [traumatic brain injury] from a hard landing in Iraq. I was discussing it with my physician who I have been with since I got there. I told him about what had happened. I had a little bit of a break, and I verbalized

X, Y, and Z, and he said, "Do you mind if I do a few little things on you?" So, he did this neuro thing with memory and it was about 5 minutes long. He was very confused and said I need you to think back and talk to me about what happened. I had had a dream about the hard landing in the helicopter and I told him about it. I told him that I hadn't told him because it was not something I choose to remember. I barely remember it. I never talk about it because it is not one of those things I want to remember. He said, "Why don't you talk about it?" I said because I don't want to. I am very stubborn. I think I shocked him with my test results and the whole story. I did the first 4 hours of the neuropsychiatry testing which was just miserable. I got an MRI and all that stuff. I did the second part of it at the end of October. When I'm in Norfolk, I go to a lot of appointments. I go to groups. I took a 2-week class which was related to PTSD and it was very helpful. I just kind of chill. I have a place to stay in Norfolk and then I have my house in New Jersey.

I am not still distant from everyone. That is absolutely better. People seem to be understanding, especially my dad. And that's the most important to me. There are others, too, who have been my support. I have definitely made a few people cry. I have been able to apologize and make amends because I was embarrassed. People would call me and say, "Let's go out to dinner and let's do this" and I would push everybody away by saying, "Oh, I'm not feeling good." What I didn't say was, "Screw you, you are interfering with my drinking." I think people started to realize what I was doing, including my father. I mean, "Who does that to a family? Well, a drunk does that to a family."

My drinking is under control now. Absolutely! I think the navy is going to medically retire me. I am angry at the navy and the VA. The system and being on med hold, I'm just done. I will probably never be able to be an ER nurse again. I don't know if I can do that. I want to travel. It will be my time. I think by telling my story to you, it's been therapeutic for me and I thank you.

COMMANDER DARBY

Darby grew up in Ohio and joined the navy after nursing school. She mentioned that she was feeling restless, having never been out of Ohio. She wanted to have some adventures.

She recalled:

I joined the navy on April 26, 1972. I am Vietnam era, but I did not
go to Vietnam. I have 42 years in the navy. I did 3 years, 4 months,
and 4 days on active duty. I was stationed at Great Lakes. After that
I got out. I married a navy doctor and we moved to the Bay area
of California where he did his residency. I wanted to stay in the
navy, but I didn't have a bachelor's degree. I was a diploma nurse.
The navy wanted degrees. So, I started working on a degree. I was
working as a civilian at the Naval Hospital in Oakland while my
husband was doing his residency. If I went to Cal State to get the
BSN, it was still more of an administrative tract rather than a clinical tract. If I did that I would have had to go back on the same floor
as a student where I had been a charge nurse in the past. I didn't
want to do that. I have too much of an oversized ego to do that.

I went back and did get a degree in psychology which was
more interesting to me at the time than nursing administration.
Then, I got divorced from the navy doctor about the time he
finished his clinical. It was 1979. In 1981, I got back in the Navy
Reserves. I didn't know anything about the reserves. I thought
they were a little like the Salvation Army people who wore a uniform and worked [*laughing*]. I made a lot of good friends and I
was in a strategic position to do a lot of incredible things. I got to
leave the country for the first time. I got to travel and be on com-
mittees. I got a phenomenal leadership job shortly after joining
the reserves. It was the type of job that senior men get and no
women ever get. I was two pay grades lower than everyone else
doing that type of work. It was a great experience. I was having
the adventure of my life in the reserves.

Darby provided details about her life:

I have four kids, not with the navy doctor. I was working as a
jail nurse in San Mateo County, CA, and that is where I met my
kids' father. It was a life-altering experience working at a jail. We
were together for 8 years and then we got married. Then, we got
divorced. We are still good friends. During that time I finished my
master's degree in counseling, and it was 1985. I was still doing
the Navy Reserves, but the Cold War was over and everything was
peaceful. There was more training for wars that might never happen, but then there was Desert Shield, it was pre-Desert Storm. I
was an ER nurse at the time, and they put me back on active duty.

I stayed active duty until August or September 1991. I got orders to deploy to the hospital ship, *Mercy*. When the *Mercy* went out originally, I think I was the only navy reserve nurse on the ship. We sat around in Oakland Harbor for a while because I think they made a tactical mistake pulling all of their doctors from a teaching hospital. They left the interns and residents standing there with their fingers in their nose. They couldn't continue the program with all the doctors on the ship, so they brought everyone back to the hospital. I opted to be on the ground and then the war was quickly over so I didn't mobilize on that.

I was mobilized to Okinawa, but we did not deploy. I stayed in the active reserves. In 2004, I went to fleet hospital training at Camp Pendleton. Then, I went to Kuwait in 2004–2005. I had wanted to go and had asked to go. My kids were older by that time, two were out of the house, and their dad was supposed to be keeping an eye on the other two. I have two boys and two girls. Their father really didn't watch them very well. I didn't call home every day either. I probably was not aware of a lot of the mayhem that was going on with my two boys.

In 2000, I hooked up with my first boyfriend ever (vintage 1978) back in Ohio and we got married. He was the love of my life. It didn't go south, it just went haywire because of me and my deployments. My navy service came first, my kids second now that they are adults, and my husband third. I told him this. When it came down to it, I was thrilled when I got the letter saying that I was going to war. I couldn't wait to be part of it. I think that taking care of our guys, no matter where they are, is simply the best job.

I came back to Ohio from Kuwait. I met with my now ex-husband about finances. I knew my bank account was hosed up because of combat pay. Surprisingly, my money was gone and his money was gone. While I was gone, he went out a lot and treated other people to dinners and drinks and gave the kids money. He went through money like crazy. I went back to my house in California. Within 6 months, I received orders to Landstuhl, Germany. I worked as an OR nurse there for a year. I worked in the same day surgical center and later in the OR. Without going to a special school or program, I acclimated well to the OR. Also, I ended up working in one of the busiest ORs in the world, which has some of the newest procedures and techniques being done because no one has seen the type of serious injuries before that are coming from these wars. I'm right in the middle of it. I'm a wound nurse. I did a lot of wound wash-outs that other people did not want to do. I had some knowledge about wounds that some of the younger doctors did not have so it worked out.

So, I was in Kuwait for a year and then at the Joint Services Medical Center in Landstuhl, Germany, for a year. I came home from Landstuhl in December and the following August, they sent me to trauma school for a month. On September 8th, I got orders to go to Afghanistan. I first had to go to Fort Polk, Louisiana, for 3 months of training. It was combat school: how to drive Humvees, how to shoot 1050s, how to assemble and disassemble automatic weapons, how to take apart Russian weaponry, and how to shoot 50 caliber machine guns. We also had language school and classes on Afghan culture. We were embedded, we were not at the American Hospital. We were mentoring at the Afghan Hospital in Kabul. Someone said, "You are lucky, you are going to the Walter Reed of Afghanistan." Well, it was just a terrible assignment.

Darby described her mental state when she returned from Afghanistan:

I came home angry, frustrated, and disappointed. I felt let-down, not listened to. I'm a commander in the navy, and I have a lot of coping skills. I saved money while deployed. But there were problems with my pay when I got home and also problems with my health care.

I met a guy online in Afghanistan. I'm in northern Afghanistan and he's in southern Afghanistan. He's been separated from his wife for 3 years and is getting divorced. He's a contractor and is retired military. I get nailed for "having a sexual relationship in a combat zone." But, I've never even met him! We texted back and forth. It got racy real quick. But I had never laid eyes on this man. His wife cites me for "alienation of affection." I get called into the commanding officer's office. I had to sign a reprimand paper. I hadn't done anything except text him.

Later, after I get home, the same guy comes to visit me in California. To make a long story short, he has a big mass on his left lung. We'll go to the oncology doctor next week. He'll be starting on chemotherapy. He's 59 years old. Everything seems to go south for me. I was taken off of active duty, and I have not been paid yet.

5

Renegotiating Roles: A Family Affair

Nurses commented on the difficulties encountered when having to re-negotiate family roles. Some were not ready to jump right back in with domestic chores, helping with homework, paying bills, grocery shopping, and chauffeuring children. Others wanted to take over their old roles right away, and were anxious to get on with their lives. Some met reluctance on their spouse's part to relinquish the routine that had been established during the deployment. Most found that easing back into a routine with a redistribution of household chores worked best.

We chose the following nine vignettes that are reflective of what many of the other 26 participants experienced on their return home after deployment. However, one has to keep in mind that some of the nurses were single or without children. Thus, the renegotiation of roles depended on a variety of factors. But all of the nurses had to do the usual household chores such as cooking, cleaning, grocery shopping, and paying bills.

LIEUTENANT COLONEL JULIE

Julie grew up in southern Virginia and attended college near her home. She joined the Air Force Reserve when she was in her mid-20s, while working in her community hospital ICU. A few physicians and nurses she worked with at the local hospital were members of the Air Force Reserve, and they encouraged her to sign up. Her boyfriend, who later became her husband, was also in the Air Force Reserve.

Julie reported:

My job was as a flight nurse. I did two tours flying out of Balad,
Iraq, and a third deployment flying air evac out of Ramstein Air
Base, Germany. I have been an air force flight nurse for 24-½ years.
When I deployed, however, I was usually deployed in a three-person CCATT [Critical Care Air Transport Team]. When we got to
our deployment assignment, we usually met up with several air
evac crews from other units and locations across the country. We
would then form a whole new unit for the deployment. I was in
Iraq in 2003 when the war began. Then I went back to Iraq in 2011.
Later, I flew missions out of Germany going to the States starting in
2012. On a CCATT, you have a critical care nurse, an intensive care
physician, and a respiratory therapist. We are usually assigned to
one to four of the most critical patients on an air evac flight.

Julie described how she and her family struggled once she came home
from her first deployment:

I didn't reintegrate well to my family at first. My husband had taken
on a whole new role while I was gone, and it was hard for me to
negotiate roles. He was a reservist, too; so, I was used to him being
gone and me picking up whatever needed to be done in the family
and household. So, I found it much more difficult to reintegrate back
into the household than I had ever anticipated. I think what made
it so hard for me in retrospect, is that I think I had some degree of
PTSD [posttraumatic stress disorder] from just seeing and caring
for too much trauma. You do your job very well when you are doing your job, and you try not to dwell on what you've just seen or
what you have just done in caring for the patient. But, later it really
clouds your mind with images and thoughts about all these terribly
wounded or burned people. I just wasn't motivated to pick up the
household chores I did before I left, and my husband was very tired
of doing everything while I was gone. I felt I needed a break. So,
there was some stress between us, and some heated dialogue.

LIEUTENANT COLONEL TONI

Toni is an air force reservist who was a flight nurse as well as a CCATT nurse.
She stated:

When I came back from my third deployment, I wasn't in the
right mindset to step right back into the role of working mother,

housekeeper, grocery shopper, and cook. My mind just wasn't there yet. I think my brain was a little oversaturated with the war and the terribly injured young people I cared for. My husband thought I would want to jump right back in, but I wasn't up to it. He told me he had never seen me like this; he said I seemed kind of withdrawn and hesitant to pick up on my usual activities. I think he wanted a break from the child-care stuff. However, I wasn't ready to jump back in. Three deployments had taken their toll. I was grieving for my patients' both living and dead. The ones that lived had some terribly disfiguring and disabling injuries. Most were between about 19 to 25 years of age. What kind of life will they have? All this took a toll on us nurses. It certainly took a toll on me. I needed time to get my bearings before I became a mom, a wife, and a housekeeper again.

LIEUTENANT KATE

Kate is a navy nurse.
  She recalled:

When I first got home, we were struggling to find our roles again in our relationship. Things got better a couple of months after I got home. My husband and I were able to sort through our issues and to communicate better. We were able to talk to each other about the things that were bothering each of us. Our circumstances as a young married couple were probably different from most. We were engaged for about 2 years, but he had been deployed to Iraq during some of that time. We were supposed to get married, but my deployment got moved up, and I had to be in California for 4 months before I deployed. So, he ended up coming to California, and we drove to Las Vegas and eloped because I would have already deployed by the date we had planned to get married.

  All in all, I was really only married for a month before I left for Afghanistan. It was a mutual decision to do it this way, but it was sort of a last-minute decision. I'm glad we did it this way because if we had waited even longer I'm not sure we would have been able to keep our relationship going while deployed. It worked out better the way we did it because I was a mess when I came back. I was angry and very disappointed in everyone when I got home. There were a couple of things that were difficult issues for my husband and me. I came home in November, and we rescheduled our big wedding with our families and friends for

March. Then, we were going to be reassigned to Guam the following June. We had a lot to do, and we both felt a lot of pressure
to get the ceremonial big wedding done for our families, and
then get packed up and moved overseas. Now, we have been in
Guam for 2 years, and our lives have settled down and everything has smoothed out to a nice pace of life.

LIEUTENANT COMMANDER ZOE

Zoe talked about her deployments from the perspective of being not only
a family nurse practitioner in the navy, but also as a wife and a mother.
She also mentioned that her husband is an active duty naval officer as well.
They are the parents of two daughters.
    She stated:

I've had two deployments. My first deployment was to Kuwait
in 2006–2007. My second deployment was to Afghanistan in
2009–2010 and that was with a provincial reconstruction team
which was a tri-service augmented role. It was an army mission,
but it involved the army, navy, and air force. We were all on the
same team.
    When I deployed to Kuwait for 6 months, that proved to
be an extremely difficult time for us as a couple. So, when I got
back from that deployment, the reintegration period was very
difficult. I was questioning who I was as a mother and who I was
as a wife. The job that I went back to at the time was very stressful with very long hours. It demanded a lot of time away from
my family anyway. Although this deployment was long ago, the
reason I reference it was because that period was so difficult. I
had to work through a lot of issues with my husband, and then
we became stronger as a couple.
    So when I found out that I was going to Afghanistan, we
immediately talked about what we would need to do, as a couple and as parents, during the deployment to Afghanistan that
would have to be so different than what had happened previously, so we could make our marriage work. We wanted to make
sure that when I got back from Afghanistan, we would not have
to go through that same period of difficulty as my first deployment in Kuwait.
    Our lessons learned from the first deployment were that
if we went into the time apart feeling disconnected because of

the distractions of work and the business of raising children, we needed to address it by communicating pronto. At the time of my first deployment, our communication was very weak. Going into the deployment to Afghanistan, we knew that we needed to communicate throughout the whole deployment. Part of that included being better at making phone calls.

LIEUTENANT COLONEL TAMMY

Tammy, an Air National Guard nurse, related her experience with renegotiating household chores once she returned from Afghanistan.

She stated:

My husband and I had to renegotiate our role transitions a bit, but overall it went pretty smoothly. My husband shared the things he struggled with while I was gone, to give me a "heads-up" in case I started struggling with the same things. I had talked to him about some things I did for the little kids before I left, like cleaning their ears and cutting their nails. He was happy to turn those chores back to me. Overall, he did a good job with the kids, and I was ready to pick up my share when I got home.

MAJOR ANITA

Anita was an air force ICU nurse who had been deployed to Pakistan and to Afghanistan.

Anita related:

Initially, it was hard to integrate into activities of daily living like cooking, cleaning, laundry, and paying bills because I just didn't want to do it. I had to change my routine, and it was funny; it was like karma. I would always get on my husband because we eat out a lot. If we go to this restaurant that we like, he always orders the same thing. He is a creature of habit. For example, there's this one Mexican restaurant that we go to all the time and I have had just about everything on the menu. He gets the exact same thing every time [*laughing*]. So when I come home, I am not dealing too well with change, and I was more like him. I didn't stay that way, but I was like that in the beginning, and it was hard. I remember day three or four after being back, I needed toiletries or something, so we went to Walmart. After about 10 minutes or so I said to him, "I can't be here anymore—I have got to leave right now." So we left and he says to me, "What's going on?" I told him that I couldn't believe the people in there, and now they have videos about the people who go to Walmart. They were the "freak people," and yet I know there are normal people who go there because my friends go there, my coworkers go there. Seeing the people in Walmart that day just bothered me and I had to leave. I was looking around at these sloppy, rude, pushy, nasty freak people. At the time I was thinking, "Really, I have just been in Afghanistan fighting for this country for God's sake and this is who we are defending and fighting for?" I said, "I never want to step foot in Walmart again." I actually went there about a month ago out of necessity, and it wasn't as bad. I think when I first returned it was the crowding that bothered me so much, not really the people.

MAJOR FRED

Fred was a longtime member of the Air National Guard and Air Force Reserve.

He remarked:

When I left for the 2007 deployment to Iraq, my boys were 7 and 4 years old. It was hard leaving them. It was hard to even get out of the house. It was hard to even think about not being there with my kids. It was helpful when I could call home. It made being away a bit easier. You had to figure out the time difference so you could call at a reasonable time. I would sometimes get up at 4 o'clock in the morning to Skype with my family. My kids were older when I deployed to Afghanistan, but I would say it was equally hard both times.

LIEUTENANT SANDRA

Sandra was a navy trauma and emergency care nurse assigned to Camp Bastion, Afghanistan.

Sandra remarked:

When I got home, I took right over with grocery shopping because they were not eating healthy. I think my husband actually gained 60 pounds while I was gone. It was because I wasn't there to cook and monitor what they were eating. I almost think they had pizza every night while I was gone.

I am an active person so I had to latch onto something to get me out of the house. I am not one to sit and watch TV. I don't sit at the computer either. I got into hiking when I got back. I loved hiking in Guam, but I didn't have that much time. I got certified in diving when I was in Guam. Hiking became my outlet, and I got people to do it with me. I think it was my contribution to the community and the command to get people out on hikes. I went to the gym, and I got others to go to the gym.

MAJOR ELIZA

Eliza hails from the Appalachian Trail of North Carolina. She joined the air force to serve her country, see the world, and gain nursing expertise. She has had eight military deployments to date. Two of her deployments were humanitarian missions to areas affected by Hurricane Katrina and to Haiti. Her other short deployments included 4 months in Kandahar, Afghanistan, serving as a ground supervisor and clinical coordinator for aeromedical evacuation flights, 2 months as a flight nurse based in Germany flying air evac flights to pick up patients in Iraq and Afghanistan, 4 months in Qatar as part of an aeromedical control team coordinating air evac missions and CCATT assignments, and 1 month of flight nursing out of Germany to Iraq and Afghanistan. Two of her eight deployments were for 6 months each. She was deployed to Afghanistan in 2010 and again in 2012. Both times, Eliza was assigned as an ICU nurse at the combat support hospital (CSH) at Bagram Air Base.

Eliza stated:

The thing that made my last two deployments to Afghanistan especially hard was the fact that my daughter was very young. I think she was 2 years old and the deployments lasted intermittently till she was almost 5 years old. She didn't like me being gone, and she lived mostly with my mom because I was gone so often. I wanted her to have some consistency. She never actually saw me packing and leaving. She just knew that I would be gone, and that I'd be coming back. She'd ask me why I was going, and I told her that as a nurse I had to go and take care of soldiers who were hurt in the wars.

My daughter stayed with my mom in North Carolina. She had to change schools twice within a year. Even with school, she was having some trouble with math. She made some progress eventually. Then when I got back from my first 6-month deployment to Afghanistan, I noticed that she had regressed. I remember asking her doctor and her teacher about this, and they both said that they frequently see this with military kids of deployed parents. They said that they often see this with addition and subtraction. They told me to "give her some time." Yet, she seemed to get multiplication and division down OK.

Not too long after that deployment, we moved again. We moved to Texas. We hadn't even been there for 6 months when I got tasked again. Luckily, it got pushed back by 3 months. I didn't leave till August, and we had been there for a year. This time the dynamics of home changed. The sitter I had left, so my mom actually moved in with us to keep the continuity for my daughter. She didn't have to change schools, and my mom made sure things were OK. She moved in 10 days before I left, and she is still currently with us. We moved here to Scott AFB, Illinois, in June. I think I'll be here for 3 to 4 years. I like it here. I like the community.

6

Painful Memories of Trauma

Many nurses could not get the chaotic scenes of wartime trauma out of their minds. Their reintegration experiences were haunted by the memories of horrific combat injuries to soldiers, civilians, and children. These images as well as the sounds and smells of war colored their world. For some, their painful memories and the stresses of nursing in a war zone impeded their ability and desire to assume family roles and household responsibilities. For others, they had difficulty taking care of serious trauma patients once they returned home. Some said they needed to transfer to another clinical area if they were to continue their nursing practice in the future.

It was evident in the nurses' narratives that painful memories of trauma impacted various aspects of their lives, such as reintegration with family, the ability to return to past clinical settings, and their ability to care for certain types of patients. Sometimes, the painful memories affected their motivation to engage in social and recreational activities. In most instances, it was the emotional, spiritual, psychological, and physical trauma of war that affected the entire reintegration process.

LIEUTENANT LORETTA

Loretta, a navy operating room (OR) nurse, described an intrusive thought of the war trauma.

She stated:

> I had one experience when I first came home that I'll never forget. We were out at a restaurant, and I had lamb on a shank. It was

91

fine, and I didn't have trouble eating it. But when I was done and
looked down at it on my plate, I had to cover it up with my napkin,
and I had the waiter take it away because looking at it, I was right
back in the OR. I couldn't look at it. That bone sitting there on my
plate took me back to all the limbs we had to amputate and all the
limbs with the skin and flesh blown away or burned away. Now,
when I think about it, I didn't eat anything on the bone when I
was over there. To this day, I don't eat meat on the bone anymore.

Loretta described the memories of patient trauma that remained vivid
in her memory:

By the time we see them in the OR, they often still have their
limbs attached and are some semblance of a whole person. The
ICU would have patients bandaged or with an eye patch on;
whereas, in the OR, I equate it with working in a butcher shop.
I lost count of how many healthy legs with boots still on that
would be put in biologic bags and would go to the incinerator the
next day. We were literally taking apart what had been whole.
An hour ago, the same guys were healthy, strapping 18-, 19-, or
20-year olds. Now, they were tragically changed forever. I can
still see the heap of biologic bags waiting to be transported to
the incinerator, and our OR floor covered in blood as a mass
casualty incident transpired. I can smell it; I can see it; and I can
hear it. We had a high profile case; a young army soldier held the
record for the number of units of blood products he received
and survived. I think in Afghanistan at the two hospitals that
cared for him, he had over 400 units of blood products.

FIRST LIEUTENANT RHETTA

Rhetta grew up on a ranch in rural Montana. An avid reader, she longed for
travel and adventure. Having read her mother's Cherry Ames series of nursing
adventure books, she went to college on an army ROTC (Reserve Officers'
Training Corps) nursing scholarship. She did her preliminary training at Fort
Sam Houston in San Antonio, Texas, knowing that her first real nursing job
as an RN would be a wartime assignment. She craved excitement, wanted to
serve her country, and didn't mind being outnumbered by men. She felt that
she grew up rather isolated in rural Montana and had not traveled much except to the state university and back for college. Her dating history was rather
lackluster which she attributed to being around farmers and ranchers most of

her life. She wanted to meet different types of men. She wanted to see New York City, San Francisco, Washington DC, and Chicago.

Rhetta was assigned to the hospital at Balad, Iraq, on a medical–surgical unit. As she was a new RN, everything fascinated her. She was a "sponge" soaking up every morsel of wisdom from her colleagues. She volunteered for every assignment possible that involved going out in a helicopter.

Although her parents supported her and the war effort, they wondered why she wanted to leave the beauty and simplicity of rural Montana. They understood her desire to become a nurse and were proud of her university education. Rhetta thought her parents would have preferred for her to work at a nearby community hospital or at most, move to Billings to work in a medical center. Her decision to join the army surprised them. However, Rhetta had three younger siblings, and her father had a large cattle ranch to maintain. Her mother helped out with everything on the ranch.

It was not long before Rhetta was exposed to the raw trauma of war. She recounted:

> In my first 2 or 3 months in Iraq I saw everything. I cared for some amputees on the ward for a day or two before they went out on the medevac flight to Landstuhl Joint Services Medical Center in Germany. They were so young, that stuck in my mind the most. The burns from IED [improvised explosive device] explosions were just awful. We had a marine vehicle blown up by an IED, and four marines were fried alive. They didn't stand a chance. We also had a family that was in a car, and it rolled over an IED. The parents died, and the three little kids were terribly burned, but they lived. Although I was often horrified with the injuries I saw, I was also fascinated with the human body and the healing process. I learned so much as the weeks went by, and I actually volunteered for more interesting assignments. I went on five helicopter runs toward the end of my tour to pick up patients. It was exciting, and I loved flying and I was able to provide the care they needed in route back to Balad.

LIEUTENANT COLONEL JULIE

Julie is an experienced Air Force Reserve flight nurse.
   She stated:

> Before the beginning of the war in Iraq, it used to have to be that patients were stabilized for flight. That was the concept of operations for air evac before the beginning of the war. Now, with the

wars, this concept has changed and patients are less stabilized. I had a guy's femoral artery open up and bleed out on me in flight at 35,000 feet. I don't know how he did long term, but he made it off the plane alive. I didn't follow up, I just don't do that. I can't force myself to do that.

The CCAT [Critical Care Air Transport] teams usually take care of two or three patients who are critical and on vents [ventilators] on the flight. But we help take care of the other 20 or 30 or 50 patients, and some of those patients need critical care, too, but are breathing on their own. We had a lot of vascular and orthopedic injuries that were splinted but needed watching, and these patients were in pain and needed pain medication. That was a real challenge because these folks were really in pain. It got better over time; because around 2005, anesthesia providers started doing nerve blocks to keep them more comfortable. They came out for the flight with the epidural catheters in and duramorph injected; so, they would be comfortable for the duration of the flight. Some were on PCA [patient-controlled analgesia] pumps so they could control their own pain meds to a point. But that being said, it is just so hard to deal with these terribly injured young people day in and day out. The burns, the traumatic amputations, the open head trauma with parts of the brain missing, the infected abdominal wounds from the desert sand, seeing this every day just gets to you.

When we flew missions back to the States, many of these folks were stable, but had significantly diminished capabilities. I felt really sorry for this one lady. She came and met her husband's flight when it was being readied to take him closer to home. She had their 3-year-old son with her. She said to me, "I feel like I have two 3-year-olds now." And she was talking about her husband. He had pretty significant closed head trauma. He couldn't do much for himself physically and also had significant cognitive impairment. I wondered what these patients lives would be like in the long run. What kind of a life would they have? Would their families be able to cope? How many will never go home again? Will a veteran's hospital become their home now?

LIEUTENANT COMMANDER ZOE

Zoe is an active duty navy family nurse practitioner.
   She recalled:

While I was in San Diego, I was able to see one of my corpsmen who had been seriously injured during our deployment, and he had survived. He was terribly injured, and the memory of "one of our own" being injured like that, in the hospital compound, really stuck with me and really "hit home" that no one was safe over there.

I was able to see him, meet his wife and children which was a really important experience for me. It had been very traumatic for everyone involved because he was actually injured on the base from a rocket attack and had essentially died at the forward surgical unit, and had been brought back to life, transfused, and medevaced out. That set a tone during the deployment, because it happened very early on. It helped me to see him, because I could see how they were surviving as a family and so that was a little bit of closure that was helpful. I am still in touch with them, and he's doing much better. He has paralysis in his right leg. His sciatic nerve was severed. At the time I saw him, he was going through a lot of rehabilitation and was walking with a cane and a special kind of foot support.

LIEUTENANT COMMANDER CATHERINE

Catherine is a navy family nurse practitioner who was deployed to Iraq and Afghanistan.

She reported:

One of the things that happened when I was in Iraq was that I wrote a very detailed account of our first few days in Iraq, and it was not meant for publication. It was not something I had done anything with. It was just a personal account of my experiences there because it became very clear early on in Fallujah that this was not a safe place to be. Two of our first casualties were medical staff. They were an army surgeon and an army medic both hit in a rocket attack, and they were killed. They were the unit we were replacing. So, as soon as we arrived, they were literally waiting for our gear to arrive by convoy; so, their unit could pack up and go home. They were within days of going home, and we had a rocket that landed right outside of our medical building, and it killed the two of them and several others became instant surgical cases. I think we medevaced four staff members as a result of that rocket attack. It became very clear how dangerous it was at the time, and we had only been in Fallujah for about 10 days when that happened. These guys were set to go home in about 3 days. It was a horrible thing, but it tested our surgical team. Yes, it was a rewarding deployment. That single event showed me the capabilities of a team to come together and do the mission. [*She starts crying.*] I guess this was the highest example of that in my career. Seeing that, I think these are lessons that I refer to in my leadership role all the time. When we are trying to get something hard done or meet a challenge where we don't have enough people, money, or supplies, it is the truest military medicine. That's the example I was left with. Nothing will be as hard as that.

In spite of the tragic losses, it was a critical thing to have happened because it showed that we were a team. None of us have ever done that before. Even if you work in surgical trauma, which wasn't the background of a lot of people in our unit, even if you had had these skills, they were not exactly the skills you needed in a place like Fallujah. In an inner city trauma center, you might deal with a gunshot wound but that was a far cry from what you get in Fallujah. There was such serious multisystem trauma. Traumatic amputations of multiple limbs, everything you can imagine, heads with chunks of skull and brain missing, everything, everything, your worst clinical nightmare!

There were horrible things that were occurring at the time I was in Fallujah. Do you remember the contractors who had been captured? They had been badly brutalized, and their bodies were hung upside down and burned. They became fodder for TV and propaganda. We were the unit that got their remains. So many horrible things were happening at that time [*crying*].

LIEUTENANT COMMANDER JUSTIN

Justin, a navy reservist, described his memories of neglected Afghan patients in an Afghan Army Hospital in Kabul, Afghanistan:

I saw patients come in with terrible injuries with exposed bone with infections that were not dealt with. Fractures were sometimes put back together incorrectly in surgery so the patient lost the use of that limb or joint permanently. When I questioned the surgeon about the placement of the screws and angle of the bones, he said "That is close enough." I am a CRNA [certified registered nurse anesthetist], not an orthopedic surgeon, but I've done enough anesthesia for ortho cases that I know when the bone alignment and screw placement is not correct. I've seen them manipulate a compound fracture of the leg of a 20-year-old policeman without administering any pain medication. This kind of stuff just breaks your heart. It just made me sick to my stomach, and it still does when I think back.

LIEUTENANT DARLA

Darla, a navy OR nurse, was deployed to the large hospital in Kandahar, Afghanistan.

She related:

There were some pretty catastrophic injuries we cared for over there. A lot of the worst injuries were from IED blasts and suicide bombers. People had burns, multiple amputations, eye sockets blown out, open head trauma with brain tissue oozing out, and brain tissue and skull parts missing. There were lots of gunshot wounds to the head and chest. We had five triple amputees that we did surgery on in our operating room suite. I had never seen anything like these injuries. It was hard to deal with emotionally, especially when the patients were little kids. Bullets and bombs don't discriminate between soldiers and innocent civilians and children. Some of this was just so hard to take, and so tragic.

CAPTAIN COURTNEY

Courtney was from a Connecticut beach community. She attended a state college there, graduating with a baccalaureate degree in nursing. She was employed at a large medical center in Connecticut. While still in her twenties, she joined the Air Force Reserve to earn extra income, see the world, and to serve her country. She was very proud to be in the air force. Her first and only deployment was to Afghanistan.

Courtney reported:

I was in Afghanistan for almost 7 months. I volunteered for deployment. I was in three different locations during my deployment. I mostly did trauma nursing for the majority of my time in Afghanistan. Then, I had 6 weeks of ICU, so it was kind of trauma "after the fact."

I got there on my birthday. I took a Blackhawk helicopter from Bagram to Bostic. We got off the chopper and went into the FST [Forward Surgical Team] building, and there was a mass casualty going on. I took my top off, I had a T-shirt on, I put gloves on, and I just started working on patients. There was a little kid they had been working on that was "expectant," but I decided to pop a line in him and give him fluids. He got shipped out to a place called Kia, it's a French-run hospital. I think it's in Kandahar. So, they accepted him as a patient. Then a month later, he came back to us, and he was good. He had lost an eye, and his head was kind of caved in, but he was neurologically intact. You have to understand that in Afghanistan, the sons are really important. The daughters are expendable, but the sons are really important. So, it was really good that the kid made it.

I spent my last 3 months in Afghanistan at FOB [Forward Operating Base] Fenti. It was a really good experience at Fenti, but every place I went there were bombings and serious injuries and a lot of amputations. In December, Fenti got attacked at the gate. The first bomb was close to our dorms. It was always the same shit; when you spend a lot of time with the army, you swear a lot [*laughs*]. My commander lived right across the hall from me. The bomb went off, so I jumped right out of bed and got on the floor. You have to wait and see if there is going to be another one exploding. When we figured out that it was clear to run across to the FST, which was a hardened facility, we took off running. We kept our "battle rattle" [protective Kevlar vests and helmets] in the FST. So, we put it on and waited for casualties. But the bombing kept going on for 4 hours. We looked out the front of the FST, and there was a gunship [armed helicopter] in view and we could see the war right in front of us. It was less than a mile away. The gunship, which was one of ours, was right there fighting back. That day, we had about 25 casualties. One of them was an American contractor who had just gotten there. He was a retired Green Beret, and he had only been there a week. He got hit. It was one of those head wounds where his pupils were blown. You knew he wasn't gonna come back, but you kept him alive so that his wife had the option of pulling the plug when he got back to the States. We saw just horrible wounds and burns at FOB Fenti. Many patients died at Fenti. We were in the thick of it.

FIRST LIEUTENANT ALLISON

Allison was an Air Force nurse assigned to the triage area and an emergency room in Afghanistan.

She recounted:

I have seen families slaughtered from car bombs. I've cared for many soldiers terribly burned from rolling their Humvee over an IED and little kids with bloody stumps for arms and legs. I've tried to console young soldiers when their buddies were killed by an RPG [rocket-propelled grenade]. Most of my memories from Afghanistan are of trauma and death. I got great nursing experience in Afghanistan, but at what cost? Will these memories still haunt me in 10, 20, or 30 years from now?

COMMANDER ROBIN

Robin was a career navy nurse who was deployed to Afghanistan. She recalled:

I was at Camp Bastion for my deployment, and I came back at the end of October 2010. Camp Bastion was labeled at the time "the busiest trauma center in the world." On a good day, we would get maybe one amputee, maybe a double amputee. On a bad day we would get a whole slew of doubles and triples. You did your best, of course, but it could really get to you at the end of the day when you would process things. Sometimes I went back to my quarters and cried at the end of my shift. I was not alone in crying. Many of us found a place to cry. Some people cried in the shower because the noise of the water dripping muffled the sobbing.

MAJOR ANITA

Anita was an air force nurse who was deployed to Pakistan and Afghanistan. She recalled:

I feel very passionate about being emotionless and having emotion because it was literally that black and white for me. Being in Afghanistan in that environment, you had to have no emotion. There was one time that I let my emotions take over. This is how it works in the ICU when it came to the active duty patients. They get blown up, and they are taken to the closest hospital, but they always end up at Bagram because in order to go to Germany, they have to go through Bagram. We were like the hub. When they get to Bagram, they are usually gone on a flight within 12 hours, usually to Germany.

We don't have them for very long in our ICU. Anyway, I had this one patient, and he was a mess. His left amputation was below the knee, his right was above the knee, he lost his right arm, and his left hand had three fingers. He also had a traumatic pelvic injury, and he had facial lacerations. Of course, he was intubated, and he was too unstable to fly, and he needed wound washouts more frequently. It would take 8 hours from Bagram to Germany on a good day. So, you have to plan for at least 10 hours and the physician said, "He has to go back to the OR for more wound washouts and can't wait that long." So, he was in our ICU for 3 days, and I took care of him for 3 days. Well, it wasn't the first time that I had called or spoken to the family of the patient. This guy was army. They were always calling for updates. They notify the family that their loved one has been injured. I got the phone number of the patient's wife, and so, I called her. I would want to know if it was my loved one. She had already been notified that her husband had been injured. She knew that he was seriously injured, and I made sure of that. She had previously talked with one of the physicians. She already knew the extent of his injuries. I decided to call her to introduce myself and let her know that we were taking care of him. She was very appreciative that I called. I became attached because there's a human element in it. These guys when they come in from the field, it's almost like a non-human. I mean it is and it isn't. It's like they are superheroes, and we are gonna pack them up and send them home. But it is different when you talk to his wife. That makes it real. She's talking to me, and she's feeling comfortable with me. I think most families are more comfortable with talking to nurses rather than physicians.

This patient's wife says "I hate, hate, hate to ask this question, but...." I said, "You can ask me anything, anything." She said, "I know about his amputations, does he have a knee?" She wanted to know specifically. I said, "I am standing right next to him and I have a cordless phone." She said, "I can do this, I can handle this." I said, "OK, the right leg does not have the knee, the amputation is right above it. The left, he still has the knee." So she is visualizing it. We go through the injuries and she says, "You're gonna think I'm crazy but I need to know. He's got this tattoo on his right leg that I hate, is it still there?" I said, "I hate to break the news to you, but he's still got that dragon tattoo." We laughed about it, and I have to tell you it was a beautiful moment. It was a beautiful conversation. She told me how I helped her deal with it. Yes, it's bad, but it could have been worse. She was comforted to talk to the person who was keeping him alive and would get him home to her. She was able to deal with it a little better. I called her every day. I said, "He's not leaving tomorrow, we're keeping him here, he'll be going to surgery, I'll be here tomorrow, and when he's done with surgery, I'll give you a call." That's how it was. The day he left, I called her to tell her he was in the air on the way to Germany. She was very appreciative. She was actually gonna be flying to Germany to meet him. She told me to keep her phone number and to call her when I got home, and she'd give me an update. During those 3 days, I became emotionally attached to him, he became my patient. I knew him by name. I knew his wife. I was emotionally invested in this guy, and it was the worst 3 days of my entire time there. I couldn't think of anything else, and it actually caused me to make a medication error. I put his ear drops in his eyes. I flipped out and started crying. It didn't cause a problem, but I was a wreck. I knew I made the mistake because I was so emotionally invested in the patient. It reassured me, that you've got to put up a wall so that you will not get emotionally involved.

LIEUTENANT SANDRA

Sandra was a navy nurse assigned to the British hospital at Camp Bastion, Afghanistan.

She recalled:

We saw so much trauma over there. I'm sure I'll never have that experience again. We took care of all kinds of troops; army, marines, navy, and the British, Danish, and all the local Afghans, too. We took care of the good guys and the bad guys.

I cried a lot the first couple of weeks after my homecoming. I think I had "survivor guilt." I would see the faces of people who would come to our ER at Bastion multiple times; a concussion here and there, then something minor, and then they'd come in with three of their limbs blown off. I'd see faces with eyes that would look at me while they are lying in the bed, and they'd recognize me. They'd be pleading in that serious condition, pleading with their eyes: "Make sure I live, save my life." They're scared, it's the fear.

CAPTAIN AMANDA

Amanda is an Air Force Reserve nurse deployed to Afghanistan.
She recalled:

> My second deployment was to FOB Wagman. I was there last
> summer. We were busy, supposedly the busiest FOB in the
> country. There were 20 to 25 of us on this forward surgical
> team. It was a navy-run FST, but there were army and air force
> troops who worked there, too. Most of our population that we
> took care of was Afghan. There were Afghan National Army,
> Afghan National Police, Afghan Uniformed Police, Afghan
> Border Patrol, and every sort of civilian you can think of plus
> numerous blown-up children. There was a lot of "blue on
> green, or is it green on blue," where they put on the other uni-
> form and try to kill the good guys. They did this multiple times
> while I was there. These guys were in the Afghan military, but
> they were killing our guys. They might have been an insurgent
> the day before or not; it was a little hairy, and they were kill-
> ing our guys. The Afghans go through the training, they take
> the oath to fight for their country, and then they just kill our
> guys. They were always considered enemies when they came
> into our FST. But, we always treated patients with the same
> respect, if you were a known enemy or not, you were always
> guarded and the nurses were protected.
>
> At the FOB we saw a ton of really nice polite patients. They
> are small in stature, and in the military just like we were. They
> were polite, sometimes the only English words they knew were
> "thank you." They understood that I was a woman without my
> head covered, but that I was nice. I helped them with pain con-
> trol and I showed them respect. I knew a few words in Dari and
> Pashto that I could say, and they respected that. On the FOB, we
> saw really, really poor Afghans, and they appreciated the care
> and were polite.
>
> In Bagram on my first deployment, we saw larger stat-
> ured Afghans who were a lot of times known bad guys. They
> were our patients, too. Sometimes over in this bay you were
> taking care of an Afghan who tried to kill your American who
> was in another bay. They were extremely close in proximity.
> We were doing everything possible to keep the bad guys alive,
> while we were fighting for the lives of the Americans over
> there. It's like this guy is dying because that guy shot him.

It was an ethical struggle as a nurse. It was so hard. But as nurses, we try to save everybody, and we'd never hurt the bad guys. At the end of the day, it was just painful that you would lose Americans because they were blown up by the bad guys who were also your patients.

LIEUTENANT DOREEN

Doreen is a navy reservist who was injured in Iraq in 2008.
She recalled:

I had a near crash experience on a helicopter. It was what they call a "hard landing." I am currently being evaluated for a TBI [traumatic brain injury]. I was attending to a pediatric patient. He was severely wounded, and we were transporting him.

It was basically almost a controlled crash. In fact, the whole trip was near impact. It was just a very bad night in terms of weather. We had to make four attempts to land, before we finally landed to pick up this kid. We were also landing in a hostile place, but it was mostly the weather conditions. There were active sandstorms. I always went out in helicopters. I went to Fort Rucker for my flight nurse helicopter training. That's an army base. I didn't know at the time that I had incurred an injury. I had been taking ibuprofen daily because it was so hot, and I had headaches. When I came home, I think I disregarded the headaches. I did not have a history of headaches. I continued working after that flight. They had called out, "Prepare for impact" in the helicopter. My patient was restrained because he was belligerent. I remember being thrown, and then coming to with a medic entangled with me and on top of me because we were all thrown. I lost consciousness very briefly. That's all I can recall. I came to and continued taking care of the patient. No one was apparently hurt, we just landed very awkwardly, and we just really got tossed. We were kneeling over the patient when we got tossed. I went on to fly other missions, and they were uneventful.

Doreen shared details of her deployment to Afghanistan:

I left in 2010 and arrived in country and was there for 6-½ months. Command structure was absolutely phenomenal; I have nothing negative to say. Never in my life have I served with a better commanding officer. He was a navy captain, and he was phenomenal. The hospital was absolutely beautiful, it was brand new. This was in Kandahar, the NATO [North Atlantic Treaty Organization] Hospital. Our living conditions were phenomenal. My first patient was a triple amputee. We waited for him to be brought in. The nurse that was training me was really good and she said, "Stand by, watch what we do and don't freak out." I said "OK, I work in a Level 1 Trauma Center, and I can handle anything." In comes this guy with two legs missing and an arm missing and even though I work in a Level 1 Trauma Center, I've never seen this, especially with a uniform intact. It was a shocker, but 2 weeks later this was normal. I hate to say that and see that, but that's how it was. Actually, I don't think it ever became normal. It was difficult. We got there at the end of August, and I was sent out on a mission very shortly after we arrived. It was a team: myself, a physician, and two navy corpsmen. I remember asking my division head, "Why are you sending me out? There are plenty of nurses who could go." It was the first mission of its kind, and they wanted to reinforce the army so we went out for about 2-½ weeks to Camp Wilson. It was absolutely horrific. It seemed like every day we had mass casualties. The two physicians out there were army docs, and there was a PA [physician assistant], too. One physician was a pediatrician just out of residency or fellowship, and the other one was family practice or primary care. Neither of them was emergency medicine, none had emergency room experience. Why the army would send them out to a FOB is beyond me, and the PA was not an emergency medical person either. Needless to say, we taught them very quickly how to do chest tubes, etc. The doc I went out with was EM [emergency medicine] physician from Brooklyn or nearby. He was phenomenal. His personality was not phenomenal, but you just had to get over him. He was a great doc. It was just very difficult to be out there, very difficult. I was not the only nurse, there was an army nurse, but he really didn't do anything. He did meds and that was it. I'm not sure what his role was when patients came in. We really didn't have enough people to handle a mass casualty. Most of the patients they brought in were dead. It was an even mixture of Afghan National Army, coalition troops, and our troops that were DOA [dead on arrival]. There were a lot that we were able to medevac out, but many did not survive, meaning NATO troops. Many died in the hospital at Kandahar. Apparently our numbers during my rotation were the highest.

When we were at the FOB, we did receive an incoming rocket/mortar that hit one of the construction battalion tents. It was very loud and there were a lot of injuries. Everyone was stable, but it shook everybody up. All night long there was outgoing fire. So no one got any sleep, and it was scary. It taught me to be humble and it also taught me to be an aggressive, assertive nurse and to stand up for what I believe in as a nurse. It was one of the most positive experiences of my life because I was part of the effort to get these guys home to their families. In Kandahar, we prepared them for the flight to Germany regardless of their brain status. If they were brain dead, we were still getting them ready to go to Germany for the sake of their families. They would eventually extubate them, of course. I was the senior nurse trauma leader. I had experience of being in a leadership position as a nurse. I am good at it. I never had any issues. My physicians were great to me; whereas, some of the other trauma teams had issues. I don't want to toot my own horn, but I never had those types of issues. I have always been one to stay under the carpet, meaning that I just wanted to keep my career quiet, do my job, play the game and retire. I didn't join the military to be known. I joined the military to do what I did in Afghanistan, and I did it very successfully.

CAPTAIN BRITTANY

Brittany is an army nurse who served in Iraq and Afghanistan.
She reported:

We were more nervous going to Afghanistan. We heard that there was so much more active fighting going on. The chances of things happening were a lot higher. There were a lot of warriors getting hit really hard. While in Iraq, we had very few mass casualty events. In Afghanistan, they were unfortunately common. The first 6 months I was at FOB Sharada with the 10th Mountain Dustoffs, and then they were replaced with the 82nd Airborne Dustoffs. It's on the eastern side of Afghanistan. It is about a 45-minute helicopter ride to the Pakistani border.

After 6 months, I moved to Helmand province in southern Afghanistan. I lived at Camp Bastion which shared the fence line with Camp Leatherneck where the marines are. I lived with the Air Force Search and Rescue Teams. Their primary mission is to rescue fallen aircraft, single events. But because things weren't happening too often, they had two airplanes and crews just sitting around. So, they decided to have a plane on casualty alert and assigned some army nurses to go with them. If people were injured on the western side of Afghanistan and needed to get to the bigger hospitals on the eastern side of Afghanistan, they would notify the Search and Rescue Teams, and they could be in the air within 30 minutes to move patients across the country. This was an air force plane with an air force flight crew and army critical care nurses.

My time in Afghanistan was very emotionally draining and very spiritually draining. We saw the worst of humanity for such an extended period of time. It is an interesting dynamic where our soldiers are trained to kill to save their own lives and to protect the mission. They train medical personnel for that too, but we are trained to save those lives. To see the results of so much violence, it takes its toll on you after a while. We saw a lot of blast injuries. There was a fair amount of amputations and a lot of gunshot wounds. We took care of a lot of civilians, too, and we had to fly them as well sometimes. There were a lot of injured kids who got stuck in the middle, especially really little kids who were not making any decisions about what was happening. Those situations were so hard. My heart went out to those kids.

COMMANDER DARBY

Commander Darby, a Navy Reserve nurse, recalled some memories of trauma that she will never forget. Much of what she described was at the hands of Afghan physicians.

She stated:

We get there and I ask the army sergeant where the hospital is and where are the marines who are going to escort us there. He responds, "There are no marines to take you there, ma'am. You just spent 3 months in combat and weapons training to be able to protect yourself. You are your own protection." I say, "That's impossible" [*laughing as she recalls this to me*]. I say, "I thought that I would only need to use my weapon if there was no one around to help." As a nurse, I really didn't think I'd be shooting people and knowing me, I'd probably shoot them sooner than later [*laughing*]. We were all dumbfounded. I then said to the sergeant, "You don't understand, I am a non-combatant." He responded, "No ma'am, you don't understand." So I have my 9 mm strapped to my leg and I have a rifle and I have all this gear on. I mean if I had tripped and fell someone would have to come and pick me up. I would not be able to get up with all of this heavy stuff on me [*laughing*].

I drew on my previous jail nursing experience. It helped me deal with some of the Afghan men. Americans are so intrinsically nice. We think if we're kind to someone, they'll be kind back. If we give to them, they'll give back.

It was so demoralizing at times in that hospital that was built by the Serbians in 1980 something. It was an eight-story hospital with 150 beds. It was used by the Afghans. There were no American patients there. We would not have let an American patient be treated there. We'd fly them 2 hours away, if necessary. The hospital was horrible. It was so far beyond horrible. The woman that I was replacing would e-mail me saying "Just get here." She obviously could not wait to leave. Her tour was 6 months, mine was for 1 year. We were the first group assigned for a whole year and we were the last group assigned for a whole year. She took me to the hospital for the first day. She had not been there in 3 months. This is how meaningless our mission was. Nobody cared if you went to work or if you didn't go. No one checked on us. She spent the 3 months back at the base, working out in the gym, reading, and watching movies. This was in Kabul. NKC [New Kabul Compound] was what it was called. We could see Gen. Petraeus's base from the roof of our hospital. But in Kabul, the traffic was awful, and it could take you a 1/2 hour to get there. It would be a 5-minute walk but we weren't allowed to walk because people were getting grabbed and others were shot. You had to drive there, and you had to have your weapons with you.

We were at NKC. We were owned by the big group, IFSA [International Security Forces Afghanistan], which was the headquarters where Petraeus was located. We were part of the medical training advisory group. They sent us to a smaller base because it was closer to the hospital. It was easier to get there, and we didn't have to go through the traffic in Kabul.

Nobody really knew us. We were located on this smaller base with Special Forces, operations people and army people, not with anyone or anything that had to do with medical or a hospital. We had no accountability. No one owned us. No one cared what we were doing. I remember thinking, "What the hell is going on here?" We were out in that community with no back-up. We had cell phones that did not work in the hospital. We had no emergency evacuation plan. We had three American nurses. One nurse did administration and was the commander of the hospital, which was a joke. So we really had two functioning nurses. There were about 250 patients in the hospital. As far as care, it depended on what tribe you were in, how much money you had, and what you had to bargain with. It was a disaster! We saw people starving to death in the hospital because they were from the wrong tribe.

Afghanistan many years ago had a medical school, and it was supposedly OK. Then the Russians came in and the Serbs came in, and they had this big war. All of the doctors were put in prison because they were smart. If they weren't in prison and weren't on the side of the Taliban, they got out of Afghanistan. The best, the brightest, and the smartest are gone.

I will say this without any hesitation; there were a lot of inbred idiots with a literacy rate of 10%. It's just a disaster and it's very tribal. You can't trust anybody no matter what. The guy who has 10 cents more in his pocket will turn in the other guy. There's no loyalty for anything. Once we announced that we were leaving, it was anybody's guess what was gonna happen. The Americans started buying and buying more of what they wanted. I didn't do it that way, and I achieved more success because I had a really good group of people with me. I had a bio-med-tech with me.

I remember my first day at the hospital taking a tour with the woman I was replacing. We were climbing a stairway in the hospital, and I see feces and urine and banana peel and garbage all over the place. There's dirt on the floor of the main lobby. The stench was awful. It was like an urban bus station or a gar-bage dump, rather than a hospital. She started crying and said, "I couldn't take it anymore. That's why I didn't come here for months."

We went to the OR. I could have probably put my mailman in charge of the OR, and he would have had more knowledge than anyone working there. The doctors there don't ever want to admit that they don't know something. The Americans could have taught them so much. They didn't want to learn. They just wanted new, shiny equipment. They believed that if they had new, shiny equipment they could work and do surgery.

Muslim doctors never work on cadavers because that is against the laws of their religion. You can't cut up cadavers. So, they only knew what they read in books. So when you cut someone open, I swear to you, there's a look on some of their faces like, "Shouldn't it be outlined in red?" I've watched these guys and if you come in with belly pain, they cut you open. I watched amputations with no anesthesia. I saw women beaten until they passed out having C-sections with no anesthesia. I saw doctors sticking needles in people's spines seven, eight, nine, 10 times where they had no idea what they were doing until sometimes I'd scream, "This is enough!"

First of all, they're all men. No women practitioners. They have a couple of females, but they never get to do anything. The young doctors in Afghanistan who are savvy because of the Internet and understand that there is life beyond Afghanistan and the financial benefits, well, they got farmed out to the boonies because the hospital did not want to compete with the Walter Reed of Afghanistan.

Darby recalled some of the upsetting things she saw at the hospital:

The anesthesia guy is taking a needle out of one guy and putting it into another guy. I've seen doctors use bloody instruments in one room and then use the same instruments in another room. They'd wipe them off on their pant leg and begin surgery. It's because they don't know, and they don't care. They don't care. They didn't know anything about sterilization. It was every man for himself. The Americans love the dogs running around more than the Afghans love each other. It was "brother against brother" and "son against father." And everyone was against women. Women are basically used for pro-creation. That's it! Maternal mortality and morbidity are very high. The homosexuality and pedophilia are unbelievable. Everything was so crooked and dirty. It was the demoralizing of life itself. We had two suicide bombers at the hospital while I was there.

Medically the hospital was such a disaster. The screams of people coming from the hospital were unbelievable. I remember a 23-year-old man in decent shape, who had a cardiac arrest on the OR table, and all the doctors put down their equipment and walked away. I yelled, "Do CPR," and they didn't. There was a lot of death and tragedy at that hospital. I saw a number of children with intentional burns and a lot of women beaten badly. The command surgeon said, "We're not gonna take care of women and children anymore." People didn't wash their hands. They didn't put on gloves or gowns or masks. I remember hearing screams from one of the ORs, and there was a woman having a C-section. She still had her street clothes on, and the baby was a girl. They wrapped the baby up, and just left her there because she was a female. They closed the mother up so fast that there was no doubt in my mind that she would not make it between the bleeding and the high possibility of infection.

I started documenting stuff by taking pictures with my camera. Also, on the maternity ward, there are no men. They have midwives. The next day, my interpreter and I visited the C-section patient who had given birth to the female baby. The patient looked "as white as a ghost." She was shocky, she was hemorrhaging internally. Her family went to get her blood. Her mother and grandmother are crying. My interpreter starts crying. I asked my interpreter, "what are they talking about?" She tells me that the patient wants me to take the baby to America to have a better life. I stood there for a long time, how could I possibly do that? I went back the next morning to visit them. I had a bunch of things to do around the hospital. When I came back to see them, they were gone. They were all gone; mother, baby, grandmother and great grandmother. No one knew anything. They didn't know the patient's name or where she lived. I still think about them to this day. I wonder if the mother died because she was not in very good shape. I'll bet the baby ended up in an orphanage, they are all overflowing with baby girls. Maybe the grandmother could keep the baby, but she was just another mouth to feed in hard times. It was the most horrible experience of my life. I literally felt like I was in a *Twilight Zone* movie. Another nurse and I screamed at people to be concerned about what was going on. I went to Army Jag [Army Legal Services] to see what could be done. I told them that people were being tortured at that hospital, especially women.

They did this mid-thigh amputation with a device that looked like a sharp piece of wire. Hundreds of thousands of dollars were spent on good orthopedic equipment. Expensive equipment and antibiotics were hidden away. Some things were hidden two or three stories below ground. The hospital didn't even have sheets on some of the beds. Also, there were not enough beds to go around. No one did anything about my reports and complaints. As a nurse, what I saw was against everything I believe in our code of ethics and patients' bill of rights. If you google the National Military Hospital in Kabul, lots of stuff will come up about torture and unsanitary conditions. No senior Americans stepped up and came in. No General Petraeus. The hospital also got blown up. During my time there, we tried to make little changes in the OR and throughout the hospital. When I think about this whole unfortunate situation, I almost shake my head in disbelief, but it really happened. Basically, you can't make this stuff up. It was unbelievable!'

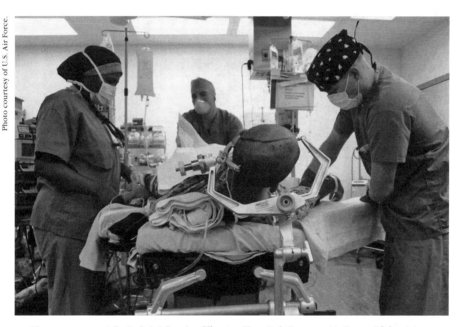

Neurosurgery at Craig Joint Service Theater Hospital, Bagram Air Base, Afghanistan.

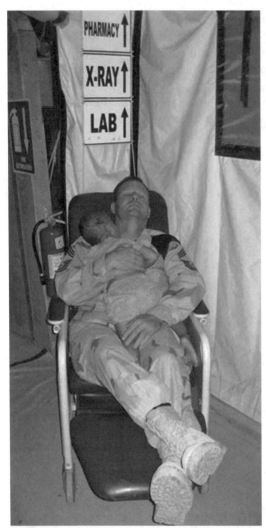

Air force chief master sergeant and injured Iraqi child.

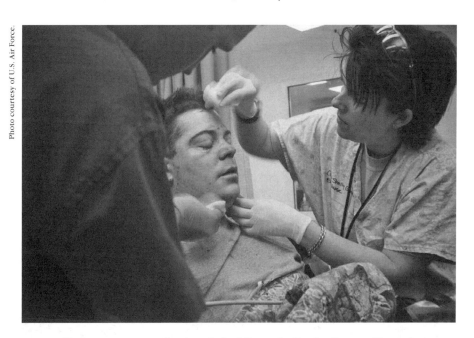

U.S. Air Force flight nurse and patient on C-17 medevac aircraft en route to Ramstein Air Base, Germany.

Photo courtesy of U.S. Air Force.

Air force nurse cares for wounded soldier at the Combat Support Hospital, Balad Air Base, Iraq.

Photo courtesy of U.S. Air Force.

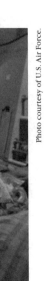

Air Force Critical Care Air Transport Team (CCATT) members from the 455th Air Expeditionary Wing prepare patient for flight to Ramstein Air Base, Germany.

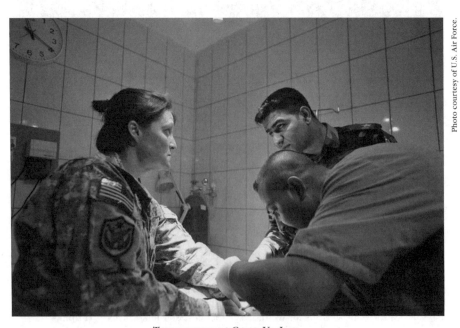

Trauma room at Camp Ur, Iraq.

7

Sorting It Out: Getting Help

Some nurses knew that they wanted to see someone in behavioral health as soon as they returned. Others decided to wait and see how their lives unfolded before making an appointment. Although they recognized the value of mental health therapy, they were concerned about the "stigma" and the possibility of interference with future assignments and promotions.

Stigma refers to a set of negative or unfair beliefs that a group of people have about something. It reflects dishonor, shame, and disgrace. In this chapter, we are talking about the "stigma of a mental disorder," which can lead to humiliation and discrimination. One harmful effect of stigma can be the reluctance to seek treatment for mental health problems. The fear of adverse career consequences can act as a barrier to a service member seeking treatment for posttraumatic stress disorder (PTSD) and similar illnesses. When available mental health services are not utilized, service members put themselves at risk for negative outcomes, including suicide.

Most of the nurses who sought mental health counseling said that they found it helpful. Some did couples therapy and others did individual therapy. Some sought suggestions to help their children. Many dealt with compassion fatigue and various degrees of PTSD. A few nurses mentioned that they went to civilian mental health care providers to avoid have things written in their military medical records. They feared breaches of confidentiality and invasions of their privacy. Some felt that stigma was still alive and well in the military. They did not want to risk future promotions and assignments.

LIEUTENANT COMMANDER KATHLEEN

Kathleen, a navy nurse, stated:

> When I came home I had trouble sleeping. I was quick to anger. I knew I needed to talk with someone but put it off because I was afraid it would affect my career. I just didn't want to put everything I had worked so hard for in jeopardy. It was very difficult because I don't care what anybody says, but there is still a stigma attached if you go to the mental health clinic. If you are an active duty service member, you are taking a big chance going for mental health services. They say it won't affect your future, but I just didn't buy that. I went to another town about 20 miles from my base to see a civilian counselor. She kept everything confidential and she was helpful to talk with. She helped me sort out my issues. She told me I had "clinical burnout" and some PTSD.

CAPTAIN EARL

Earl was a paramedic and registered nurse, who joined the Air Force Reserve a few years after graduating from college. He was raised in the Pacific Northwest and still resides there. He and his wife both had deployed to Iraq as flight nurses, although they were prohibited by regulations from flying on the same aircraft.

Earl reported:

> My wife and I were both flight nurses. We came home within a week of each other. At the time, she was fine, and I was not. I had anxiety and anger issues. It seemed like anything I enjoyed before, I didn't enjoy anymore. Finally, my wife said, "Your behavior is way out of line. You need some kind of help."
>
> Here's my story. I was recalled to active duty during the initial invasion of Iraq in March 2003. I was part of the first squadron for aeromedical evacuation to fly the wounded out of Iraq and Afghanistan back to Germany to Landstuhl Hospital. We had to build the squadron up from scratch. There was no system in place. There were no theatre hospitals in Iraq and Afghanistan so all the casualties were flown back to Landstuhl, until they could get a theatre hospital set up in Balad and Bagram. It was very difficult because we were a small squadron, and we only planned on the war being 6 weeks long. Our workload actually increased. It was a very difficult environment because on some days we didn't

have enough crews to stand alert to fly urgent missions. We got beat down pretty bad. I was on the flight schedule for 115 days and evacuated 800 casualties on 56 different sorties. Our biggest patient load was 78 patients split between three nurses and four medics. It was very difficult, and then they didn't have ground support. So, days when you were not flying, you'd be out on the flight line loading and unloading planes. There could be three or four planes a day. So, about 6 months later they replaced my unit because they knew we were all getting burned out. And in the 6-month period, we had evacuated over 7,000 casualties from Iraq and Afghanistan to Germany and then another 3,000 back to the States. Literally, that squadron of 150 people experienced a tremendous number of casualties in a 6-month period.

Earl talked about returning home:

When we got home, no one really asked us how we were doing. I think they assumed we were nurses and that is what we do. People thought your special training immunized you or made you exempt from combat trauma. The term "compassion fatigue" did not really exist back then, and PTSD was not really discussed. I recognized that my crew was having some problems, and I was having trouble with sleep. I went to the flight surgeon about my sleeping problems, and he grounded me for 3 months diagnosed me with "combat fatigue." There really wasn't a process. My wife was also deployed in two different countries. She was in Oman and then in Pakistan. She came home after 6 weeks and was fine. She was still the same person.

My reintegration was a problem, and we were both flight nurses. She was fine, and I was not. I started thinking that something was wrong with me because we basically did the same thing. I had anxiety and anger issues. I couldn't even put on a life jacket for water skiing, which is something I always liked to do without experiencing anxiety. It seemed like anything I enjoyed before, I didn't enjoy anymore. And finally, my wife said, "Your behavior is way out of line. You need to go and see the flight surgeon. You need some kind of help." We were having all kinds of fights. The air force was not doing anything to help. They gave us 2 weeks off, and they said, "You better start preparing to redeploy. And you'll be going for 6 to 9 months." Well, the last thing I wanted to do was to get back on a plane. So, that created additional anxiety for a lot of us because the war wasn't over, and they were telling us that we'd probably have to redeploy.

I was mobilized in January 2003, deployed in March 2003, and came home in August 2003. The air force jumps back and forth between 4- and 6-month deployments. They never do a year. It seemed like every week the air force had a different plan for us. Nobody was accepting that this was gonna be a long-term war. They kept coming up with these short-term fixes. There was such a lack of planning.

LIEUTENANT KATE

Kate, a navy nurse who served in Afghanistan, reported:

I tried once to go for counseling. It took me a while to realize that I was having difficulty dealing with people when I got home, and even with patients once I was home. I was having a real hard time with people and relationships. I only went for counseling once, and since it didn't seem to help, I quit going right away. Even though they say there is no stigma in going for counseling, I think there still is. I was uncomfortable with getting help from naval mental health services because I was also a health care provider. When I went for my counseling session, I was guarded in what I said because I didn't want stuff going in my medical record. I didn't want my medical colleagues to have access to my health record pertaining to mental health and coping issues. So, my husband and I decided to try to iron things out on our own.

LIEUTENANT COLONEL TONI

Toni, an Air Force Reserve Critical Care Air Transport Team (CCATT) nurse, described her family situation:

I'm married, and we have five children. Most of them were teenagers when I deployed. We are very blessed that they are all good kids. The youngest is now 19. My husband and I ended up going for counseling shortly after I returned from my last deployment in Afghanistan. The counselor gave me some tips and topics to talk with the kids about. It actually worked out really well. The counseling with my husband was weekly for 11 weeks. My husband was in the air force in his younger years, but he had never deployed. So, there were some things about my behavior that he didn't understand. I was upset by loud noises when I returned.

I also had trouble falling asleep and staying asleep. The counseling was really helpful for both of us.

LIEUTENANT COLONEL JULIE

Julie, an air force reservist who served as a flight nurse and as a CCATT nurse in Iraq and Afghanistan, described why she went for counseling after her third deployment.

She stated:

I went for counseling shortly after I got home from my last deployment because I felt kind of numb inside. I didn't feel up to taking over my share of the household chores, and I was having words with my husband about "the division of labor" in our family. Well, the counselor said that I had compassion burnout, a form of PTSD. It is when you have suppressed your own feelings, your own anxieties, and your own fears. It was a pretty natural thing to do because you had to take care of people, and you had to do it very well. There was no time to let your guard down, and to not be that way. Then, when you come back, all those feelings, all that internalization comes to the surface, and I think it led to depression for me. This stuff all came to the surface when I got home. You start thinking about all the stuff you experienced in Iraq, and start talking to your peers in the reserves, there are five of us that are pretty close. We are there for each other, and even though we don't live close, they are only a phone call away.

The counseling helped me because I was kind of spiraling the wrong way. I was self-medicating with way too much alcohol and just really not doing well. It brought me back to who I was. A lot of the therapy was just talking. Realizing that what I was feeling was OK. I wasn't a bad person for feeling this way. We tend to beat ourselves up very badly when we think we have taken too long to adjust, or we think we didn't do enough for patients, or we let our family down. It took me about 2 months of therapy going every week to a private therapist. I wanted to do it without any antidepressant meds, and I did. I wanted to be able to think clearly. They suggested an SSRI [selective serotonin reuptake inhibitor], but I wanted to try therapy without meds at first. That's just the way I manage things, I wouldn't say that would work for everybody. I couldn't continue my career as a flight nurse if I was on an SSRI. Flying personnel are very limited on what meds that are authorized to take.

LIEUTENANT COMMANDER ZOE

Zoe was a family nurse practitioner, deployed to Afghanistan in 2009 as a member of a provincial reconstruction team, which was a tri-service augmented role. She returned home in time for the 2010 Thanksgiving and Christmas holidays. She stated:

> Although I was excited about the holidays, I was also worried. It can be such a "false" time for people, being stressed, but at the same time you are supposed to enjoy things and be thankful.
>
> I found that I felt so emotionally labile. I remember going to my daughter's holiday performance [*starts crying while talking*] and seeing these beautiful, carefree children, so joyful. I remember I started crying. I remember being so glad that children in the United States could be so joyful and free. I was happy that the people there were so happy and safe. But I was so torn because I knew at that very same time people half a world away were still facing danger every day. I kept thinking of the military people who were friends of mine and the Afghans who do not even have the ability to feel so much joy and for their children. So, that was hard for me. I remember feeling thankful and feeling so much appreciation and love, but also guilt and sadness, too.
>
> And people didn't understand. My older daughter would look at me and say, "Mom, why are you crying?" I would do my best to explain, and my husband would just hold my hand. I don't think people really understand unless they have gone through that type of experience, where they really realize how blessed they are [*crying*].

Zoe talked about feeling cheerful, but having guilt. She mentioned that Facebook was helpful in keeping in touch with some of the people with whom she was deployed. She stated:

> Facebook was helpful but some would post things saying, "I am really struggling, I can't find a job," and I would feel a level of responsibility, like I need to continue to take care of them, like what I did when I was over there, you know, physically and mentally I took care of them, like when someone was dealing with immediate trauma or when we had a vehicle roll over. For example, one of our guys lost his hand and another is paralyzed from the waist down. They were on my team, and it was my responsibility to help them when they were going through these things.
>
> So when people were all the way across the country and they'd post something that sounded desperate, I had no real ability

to help them, and they were struggling. Some said they were struggling at the VA [Veterans Administration], you know, they wrote, "I spent 3 hours waiting at the VA, and they told me that my appointment was cancelled." I just felt so helpless, but still so responsible. Even within this last month, a guy I was stationed with posted a link to a YouTube video about one of the navy mobilization augmentees who deployed with us and worked with our civil affairs team that was with the provincial reconstruction team. I learned that she had gone through severe depression and had attempted suicide. I just found this out a month ago, and my initial reaction was, "How did I not reach out to her? What did I miss when we were deployed? What did I not recognize? Did I not help her get connected with mental health when we got back?" I feel a level of responsibility when I learn that people from our team have struggled. I guess I'll always have that feeling to some degree.

So, while social media and those type of connections are really helpful, it's difficult because you wonder what your responsibility is when you read someone's status update, and it is troubling. You see that someone is threatening in some way to harm themselves. What do you do with that information? That has happened to multiple members of our team. Basically, what I have done is write to them online to tell them to get help locally. You have to ease up on that sometimes which is hard for us as nurses because we connect with people. It's not just intellectually, it's a deeper connection, a holistic, caring connection. And when you read what they have written, it's really a call for help, and you know that when you read it. What do you do with that? You can't just scroll down through it and say that it is an obvious call for help, he's struggling or she's suicidal. The guilt and the responsibility have been difficult to this day. It's been 3 years back, and people still have issues. The postings can bring me right back. I've noticed over time that those who seem to be struggling the most are those who were single at the time and without kids and maybe they didn't have a home command. I know that our Guard guys have struggled a lot and some of our reservists.

LIEUTENANT COMMANDER CATHERINE

Catherine is a navy family nurse practitioner.
She recalled:

When I got home one of the most surprising things to me was how angry I was. Anger was an emotion that I felt strongly. I was glad to be home. My anger was not at all directed toward my family, or friends, or coworkers. It was undirected anger. I didn't have a focus for it. It was just anger! Politically, I tend to be far left. The politics of war was complicated.

I certainly did not believe in why we were in Iraq. The whole country had been whitewashed in terms of thinking about these weapons of mass destruction. It was the 9/11 disconnect. Iraq wasn't the source of the terrorists that brought down the World Trade Center and the Pentagon. I remember feeling what the country was thinking, that part I had to resolve somehow because there I was, and so the easier part was to think, there are hurt people, and they need care. And so, that just made it easy. I think for our unit, the politics of war weren't often discussed because I think we were so focused on taking care of our patients that you didn't have to care about the politics. Let somebody else worry about that. That part was easy to reconcile even though I could say that the politics would have been a source of anger. Except when I came home, I can't say that I was pissed at the president, I couldn't say that I was mad at George W. Bush. That could have been in the mix, but I can't say that was why I was mad, maybe it was collective or cumulative. I don't even know. I can't even describe it. It was a surprising emotion for me. It was unexpected. I'm pretty optimistic and levelheaded, and I don't like to be angry [*laughing*]. So, I don't stay angry for very long about things [*laughing*]. It was kind of an overwhelming emotion.

I remember being at a restaurant, and there was this man, and he was smoking, and smoking was not allowed in the restaurant, and it was very offensive to me. I don't like to be in public places where people are smoking. And so I remember asking the waitress to ask him to put out his cigarette. He wasn't sitting close enough for us to talk. He carried the cigarette over to a booth that was near us, and it was almost like passive-aggressive behavior. He kept the cigarette lit for quite some time, and I'm sure that he knew that I had asked for him to put it out. I just felt like he was such an ass [*laughing*]. I had to really fight the urge to just verbally unload on this man. I knew, if I opened my mouth, he was going to get the full brunt of that anger. So, I really had to squelch that because I knew that I would have not been a good example.

When I came back from Afghanistan, my son at the time was the age of most of the casualties we were getting. It's hard not to identify with that from a maternal perspective. I also think what helped me was my age, my maturity, my experience, and my stable marriage. The fact that I was a parent and my professional roles were things that have helped me. I have had a lot of friends who have had terrible PTSD to the point of incapacitation. I acknowledge my emotions, I'm OK with them. I give myself permission to feel my feelings, and I'm a talker, and I think those things have helped me process a lot of deployment experiences. And, I have great family support and understanding. Anger and rage were big things that I came back with. Again, they were not directed toward anybody.

Catherine related that coming back from her second deployment, which was to Afghanistan, she felt that she knew what to expect emotionally. She didn't consider herself angry. She wasn't doing combat trauma; instead she was on a provincial reconstruction team that had convoy operations every day. She stated: "The risk was very great." She reflected that being on this team was challenging from the length of time involved to the "risk and vulnerabilities." She added:

A lot of people do not go outside of the wire. I did 80 missions in full gear, two weapons—a 9 mm and a rifle and a full combat load of ammunition. To do that, I am riding in an armored vehicle, an MRAP [mine resistant ambush protected], and I'm carrying 60 pounds of gear.

LIEUTENANT COLONEL NATASHA

Natasha, an air force nurse, remarked:

Before I got my antidepressants, loud noises and crowds bothered me a great deal. I couldn't handle these things, they made me very, very anxious. Once I got my medicine, I was doing great! I call it, "Better living through chemistry" [*laughing*]. While I was deployed, a biomedical technician committed suicide. He was one of my 17-member team and thought his problems were insurmountable and killed himself while we were there. That was tough. It may have had some effect on my depression, you never know. I think I recognized my depression fairly early and made the decision to try the medicine because of my family history. I saw my mother suffer for years with untreated depression, and I knew how bad that could get. I think I was pretty proactive.

You know how it is at times, you second guess yourself wondering if you jumped the gun with meds. But then you remind yourself how bad you felt before you started on the meds. When my mom passed away, I remember traveling cross-country for 3 days and forgetting my medicine and again witnessed that darkness again that I forgot existed. I'm pretty happy with my pills. I have an anxiety-based kind of depression, and I had panic attacks. I'm much better now.

LIEUTENANT COMMANDER JUSTIN

Justin, a navy reservist, described why he went for help after he returned from Afghanistan:

So, coming home my family didn't know what to do with me. I didn't want to be in crowds or around most people. My now ex-wife really couldn't deal with any of this. A friend of mine came by with his wife, they knocked on the front door, and I ended up hiding under the kitchen table. I developed a very close relationship with another U.S. service member while I was deployed. The question when I got home was do I want to work on my marriage, or continue with a relationship with this other person. I knew that there were some serious problems with my relationship with my wife. There was a lot of "her-way-or-the-highway" kind of thing. When I came back I wanted to work on our relationship, yet it had to be on her terms. I couldn't deal with that. I went to see a therapist because I needed to calm down. I had to get this hyper-alertness out of my system. I couldn't spend the rest of my life in the apartment or under the kitchen table. I couldn't ask my 18-month-old son to decide what kind of cereal to buy because I couldn't make a decision, and I was the grown-up.

LIEUTENANT DARLA

Darla, a navy operating room (OR) nurse, explained why she sought help:

I went and saw deployment mental health when I got back because I had only been home for a few days, and things were not going well with me and my boyfriend. He had been very supportive while I was deployed, but he was kind of cold and distant when I came home. My boyfriend had complained that

I was forgetful since I came home. I said, "That's kind of me." I am a multitasker and think about a lot of things at the same time. He disagreed. The first day I was supposed to go to work, I accidently left my keys in his truck, and he had left earlier that morning. So, I couldn't drive my car because my keys were in his truck. I had to take a taxi to work, and later I got my keys from his truck. He was pretty impatient and annoyed about this happening. He's pretty impatient. He was particularly impatient and easily annoyed since I came home from deployment. His fuse seemed much shorter than I remembered. He didn't like being inconvenienced with anything. The mental health counselor listened to me and helped me problem solve. I went to see her a couple of times. I decided to leave my boyfriend.

CAPTAIN CORABETH

Corabeth grew up on a cattle ranch near Taos, New Mexico. As a young girl, she cared for the newborn calves and thought about becoming a veterinarian. In her teen years, she became more attracted to a nursing career and joined the future nurses' club in her high school. After graduating from college, she began working on a medical–surgical unit near Santa Fe, New Mexico. After a few years, Corabeth joined the Army National Guard.
Corabeth related:

I was deployed to the Abu Ghraib prison hospital in Iraq. We closed it down and moved the detainees to Camp Cropper, Iraq. I was in Iraq for 1 year. I was there from April 2006 to April 2007. Our mission was detainee health care. I maybe saw about 5% U.S. or coalition troops, the rest were detainees or local civilians. At the time of my deployment, I was stationed at the 2nd General Medical Center in Landstuhl, Germany. The reason I volunteered for Iraq was to gain experience and better understand war injuries we were receiving in Germany. I wanted to relate better to the troops I was caring for at Landstuhl.

Four nurses from Landstuhl deployed at the same time to Abu Ghraib. When I returned from Iraq, I came back to an ambulatory care and day surgery position. It was hard to return to Landstuhl because no one knew about our mission with detainee care. Some people had difficulty relating to it. They thought that it would be better for us returning not to go back to a regular floor right away. I would say that about 6 months after deployment, the real challenges began. I don't know if it's because the "honeymoon phase" was over, or if that's just when things catch up with you. After the deployment, I was still on active duty and was sent to Fort Bliss in El Paso, Texas. When I was in El Paso, I was all alone living in an apartment by myself. I was a captain in charge of all these lieutenants. I didn't have any friends. I was totally isolated. The guy I had met while on leave became my fiancé. But he was not in El Paso. It was hard.

When I was released from active duty, I left El Paso, and I moved in with my fiancé, who is now my husband, in Albuquerque. And then I had therapy, about $7,000 worth. I'm cured and life is great now. I was still in the military reserves, and I could have waited and tried to go through the Veteran's Administration [VA] for mental health counseling. If I went to the VA, I could have received some disability. There's a girl I know who went through the VA and received disability for PTSD.

With 5 years of active duty, I guess I could have asked for VA benefits. Being screened and interviewed gave me a boatload of anxiety. My PTSD was totally linked to the mission of detainee care. I got myself in trouble working 60 to 72 hours a week for a year. All of us had volunteered to take care of soldiers, not detainees. Where I got myself in trouble probably goes back to my codependency and inability of establishing boundaries. What I will and will not do to take care of someone. I think all of us nurses felt "all children are God's children" and you should treat them as such. It was challenging, and I think I tried to overcompensate for some of my colleagues. You give, give, give, give, and give. Our mission changed the hearts and minds of the Iraqi people. And at some point, you realize that all you did, did not make a big difference. And then, you feel like you were not good enough to make a difference. I had severe depression. It was one of those dumb things. I put my mind and my heart into something, and it still did not make a difference. So anyway, that's what it was for me. It hit me while I was over there. Also, about three-quarters of the way through the deployment, my roommate shot herself. She was not a nurse, she was a medical service corps officer, who was with an ambulance company. She survived. She shot herself in the chest. I had a lot of guilt about this. She's disabled. She had threatened to go out and shoot all the nurses. It was all over the news. Everybody cracked. I just cracked later than everyone else [*laughing*]. I'm proud of that. Doing detainee health care for a year was about 3 to 6 months too long.

With my experiences in Iraq and being a nurse, I feel I'm respected. Once they know I'm a veteran, people respect me for what I know, what I was able to do, and for my opinion. Working for the VA has been a warm experience. I try to see things as positive. I am grateful for the respect I get. Being in therapy for 1-1/2 years was an absolute growth experience for me. The cost was worth it. I really learned so much about human nature. I take my deployment experience, and all that I learned through therapy, and integrate it into my clinical practice as a nurse practitioner. I feel like I am an effective and compassionate practitioner. I feel like I've taken a negative experience and put a positive spin on it, which has benefitted me and my patients.

CAPTAIN COURTNEY

Courtney is an Air National Guard nurse.
She stated:

I felt that they were very, very good sending you to war. I felt very prepared. But, you were not prepared to come back. You are hypervigilant. I was always alone in Afghanistan, but I was never by myself if you know what I mean, if that makes any sense.

My husband took some time off, but then he had to go back to work. With me, they make you take a month off. You can't just go back to work. So, I'd be alone in the house, and I'd hear doors closing. I was afraid to take showers. There was really bizarre stuff. I couldn't sleep. Ambien didn't work. That took a long time. I still have occasional problems with sleeping, but it is much better. I knew it was psycho-processing, and you just have to go through it. Loud noises were bad. I wanted to get a weapon [*laughs*], and I'm such a democrat! I said to my husband, "We have to go buy a weapon" and he said, "No, we don't" [*laughs*]. I don't even know where that came from except that I carried a weapon with me for 7 months, and I felt naked without it. We have a "Louisville Slugger" by our bed now. This baseball bat is my weapon, but I can't put it in my pocket. So it does take a while to transition back. In the air force, they have mental health people that call you to check in with you after you've been back for a certain amount of time. Well, I never got called. It is easy to fall through the cracks when you are one-zees/ two-zees in the [Air National] Guard. There were just a bunch of things that I needed to get off my chest. So, I talked to the chaplain at the base. He's a

full-bird [colonel]. I also talked to a lot of the nurses who I went
to combat skills training with because I knew them all very well.
We kind of, among ourselves, talked through a lot of stuff. They
were all air force, and most were active duty. I was one of three
Guardsmen. I don't think there were any reservists in my group.
There were doctors, nurses, shrinks, and a nurse anesthetist. It
was a mix of people. We went to combat training skills together,
and it was about a month long. It was classes and literally learning
what to do, how to defend yourself. We lived in dorms and it was
at Fort Dix, New Jersey. But, I also had classes in San Antonio,
Texas. I mean they really prepared you. You knew how to break
down your weapon and load it. You really learned what to do.

CAPTAIN TENLEY

Tenley is an army nurse and veteran of two deployments to Iraq.
She recalled:

Both missions were detainee health care to Abu Ghraib and
Camp Cropper. I am active duty. I spent my first year in Iraq
shutting down Abu Ghraib and opening up Camp Cropper. So,
we were dealing with detainees the whole time. Fallujah was
still the wild, wild, west; so, we got a lot of marines in and a few
army people that were injured from that. A lot of stuff we saw
was medics bringing in a detainee saying, "This guy killed my
buddy, my soldier, my medic." And so, that was most of the hardship we saw. The detainees somehow figured out how to push
every button we had. This was 2006–2007.

We saw a lot of suicides. There were three of us in a bar-
racks room. At one point, one of my roommates (not a nurse)
held a behavioral nurse hostage, and she eventually shot herself.
We had to deal with her. She didn't kill herself, she actually survived, but it brought a lot of emotional trauma. She opened up to
us a little during the deployment, but it wasn't until near the suicidal situation. She wasn't in our unit, she was with an ambulance
company. But our unit wanted her to do X, Y, and Z, and her unit
wanted her to do other stuff. So, there was a conflict. She wanted
to do the right thing, what was best for the soldiers. But she was
really torn between what our unit wanted and what her unit
wanted. I guess that one of the executive officers was not a very
nice person to her. So, she was just terribly frustrated. I guess
this XO [executive officer] was mean and didn't understand and

didn't care. Come to find out that this suicidal person had a psych history and probably just reverted back to what she knew.

About a year after I got home, I received a phone call from an attorney's office saying that the troubled roommate had been court marshaled and that I needed to testify, me and my other roommate. We had to testify in her court martial case. This brought a flood of emotion when we heard this because we had done our best to move past the situation. So, a flood of emotion returned. It led to anger. It was very sad because I think suicide is a very selfish act. A lot of anger went along with this. It was probably the last thing we wanted to talk about.

Tenley talked about her experience of taking care of detainees:

Taking care of detainees, we had the faces to go along with the hostile actions toward our troops who were just trying to do the mission. We had to take care of the enemy who killed our soldiers and our medics. It was horrible! This wore on us while we were deployed and after we got home. We all made it through, we all survived, but we were just left with a lot of emotional frustration. It was hard taking care of detainees for a year, the bad guys, the enemy.

Tenley shared details from her second deployment to Iraq. I was in Fort Bragg, North Carolina, working in the ER. I knew what to expect from deployment, and I knew what was normal. I was still a little easily angered, and I referred to it as my "Iraq mouth." My second deployment was not nearly as traumatic or had as dramatic a return as my first deployment to Iraq. This was 2009–2010. I did the exact same mission, detainee health care. I went back to Camp Cropper. I probably cried for a week when I found out that I'd be doing the detainee health care mission again! I felt barely emotionally OK.

I got my orders and it was the 14th CASH [Combat Army Support Hospital] out of Fort Benning, Georgia. I was hoping for Afghanistan, something new. I couldn't believe that I got the detainee health care mission in Iraq twice! It was such a curse! I don't wish the detainee care mission on anyone twice. You can handle it once, but twice is ridiculous!

By the time I went back, the mission had changed in Iraq. So we didn't see the wild, wild, west. We didn't see gunshot wounds. We didn't see that. It was like, "This guy's got a lipoma. Are we gonna ship him out with this because the general surgeons are bored?" That was the attitude this time. I kept thinking,

"We are wasting taxpayer's dollars" [*laughing*]. I think I saw five traumas during my whole second deployment. I was there 7 months. I think a 6- to 7-month deployment is much more emotionally stable than a year's deployment. After 9 months, all you want to do is go home. Once I got there the second time, I was fine. I met great people, friends for a lifetime. Because the mission was not that much of a hardship, it was a lot easier to come home because you knew that the war in Iraq was winding down.

CAPTAIN MARLEY

Marley talked about her anger when she returned from Iraq.
    She recalled:

When I was in Iraq my mom actually bought a "flipper" house for me with my money. So, for 3 weeks, I worked on remodeling the house where I didn't have to deal with many people. I could just work on the house and take out my frustrations. It was really good for me. I was very angry at having to do the detainee care mission. I think that caused my postdeployment fog. You kind of remember things, but there a lot of little things you forget, like if you have an appointment or you tell someone that you are going to do something, but you forget. It is not something that regularly registers in your brain. If you do not write things on a "to-do" list, you'll forget. For example, I remember going out with friends, and we went to this after-hours place to get something to eat. Someone shot a gun outside, and I had a mental breakdown. I remember pulling my friends down in the parking lot below the car and thinking, "I don't have my gun with me or my body armor or equipment." I couldn't believe this was happening. Then, one of my friends said, "We have to get her out of here." We were all dressed up because we had been out. But, my mind went right back to the wartime mentality. I just started crying and babbling. I went home, and my mom saw that I was upset. It was hard because I had not told my mom very much about my deployment because I didn't want her to worry. It was a hard night.
    Sometimes you can't tell your mom everything you do over there, especially because I was taking care of the 10 most dangerous detainees. My mom would call me on my cell phone while I was in Iraq. Once in a while, she'd hear a rocket go off or a mortar blast. She'd be upset or cry. Medical-wise she got it because she is an open-heart surgery nurse. She works in the ICU. But, I tried

to downplay the danger to spare her more worry. On that deployment, I tried not to tell her everything. The deployment violence was scary and hard for her. We got rocketed a lot because of taking care of detainees. I remember one flying right over my head. I thought, "Well, I'm alive." I remember one time telling my mom about the rocket flying over my head and telling her I was fine; I'm alive, and I had a rough day, but I'm taking care of others. And, I remember her crying on the phone. My mom is a beautiful soul, and she's good for me. Otherwise, life could be dark. We were angry at having to do the detainee care mission. We found out our mission when we were helping out during Hurricane Katrina.

Marley talked about the aftermath of Afghanistan for her:

When I went back to the hospital in San Antonio, my friends had moved. Most people move every 2 years. This time I didn't come home with anyone that I had deployed with. I had done so much trauma and so much sick call and so much real world stuff. But when I was back at work in the ER, there would be all these residents jumping in and doing stupid stuff and not knowing how to do what I knew how to do. I was angry.

My boss who had deployed before said that she had this rule that anyone who had deployed before was not allowed in the trauma room for a month. I flipped out. I said, "It's not fair, I'm better in the trauma room than any of the people you have." My saving grace was that Major W. was the assistant head nurse, and she was my boss in Germany, and now she was in San Antonio. I could tell her anything [*crying*]. It was so hard because all I wanted to do when I came back was to take care of soldiers. That's the one thing you know.

I have a dog that I want to hangout with named "Trixie." I had to walk the dog and go to the grocery store to get food for the dog. I dropped down from 170 lbs. to 130 lbs. Major W. told me that I should go for counseling. My mom also said that it would be a good idea. So, I started talking to this counselor. I thought it might help me with the anger. Also, my mom got interviewed for an article for the newspaper, and I walked past the room, and I heard Mom say, "She is different after this last deployment." I overheard it. I went to counseling while I was getting out of the military. Then, that horrible shooting situation occurred at Fort Hood when my troops were there. I said to my counselor, "How can I have confidence in you, when this horrible thing happened with a psychiatrist shooting people at Fort Hood?" When I heard it on the radio that day, I was driving, and I had to pull over to the side of the road because I was bawling my eyes out. I couldn't drive. I had just gotten home from Afghanistan, and I couldn't believe that this had happened. This person was supposed to be helping people, and he turned on them. He had never deployed before. "Why is it that I feel safer sleeping on a cot in a tent with 18 guys, and I'm the only female than being back here in San Antonio?" I don't feel like I can do trauma anymore. I transitioned out of the army. I applied to the University of New Mexico, and out of 50 applicants I was one of the eight selected. I did well, and I promised myself to keep doing well. I also joined the "American Women Veterans" organization.

I had gotten out of a bad relationship. I don't need anyone but myself. The counselor that I didn't like turned out to be very helpful. She made me do my homework. I was really depressed about all of the people who had died in front of me. She brought up a lot of good points. And she said, "Do you believe in God?" And I said, "Of course, yes" [*crying*]. She asked me if I was better than God, and I said, "What are you talking about?" She said, "God has forgiven you, why haven't you forgiven yourself?" She gave me a lot to think about. I like her as a person now, but I didn't like her then. No, I don't see her anymore. I think my other therapy is just helping other people, especially women.

I think I've also had a pattern of dating people who need something. Then, when I finally met someone who didn't need something, it was really different. I worked at Brooke Army Medical Center in the ER. There were many people who had deployed; so, it was easier to be around them and share some common experiences. They understand you, your feelings, and frustrations.

COMMANDER ROBIN

Robin is a navy nurse who served in Afghanistan.
She stated:

I came home in late October. I was able to get a lot of things done and "be a mom again." I checked into the hospital toward the end of the year and that's what was harder because I had had migraines before I went to Afghanistan. I had been diagnosed with migraines. So, I had a lot of apprehension coming back to the command. It was the same command I had left. I could not put my finger on it, but I was having palpitations, migraines, and I was really, really anxious about coming back to work in the hospital. I had no idea where I was going to work. I can't say that I had any major negative experiences there before my deployment. Of course, everyone has ups and downs, but I could not pinpoint the cause of my symptoms. I had been at Portsmouth before working in the hospital since 2003, and I deployed in 2009. So, I had already been there for 6 years.

Before I checked into work, I took a week to myself and flew to Santa Fe and did massages and body treatments, and I had my first acupuncture treatment. I remember that the acupuncturist had put all these needles in my ears, and I asked her what they were for, and she said, "They are for PTSD." So, when I got back to Portsmouth, I found another acupuncturist, and I have been seeing her for 2 years now. I don't have migraines anymore. I occasionally have other minor headaches, but no more migraines.

I originally wanted to see an acupuncturist for shoulder pain after all those "bag drags" and carrying gear. My shoulder was bothering me, and I didn't want to have surgery. In Afghanistan, we had to take Doxycycline every day to ward off potential malaria, and I was also taking my migraine meds. I was so tired of taking medication that I wanted to try another approach. Acupuncture helped me a lot, and I established a good rapport with my provider.

In terms of work, I had a hard time initially so they made me the division officer for the same day surgery unit. The directorate for surgical services is huge. Our unit was pretty big. We had a lot of GS [government service] employees, and they had just gone through an intervention because there had been a lot of complaining, you know EO [equal opportunity] complaints and the like, and that is where I was put in. It was doable, but at the same token, they also gave me this collateral where I was the EO officer for the whole command of 6,000 people. I learned a lot, but felt very overwhelmed. The weeks that I didn't have my kids, I would be staying late at work, like tonight with flu immunizations. I told them, "I got that collateral by default because nobody else wanted it, and I had just gotten here." I felt I struggled a lot initially, and when people asked me how I was doing, I told them that my blood pressure was really high, and at times I could feel my heart racing. I did the postdeployment health assessment and the mental health assessment right away, and they told me, "Yes, you sound like you have some symptoms of depression." I would be sitting on the couch or getting ready to go to bed or lying down, and I would have this wave of sadness that would come crashing over me, and I would start crying, not sobbing, just crying quietly and being tearful. That was often; and eventually, it just tapered off. Sometimes, I would just be watching a sentimental commercial on television. It was more than PMS [premenstrual syndrome].

You have to recognize that people who have been deployed all acclimate differently. I had had therapy when growing up for various inappropriate father figures, and that didn't work well for me. So, I don't feel comfortable going and talking to a psychologist or psychiatrist, and I didn't want meds. Everyone said, "You need to talk to somebody, you need to talk to somebody." So I talk to my friends. I'm not asking them to "fix it," but I can talk to them. Part of me knew I should probably talk to a therapist because of the headaches and anxiety and the nervous palpitations. It was hard. It was hard to focus. I finally did my postdeployment mental health assessment, and this was about 3 years out. I had taken the survey online, but I never validated it with an appointment [*laughs*]. You are supposed to do the physical assessment within 3 months, and then 6 months, and then a year. I was supposed to go see psychology within 2 to 3 months, and I did make two attempts to call and make an appointment and was told, "We are completely booked, we don't have the schedule out for 4 weeks; so, give us a call back." And I thought, "OK, forget it."

With my immediate leadership there was never an official, "How are you doing, how was your deployment?" There was no official acknowledgement, like "Are you doing OK?" There was the basic, "Hi, how are you?" and I'd respond, "I'm having migraines pretty much every day, and I can feel my heart and my blood pressure pounding." It would be like, "OK, noted. However, you still need to be at this muster and hand this in and do this and that was due yesterday." So, I'd reply, "Yes sir, noted, I'll get right on it."

Robin talked about her plan, stating:

I will finish my time and will go out quietly. I appreciate the experiences, but I can't keep playing this game. It's just too much. I feel like I don't need to be at work till 7 or 8 o'clock at night trying to get stuff done. On the weeks I have my kids, I have to be out at 5 p.m. to pick up my youngest. On the weeks I don't have my kids, I'm easily there till 7 or 8 p.m. I'm looking forward to not having collateral upon collateral, and not having to do all this extra stuff, and just do my job.

I finally had the postdeployment mental health assessment and evaluation, and they referred me to an integrated health behavioral analyst. There's a medical cohort through your PCM [primary care manager] where they look at everything collectively with your symptoms, and then, if they need to, they refer you to a psychologist. But honestly, just getting back into yoga again and trying to make time for myself like this weekend, helps a lot. I just took a weekend to myself, and I went to a wooded area with deer; it was my reset button.

I am looking forward to getting out in many respects, but I've worn a uniform for so long, just the thought of wearing clothes [*laughing*]. I'm looking forward to being able to focus on less. After 8 hours, I need to go home instead of all this stuff with meeting deadlines. It's bittersweet. It has had its pluses and minuses. It is unlikely that I'll deploy again with 18 months left. However, I'd go back to Bastion in a heartbeat. I would have no problem going back there, and doing what I did again.

MAJOR ANITA

Anita is an air force nurse who served in Pakistan and Afghanistan. She recalled:

My overall experience was very positive. I loved everything about it. I loved taking care of the troops. I thought the hardest part of it would be to take care of the bad guys, and it was a little difficult at first because you just don't know how you should really interact with them. Because as a nurse, you are a caring person, and you love your patient, and you want to do everything possible for your patient, and now you have someone who killed some Americans and you think, "I'm supposed to take care of you." It was hard in the beginning.

The mind-set you get into is kind of like putting up this screen or wall in front of you, which allows you to function and do your job without emotion. In that environment, you cannot have any emotional ties to any of your patients, even the Americans. If you allow your emotions to sink in you'll start thinking, "Oh, this is so sad and traumatic, he's married and he has two kids. Blah, blah, blah," and then you get caught up in that, especially for me and especially for a woman. You let your emotions take control, and then you set yourself up for failure, accidents, and mistakes. You could miss clinical things that you shouldn't miss, and the whole scenario is hard on yourself. You learn very quickly that you can't get attached or emotionally involved, because it will do a number on you. You create a very hard shell and get tough. "You know, I'm this tough girl" [*laughs*]. And as a tough girl, I wore my body armor all the time, and I lifted weights. It's the mentality you develop when you are over there, but it also protects your inner self. Otherwise, you wouldn't sleep at night; you'd worry about what your patients would be dealing with when they got home, and it would be too much for you to take. Since I developed early on the ability to emotionally detach, I was able to enjoy myself. I would go in; do my job, and do what I had to do. I was great at my job. Sometimes, I would pick up on things that maybe someone else didn't pick up on. When traumas would come in, they would go to the ER first; even though, we knew they'd end up in the ICU. We would go to the ER and help. They appreciated it. We'd get them stabilized and to the ICU. It was fun; so, when I left work, I would not think about my patients. I would just enjoy my time. We had movie night every night, and I would socialize or talk to my family. I am a big reader; so, I would spend a lot of time just reading. I was able to shut my brain off. Because of that shell I created, I could enjoy my book or the movie.

I actually had to give advice to a few other people who were struggling in the beginning, I told them, "This is how you've got to do it. We're still expected to do a job no matter what, no matter how hard it is, no matter how devastating the story is, we're still expected to do our job, and to do it well." Everyone has to find a way to do it. So, I'd have coworkers come to me because I have that personality where people would come to me, and they'd say, "Oh my God, I can't believe this happened. I don't know how to deal with this." I'd say to them straight out, "This is what you need to do to protect your inner self, and the only way to do that is to build this shell around yourself." I would explain it, it is simply a coping mechanism, that's all it is, and my advice would help them. They had to work hard on it, and then it came naturally. In the beginning, you had to tell yourself, "I'm not gonna emotionally attach to my patients, and I don't want to know about their family at home." In the beginning, you had to make yourself do this, but over time it got easier. I was just trying to help my coworkers by telling them what worked for me.

Anita talked about taking leave when she came home:

I took almost a month off. I flew in on a Saturday. So, you have to report in on Monday just to sign back in; so, your commander can say, "Welcome, hey you made it back!" Then you go on 2 weeks of leave. That's the R and R [rest and relaxation] they give you; so, it is not your leave time. It doesn't take away from the leave time you have accumulated. Then, you have to go into work for at least 1 day; so, you can take leave again. They do that because of the high suicide rate, just to do a little "face to face" and "Are you doing OK?" I spent the first 4 months angry, and I'm a happy person; I'm a "go with the flow"; I'm spontaneous; I'm the happy-go-lucky "Dancing Queen Girl." The first 4 months I was back; I had anger issues. Everything made me mad. My husband made me mad. Work made me mad. I honestly think that it just came to a head one day. We were at Chik-fil-A, and I just got angry, and I started yelling, and I had this moment of clarity. I was thinking in my head, "Why is he this way? It's all his fault." And then it dawned on me, "Is it his fault or is it my fault?" That's when I came to the realization that "Holy Cow; it's not everybody else; it is me! I'm the problem here," and I kind of had a little breakdown here, and I started crying. I told my husband, "Oh my God it is me. I'm the bitch!" I was accusing everyone else of being the instigator. So, I had to really reflect and really take a step back. I came up with a "safe word" to help me not get so angry. So, if I started feeling angry, I say the "safe word" in my head. I can tell you my "safe word"; it's not a secret. It was "Bruce Banner," who was the Incredible Hulk on TV. He was the superhero who was the Hulk. He was a doctor who would turn into the Hulk when he got angry. It became a running joke. With my iPhone, I made a picture of me imitating the Hulk, and my husband used Photoshop and made me green [*laughing*]. It was hilarious, but it helped. It worked for me. Everyone has to find their own "safe word."

I am such a jokester. Everything I do is a joke. I had read *Fifty Shades of Gray*, and in that book, there were some sexual acts and stuff that the main character didn't know if she was comfortable with because she had never experienced it. So, she had to come up with a "safe word" that she could say in the middle; so, he would stop. That's why I call it my "safe word" because it's funny to me. To be honest, it wasn't a great book. It was actually a raunchy book. Most people read fiction to escape reality.

Anita went further to think about her anger issues after returning from deployment:

> Upon reflection after my anger issues and hating work and tak-
> ing care of people who aren't gonna change their lifestyle, I
> had to really reflect on why I was so angry. What I came up
> with was for the 6 months that I was there, I put up that screen,
> that wall, that shell that I told you about to keep myself from
> being emotionally attached to anyone. I was emotionless. So,
> when I come back to the real world, I am expected to have
> emotions, and I don't know how to deal with it. You can't just
> turn it on and off like a switch. Somebody would say, I have
> this scratch on my leg, and I would say, "You need to suck it
> up, dude." I still had that wall. I had to slowly let myself take
> emotion back in. I had to work on it. I finally figured it out, and
> I told my husband about it because we were struggling for a
> while, not on the verge of divorce or anything, it wasn't that
> bad, but we were struggling. It was rough. Fortunately, he was
> a good support system for me. The key was figuring out a way
> to slowly allow myself to feel emotion again. I had to be careful
> to not get overwhelmed with emotion. I was expected to have
> emotion. I was expected to care. I was expected to love. And
> I couldn't do all these things. The first thing was to recognize
> what the problem is and understand it. That wall that kept me
> strong in Afghanistan needed to be knocked down. That wall
> that let me do my job in Afghanistan was killing me at home. I
> slowly knocked it down and found a way to let emotion come
> back.

MAJOR FRED

Fred talked about spending many hours alone in his room when not working during his deployment.
He recalled:

> The navy treated their people a lot different than the air force.
> My medics and I tended to spend a lot of time in our rooms away
> from everyone when we were not needed to take care of pa-
> tients. So, when I got home, I had a little trouble dealing with
> crowds for a while. It doesn't really bother me now. For 6-½
> months, when I was not busy at work, I was in my room watching

movies or reading. In the morning, I would go to my office and do the necessary paperwork, but then I could spend another 20 hours in my room by myself. So, when I came home, being out in public and being around a lot of people was a big adjustment for me. I didn't go for any counseling; I just worked on it myself.

LIEUTENANT SANDRA

Sandra is a navy nurse.
  She remarked:

About 3 months into the deployment I was not coping well because we were working day, night, day, night every day. You'd work a day shift and then be off for 24 hours and then work a night shift. Then in the middle of that you are on call for 12 hours. So our sleeping schedule was terrible, just awful. It wore and tore on us. I think people respond differently and cope differently and have different relationships with people back home. I'm a really optimistic person. I love life, and I love what I do. I had a really tough time about half way through, and there was really not anyone I could turn to while I was there to make it better. I was close to one girl, and others started to see me go downhill. I wasn't as chipper and nice and with the Brits; they expect you to behave a certain way, regardless of how you feel. It's that "stiff upper lip." So, even if you are having a bad day, you have to suck it up. We tried to change the schedule.

She talked about the difficulties she faced returning after deployment:

After coming home, another problem was trying to sleep again. Traveling so much and sleeping in a bed with another person again, after you've been sleeping on a terribly uncomfortable cot for a while, contributed to the problem.
  I only got to make phone calls rarely. The connections were terrible. Also, when someone died, they called for silence on all the lines, and the Internet would be completely down. The phones would be down until they lifted that security measure and contacted that family who had lost someone. We didn't get to talk as often as I would have liked to. I mean I would have loved to call them every day. It was probably once every 2 weeks. It got less frequent near the end.

MAJOR ELIZA

Eliza, an air force nurse, shared some details of her deployments.
She recalled:

The first deployment to Bagram was not too bad as far as coming
back home. Everyone was in their place. My daughter was with
my mom. I don't think it took me that long to reintegrate. The
second deployment, there were so many things going on at the
same time. It was pretty crazy. Even the nurses who work for
me were asking, "Are you OK?" They said they didn't want to
say anything to me at first, but they finally told me that I seemed
very quiet, and that I didn't seem happy. I said, "Oh, I didn't realize that." I had a lot to think about. I found out while I was gone
that I'd be moving again, and I knew that my daughter would
have to change schools. We'd have to move earlier to get my
daughter settled. Plus, this last deployment was really rough
emotionally because of all the dynamics of the leadership down
there. The patient load was actually not as intense as when I was
there before, when we were just moving patients over and over
and over. I remember thinking, "Oh my God, enough already,
can we just stop, every night moving four and five patients out
who were missing limbs and had traumatic injuries." But, you
get into that routine, and you are doing your part, and you are
making it happen. You are exhausted, but you keep going, you
keep going, that is what you do. You are making a difference,
and you are basically doing OK. There were little personality
crumbles with some of the people I worked with, but overall
we worked really well together. It made the environment OK.
I had a really good outlet with church. A chaplain was always
available to talk. I remember telling her that I was having trouble
taking care of these types of patients. It was the prisoners that
we sometimes had to take care of. I just had to put myself in a
different place mentally when I took care of them, because some
of the other staff members were saying troublesome and inappropriate things. For example, some said that enemies "were not
human." But because of my faith, I was able to realize that it was
not up to me to judge them. I was there to do a job, and I treated
everyone the same. I did not pass judgment. I was there to take
care of everyone equally. The chaplain told me that I was not
the only one to come to her with this issue. She had me look at
a passage of scripture that made it clear to me that I was doing

the right thing. I did so much better after that encounter. Things went well for me; even though, it was challenging. I was OK. I was grounded. Some of my coworkers had PTSD from everything they saw and did. I was fortunate to be OK.

However, when I got back some of my coworkers sat me down and told me they were concerned about me, because I seemed very quiet and seemed like I had a lot on my mind. I am not a really vocal and loud person by nature. But, I guess I seemed unusually quiet and maybe withdrawn a bit because I did have a lot on my mind. A close coworker said, "You're not really here. You are here, like present, but you are not here like you are normally here." I said, "Oh, I'm sorry, I do have a lot on my mind." She said, "You are different."

I had warned my mom, before I came back from this last deployment, that the deployment had taken its toll on me and that I was exhausted. I had to deal with a lot of personal drama with my coworkers and the leadership. I told my mom that I was not sure how I was going to react to coming home this time. I told her to be patient with me and just to give me some space. She said, "OK, not a problem, we'll just let you be, and we'll give you some space." About a week or so after being home, I felt like something was just different. My mom sat me down and said, "Do you hate me?" I said, "What are you talking about?" She said, "You look at me like you don't want me here. You are so evil." I said, "What? Am I giving you that impression?" She said, "Yeah, are you OK?" I said, "Yeah, yeah." So, we talked, and I just needed to take a little time because I was internalizing things, and I also needed to look at how I was coming across to others. I was not aware of it, and I guess I needed a little more self-awareness. It took a while. You get into that mode of thinking, I just came back from a deployment that was really not great, and as soon as I get home within 90 days, I have to pack up and leave and go again. I was in overdrive. Plus, you are back at work. There was drama there, too. I remember going to a staff meeting and thinking, "There is some weird vibe, some weird tension in the air." There were things going on at work with coworkers that I did not know about, but I could just sense something was different. This was in Texas. Then, everyone was mad at me because I was leaving. I was reassigned, and no one expected it. I didn't expect it either. They said, "We finally get someone who cares about us and who cares about the unit and who wants to make things better, and now you are leaving. We are so mad at you." I was like, "Yes, I put in for the fellowship, but I didn't know that I actually was gonna get it." That's where I am now. I got the "Headquarters AMC [Air Mobility Command] Air Crew Training and Operations Fellowship." That's why I was sent to Scott AFB [air force base] in Illinois. I put my name in because I knew that was something I wouldn't mind doing at this point in my career. And, I got selected. Then, I felt like I was on a mission before I left Texas to make things better. It took a lot of my personal time and energy. I just wanted to leave things with more order and leave things in a better place. From what I hear now, it didn't make much of a difference. I had a good rapport with everyone, and they could come to me about things that were going on. I did whatever I could to make things better. People would say, "You actually care." Of course, I did!

I wanted to make some changes and actually have some impact. This was Fort Sam Houston, Texas. It is the new combination of the air force and the army hospital. The new official name is San Antonio Military Medical Center. They still have Wilford Hall for outpatients. They still have the old building, and they are building the new ambulatory center out in front.

CAPTAIN AMANDA

Amanda, an air force reservist, reported: "Sometimes I was scared out of my mind on the FOB [forward operating bases]." She told how she tried to distract herself with exercise and by looking forward to meals. She went further to say:

I paid all my bills online and took care of all my finances. I lost 20 pounds on the FOB. I used the exercise bike. I ate veggie curry almost every day for the whole 6 months. I did appreciate food over there because we didn't have a lot of it. When I got home, I was so happy to be home with coffee. It's weird on the FOB, you can't go to the bathroom at night because you'd have to wake up someone else to go with you. It's a blackout FOB; so, you can't bring a flashlight, you might have a little red light. I had a gun, and I had my husband send my MACE. It was insane how unsafe I felt on the FOB. You worried about getting raped by a contractor or local nationals. I always thought I was gonna be sexually assaulted. I didn't drink a beverage after 6 o'clock at night because I didn't want to have to go to the bathroom. When I got home, I loved to drink liquids at night. It was such a relief, such a glorious thing. If I was desperate, I would pee in a container or on towels and, then throw them away during the day [*laughing*]. Then, I ran out of towels. I would try to clean them, but sometimes it was a mess [*laughing*]. At the end of the deployment, the people at the FOB completely changed. Three of us living in a hooch together would stay up late and go to the bathroom together one more time as a group. It was a navy lieutenant, and army captain, and an air force captain; so, we were all 0-3's. It was awesome; it was our Christmas card; it was awesome living with those ladies. Urinating was a big concern for us over there [*laughing*]. I would bring a Gatorade bottle full of urine in my shower bag and dump it out in the shower [*laughing*].

LIEUTENANT DOREEN

Doreen was a navy reservist who served in Iraq and Afghanistan. She talked about a situation that proved to be very problematic for her in Iraq.
She stated:

My issues were change of command issues, not very positive, and it was very stressful. We had a navy 0-6 [captain] MD who was a reservist. We were actually serving with the Marine Corps in a "shock-trauma platoon." This navy captain was removed from his position. I was a lieutenant in the navy at the time, and I actually had to call a Marine Corps EO representative from the headquarters. I wouldn't say that this navy captain physically assaulted me and three enlisted people, but he poked with his fingers very hard in our chests. After that occurred, I called the chief who was at headquarters out in the FOB. They didn't do anything about his behavior or see if we needed anything. I finally said, I'm gonna call the IG [Inspector General] because this is ridiculous. I finally had to take away one of my member's weapons because he threatened, not necessarily suicide, but he was not safe. We were a very small unit of 16–17, and it was two of them that were problematic. It was the captain and a petty officer who was an E-6. Eventually, they were both removed. The petty officer was removed from the camp for having sexual behaviors with a marine who was part of our chain of command. The navy captain was removed from his position because of his inappropriate behavior. This was all on the ground and did not take place in a helicopter.

The captain threatened us all the time that he was gonna send us home. We were all terrified. We would go to sleep at night locking our doors. We were all afraid of him. He was a reservist. His regular job was taking care of severe diabetics, which was interesting because one time we had this Jordanian or Syrian truck driver come in, and he was obviously in severe DKA (diabetic keto-acidosis), and this captain MD didn't know what to do with him. I mean it was obvious to me as an ER nurse. He said that he "didn't know how to manage this," and I said, "Sir, I can stay up all night and chart his blood sugars every half hour and give him the insulin on a sliding scale," and he said, "that's too much of a risk." I reminded him that that's what nurses do. He was supposedly an experienced physician and was about 64 years old.

My deployment was a negative experience and an angry experience. How does the military allow this to continue? How do they allow this man to practice? How do they allow this man to assault enlisted people? It was like this my whole 6 months. I couldn't wait to get out of there. My anger was because of the command situation over there.

CAPTAIN BRITTANY

Brittany is an army nurse.

She related:

I deployed two times, once to Iraq and once to Afghanistan. Coming back from Iraq was pretty easy for me. About 2 months after I returned from my second deployment, I started to notice a big change in myself. I was super angry; jokes weren't funny anymore; there was no laughter, and my resiliency was on its last leg. I just didn't bounce back like I used to. When I got home, I realized how exhausted I was. I knew I was emotionally and spiritually drained, but I was also physically exhausted. Your adrenaline just kept going over there, and then when you get home you realize just how tired you really are. I didn't have supportive army leadership that I could talk to because we were geographically separated. I did try to contact my leadership for advice and guidance, but they were not helpful. Not getting guidance was one of the hardest things; I almost felt abandoned. Luckily, the air force leadership that I was working with at the time in Afghanistan was really good. I felt comfortable talking to them. Eventually, I got help from a therapist.

My homecoming from Afghanistan was just very different. In April I started e-mailing my leadership back at Joint Base Lewis-McCord, letting them that I wasn't doing so well, and that I wanted to see behavioral health as soon as I got home. When I got home, everything just fell apart. I didn't get to see anyone in behavioral health until August, and I got home in June. My sister was supposed to get married while I was in Afghanistan, but she moved the wedding back, so I could be there. So, 3 days after I get home, I'm in California for the wedding, and then back up to Lewis-McCord and not feeling right. Something just felt wrong. A lot of people try to tell you they know what it's like they've been there, but everyone's deployment is very different. My emotions are different than yours. We could go and see the same thing and do the same thing, but my interpretation might be very different. My leadership was far less supportive than for my Iraq deployment. The level of help wasn't there. It took 2 months before I could see someone in behavioral health, and that only happened because I ended up coming home early from leave. I started to think I was becoming a danger to myself. I came home 2 weeks early from leave to see behavioral health, and they said they wouldn't do anything for me for another 2 weeks. They said this was because I already had a scheduled appointment. Because I came back 2 weeks early, the social worker who did my intake said that they couldn't do anything for me because I already had an appointment. It was unbelievable. I let my boss know, and she let her boss know. I had a meeting with the assistant chief of behavioral health. So, I met with him once a week for 3 weeks before I was actually able to start with my therapist. They changed my medications and all kinds of stuff like that. It was definitely a story of a soldier falling through the cracks. They could have made it so much easier for me. I think this is a classic case of the army leadership not knowing what to do with someone coming home so broken, and I was admitting that I was coming home broken. I've really never known much about depression or anxiety or PTSD. I've taken care of patients with things like that, but no one in my family has ever had that. I've had no close contact with things like that. It was a totally new experience not only to grasp what was going on, but to accept it. I knew with help it would get easier, but I also knew it was something I'd have to live with. My leadership really didn't know how to help with that. They completely isolated me from everyone. They put me in an office with no windows doing paperwork. I would go almost an entire week without any human contact. When I first got back, I requested that I have a couple of months before I would go back to the bedside, just so I could breathe. I knew that I was quick to anger, and I didn't want to get angry at a patient or a team member. I asked for a break for a couple of months, and they said that was OK. That break had turned into a punishment in some respects, and that's how I felt about it because they wouldn't let me go back to patient care. They kept trying to keep me from going back to patient care. They didn't give me an explanation. My rater and my head nurse kept trying to create reasons why I couldn't go back. She'd say things like, "If I'm going to let you go back, here are the things you are going to have to do." I would do whatever she told me to do, and then she would just find something else, a benchmark for me to meet. I finally got to the point in December that I wrote a response to a counseling statement she had given me. She sent it up to her boss, who sent it to her boss, etc. I got called into the big boss's office after that. That relationship was deemed "a hostile environment" between myself and my rater. In my memorandum, I had pointed out the lies that my rater had been spreading and the choices she had been making to keep me away from patient care. So, the decision was made to immediately pull me out of that ICU; so, they moved me to the other one. So, I started patient care the next day. There was just one person who was so afraid for me to come back. They didn't understand what it was like to come home different, and it scared them. I don't think they were really truthful with the chain of command about what was really going on.

I am still at the other ICU now. We had a very junior person as our OIC who made it difficult for everybody just because she was so inexperienced. I told the higher up leadership right then that it was not gonna be a good change because there would be some huge conflict between myself and the leadership in that unit. There was the same rank and the same time in service, and I am far too strong of a personality, and they didn't believe me. I had a fair amount of experience too. It was a difficult few months, but now the leadership has changed, and the leadership now is very "pro" the soldiers and very "pro" the nurses. They want us to succeed, and this is a breath of fresh air to succeed. It's a lot better now. It's over a year since I have been home, and I'm finally enjoying going to work again, and my teammates enjoy going to work. There are still things that make it difficult, and there are anniversaries that hit home. There were some big events like mass casualty events. For example, about a month after I came home one of the medics I worked with was hit and died, and one of the crew chiefs that I worked with was injured in the same attack. It gets to you if you don't have any resiliency left. I was back here, and they were still in country getting ready to come home.

It's been nice to have conversations with someone. My therapist has been deployed; so, he knows. He listens to me and has made a safe environment where I can talk. Therapy has helped me realize some stuff and has helped me make some better decisions about things here and there. I still have a long way to go. It's a bummer that it took as long as it did for me to start the healing process, especially when I started contacting my leadership 3 months before coming home saying that I am gonna need some help. And then it took 2 months before I got that help, and it took a pretty significant breakdown before that happened. I was not hospitalized, but I think I got pretty close to that though.

Brittany recalled the events leading to her mental health issues in Afghanistan. She stated,

In April, I started feeling mentally exhausted and the adrenaline started to wear off. That's when I took 2 weeks R and R, which was nice. I think coming back from that I knew something was off, something was wrong. I went to Australia for R and R in March. It was good to get away, but it was something I should have done earlier in the deployment. Since they saw me day to day, they could tell good days and not so good days. They were helpful. I made lifelong friends out of that air force group. They became family while I was there. We hung out together. There was almost no army where I was. They were all aviation people, pilots and navigators. There were just two nurses and two air force general medical officers, and the flight surgeons were 2 years postgrad. In their minds they knew everything which was an interesting dynamic [*laughing*]. It was very eye opening at times. There was some butting of the heads periodically, my thought process on treatments versus the physician's thought process on treatments. My decision would be involved when the attending physician and anesthesiologist said what they wanted to have done on the flight. They had known the patient far longer than I had in the OR, and how the patient had responded to treatment. I would take their lead to make sure that the soldier, marine, or airman got to the next level of care.

The second 6 months was actually more fun. I think that was because of the people and because of the mission.

The AF aviation team was such a tight-knit group, but they were also very inclusive. When I was assigned to a crew for a 24-hour shift, we'd all go eat together, and we'd do stuff together. There was hangout time. I loved to get to know my teammates, and we ended up having a common bond. That made it a lot more fun. Also, the flight crews had just gotten there; so, they were full of energy. So, for a while it gave me more energy. I got to see Afghanistan through their eyes. I had forgotten how beautiful the mountain tops looked when they were covered with snow. They kind of invited me to stop and smell the roses.

MAJOR COLLEEN

Colleen, an army nurse, talked about her deployment to Herat, Afghanistan. She recalled:

My friends were people I deployed with or who were in my unit. My civilian friends have never understood my deployment. My parents were fine. I am the type of person who is always busy; so, even when I have something bad happen, I just keep moving. I didn't really deal with anything that I saw or did down range. So, when I came back, some things would trigger me a bit. I remember right after I came back, it was New Year's Eve, and I was in El Paso, and I hadn't gone home yet to see my parents. My husband was at work and was overnight that night. I had decided not to go out; so, I stayed home and was watching movies, and I saw something about a young girl who had died, and I couldn't sleep the rest of the night. I literally thought that I was gonna die. I stayed up all night; I was falling over tired. I remember calling my dad. My husband had told me I was crazy. I called my dad, and I was crying and I said, "I think I'm crazy." He said, "You are dealing with it, and you are going to be OK." He listened to me. He had never been deployed. He had been in Turkey during the first Gulf War. He was in a combat zone, but he was never under fire. He's not medical, but he understands that reintegration is difficult. My parents were really good. My husband was a reservist, and he had deployed. He wasn't very helpful to me. He's a very narcissistic person. I'm glad I realized that eventually. Before I deployed, it wasn't that apparent. When I had met him, I was this brand new girl in the army who had just gotten out of college and here was this guy, who is a couple of years older than me, and who knew everything. I was a little star struck. Even before I deployed, he told me that he knew I couldn't handle it. But I did really well. I even came back with an award, and he did not come back with the type of award that I had. I came back with a bronze star, and he did not. That might have contributed to some of our problems [*laughing*]. I did my job. It was always about him. That was one of the things that made me angry when I came back. This included his family. I was gonna move up to Michigan with him to be close to his family. It was always about him. I'd be introduced to people as Alvin's wife. The attention was always on Alvin, you know, "Alvin did this and Alvin did that." His wife is a nurse in the army, and she has deployed too. It was never recognizing what I had done. Even to the point where I was down range, and he'd call and complain about work. He had been doing some overtime here and there. He'd call me and would say "How was your day?" I'd say, "Not good, we've had some traumas." He'd say, "Do you want to talk about it?" I'd say, "No, let's talk about something happy, let's talk about the future." Then he'd go into this rampage about how much he hates work and that he had to work an extra hour. You can't have a whole lot of compassion when you just watched someone die. He just didn't care; it was always about him.

Colleen talked about her decision to go to Korea after Afghanistan. She stated:

I think going to Korea, I kind of knew that they had been shooting off missiles. I liked being down range; I liked the excitement. I liked focusing on the patients and could put the other stuff aside. I feel like my decision to go to Korea was my continuation of pushing that stuff aside. I went to a counselor in Korea, and I said, "I want to make sure that I've dealt with all the stuff I've been through in a crazy place and even before that and my crazy ex-husband and my deployment." The counselor basically told me, "You are completely fine, you've dealt with everything."

I think part of my reintegration happened when I came back to the States a year ago. I really started to deal with stuff in all honesty. It was terrible. I got into a relationship in Korea, and then I was planning on coming back and getting married. But I requested when I was leaving Korea, that I be near family. I put on my list Fort Lewis where my fiancé was, Fort Carson because my brother lives in Denver, and I have a lot of friends there, and I put going back to Fort Bliss. I had been on two long tours at this point; so, instead they sent me to Fort Huachuca, Arizona, which was my fourth choice. I didn't even know they had nurses there. When I got there things were quiet, it's an outpatient facility. I was put in a head nurse position, and we had high ratings on everything. But, there were some things about it being a hostile workplace environment. So, there was stuff going on. I was lonely and things just started coming up. Then, my fiancé broke up with me.

Here I was at Fort Huachuca, and the plan I had made was gone. It was really, really hard. I didn't know anyone, and most of the people here are civilians. So, I was basically alone. Most of the people here are married. It's a very small post. I was really on my own. One of my friends from Korea came a few months later. She was actually deployed with the same unit as me, and then ended up in Korea as well. I found out there were some jealousy issues, and that she had backstabbed me pretty bad. I was alone again because my best friend had really backstabbed me. I am still stuck here with her. I had one person who I could kinda confide in, and she was a lieutenant colonel. She just retired a few months ago. She thought that this was a bad place for me being single, being away from everything, and that the place is so quiet. She advocated for me to move to a bigger post such as Fort Bragg, Fort Lewis, or Fort Carson. I was turned down. Then they told me that my 2-year assignment had been extended to 3 years. I went through 3–4 months looking at ways to get out of here. I talked to my mentor from Korea, and basically said that I can't do this anymore. I think he called some people, and I got a call a few days later, and they offered me a job in DC, the office of the surgeon general. I think it was a reward job to keep me from getting out. I accepted it, and said, "I'll give the army another year and see how it goes." It would be a 1-year internship. But, a few months later the job was cut. They said, "Sorry, you are gonna be here for 3 years." They allowed me to move to a different position. But my current chief nurse is pretty hostile. She's not a very nice woman. We had an investigation of my unit that I deployed with. That was a bad couple of days. I wanted to go and get my nurse practitioner degree, and they were not supportive of letting me leave to do that. I feel that I am single; so, I might as well go and do it now before I have kids. The army is not gonna be the best place for me at this point, and I got accepted to the family nurse practitioner program at Georgetown. I'll be getting out, and I'm not entirely happy about that. The army has not let me do what I need to do to take care of myself. I'll be getting out in May. I actually already started the program. It's an online hybrid program. I started it on

September 9, 2013. I am about half way through my first class. I am only taking one class right now. Next year when I get out, I'll go full time. The chief nurse also told me that she would not support me because she doesn't believe in online programs.

Colleen went on to talk about her issues after deployment and her assignment in Korea:

With my deployment and the assignment in Korea, I learned to just push everything away and not deal with life. My first reaction is just to do that. I guess it is something I have to work on, and I am. I also have some difficult stuff left over from college. I was not actually raped, but I have some traumatic experiences left over from college. It's a combination of things, I think. The biggest issue I have at this point is the relationships I've had with men. In Afghanistan, Korea, and even here in Arizona, there are very few females. And there are very few attractive young females. So, guys are just not good about it [*laughing*]. Also, I moved around a lot as a child, and I've always had this tendency to "move on." I'd close one book or chapter and open another one. I've done that my entire life. So, not being able to run away from here has been difficult. But, I think it is needed. It isn't easy, and I hate feeling weak. Other people haven't been through what I have been through. I've moved six times in 7 years.

I used to love shopping. I was a big shopper, and I used to love to go to the mall with my friends. Now, I don't go to a mall and walk around anymore. Plus, I was probably home for a month or more before I felt like I could go to a mall. I go to the store that I want to and buy what I want. I don't go to Walmart, it overwhelms me. There are too many choices. I remember it took me 20 minutes to pick out what kind of deodorant I wanted.

She continued, I also had a hard time eating regular food. I had been eating Spanish food for a year. When I went back for R and R, I would eat American fried food. When I got home, I would do this, and sometimes I'd throw up. My diet has changed pretty drastically. I ended up losing 50 pounds when I got home from Afghanistan. I went from being the person who was overweight all the time, to being the person who was almost underweight. People would tell me that I needed to eat more.

I did a lot of thinking when I came back about what I saw and what I did. I ended up doing rock climbing. I wanted to have an adventure when I came back from Afghanistan. I went to

Joshua Tree. It was something I wanted to tell my future grand-kids about. One of the things that helped me in Afghanistan was to stand back and look at a trauma, where they were missing an eye and missing a leg, and I would take a deep breath and focus on the tasks that I needed to do rather than the horrific nature of the wounds. I would step back and say, "I need to put in the IV, I need to get the labs." Then, I would step back again and think, "I need to do this and I need to do that." The concentration would clear my mind. I could then think about home and the issues with my husband more clearly as a result of the way I approached trauma care. I was almost scared to come home because I was afraid that I would never be able to think clearly again. I thought I could not get that level of concentration. So, the first time I rock climbed, I got up on the wall and realized I could do the same thing with my mind. You have to have concentration with rock climbing. It is all that matters. You can't be thinking about problems with your husband. All that matters is that you put one hand here and move it to there. I got some rock-climbing friends. We'd go out to the middle of nowhere on weekends and just climb. I became an out-doorsy person, a hiker, a rock-climbing type since Afghanistan. It gives me that clarity and is therapeutic for me. It's my therapy. I developed a little bit of an eating disorder from things that people said to me when I was younger and also being in the unit I was in. The commander was so obsessed with weight. I started having some problems with eating down range, but then my weight loss was also due to the different food. When I got back to the States, I did seek some treatment for bulimia. All the trauma and stress didn't help. I went to my facility when I got back, and I kind of got a little scapegoated to the point where I will not talk about my problems anymore with anybody at work. Absolutely not! They were not good to me. I went to talk to someone because my fiancé broke up with me, and that I was fat. The social worker asked me if I had ever done any trauma therapy, and said, "I think you need it." I did EMDR [eye movement desensitization and reprocessing] for a little while. Because it was the facility where I worked, it ended up being a conflict of interest. It was just a bad situation. I will never, never, never, never recommend that someone go to be-havioral health in the military. It was not a good situation for me. I work with these people all the time. My chief nurse had never been deployed, and when I told her I had been through a lot, her response was, "Everybody's been through a lot." She was not sup-portive. She said that I couldn't handle the stress in my life.

FIRST LIEUTENANT RHETTA

Rhetta, an army nurse who was deployed to Balad, Iraq, said:

> I really can't complain because the only health problem I had while over there and now occasionally back in the States, is trouble falling asleep. I handled things great while at work, but occasionally at night, I would not be able to shut my mind off. I'd have racing thoughts or my mind would wander thinking about my patients, and what their lives would be with their injuries and disabilities. A doc that I worked with prescribed a minimal dose of Klonopin to calm down my anxiety at night. We decided that I would only take it after tossing and turning for more than one hour. I am not a pill person, but I needed my sleep to function. It helped. Now back in the States, my primary care physician has prescribed a low dose of Xanax for the same thing when my mind takes me back to Iraq. I figure if that is the only problem that I have after being in a war, and it's a very minor one, I'm OK.

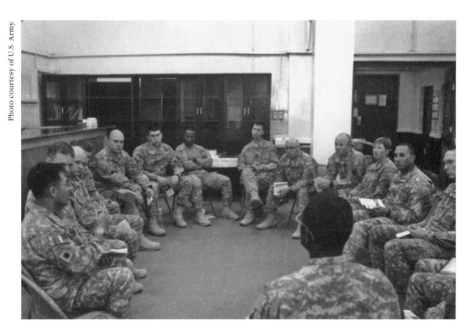

Photo courtesy of U.S. Army.

Army reintegration discussion group led by army chaplain.

DailyNurse™

THE PULSE OF NURSING

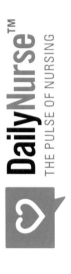

DailyNurse™

THE PULSE OF NURSING

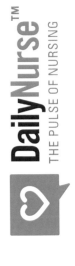

8

Needing a Clinical Change of Scenery

A clinical change of scenery may be a change in geographic location or a change in one's nursing role or a change in one's clinical setting. Some nurses may desire to work in a different hospital postdeployment rather than return to their previous hospital. Others might want to become involved in administration or teaching and take a break from the clinical nursing role. Some may request a transfer to a different clinical area within their hospital such as working on the maternity unit instead of returning to the emergency room (ER) or working in the outpatient clinic rather than working in the operating room (OR).

After serving in a war zone, it was not considered unusual for nurses to request a break from the trauma intensive care unit (ICU) or ER. Some nurses who saw a lot of injured children elected to work with older patients on returning home. Requesting a clinical change of scenery was often an attempt to remain as a practicing nurse. Conversely, there were always a few nurses who missed the adrenaline rush of the combat environment and were bored with taking care of retirees and dependents and decided to remain in the ER or ICU.

LIEUTENANT COLONEL JULIE

Julie, an air force reservist, described how she changed her clinical area after returning from Iraq.

She stated:

> As a civilian nurse I worked in a Level Two Trauma Center before my deployment. I was a trauma emergency room nurse. Now, I

work in the recovery room. When I came home from Iraq, I was burned out on trauma. I saw enough trauma to last a lifetime. It simply took too much emotion out of me. Luckily, my superiors understood and valued the work I do. I'm doing OK in the recovery room.

FIRST LIEUTENANT ALLISON

Allison was an air force ER and triage nurse who served in Afghanistan. She remarked:

What frustrated me when I returned was the type of patients we take care of back in the States. They are mostly older people with chronic problems. I really miss the deployment mission and trauma care we provided. It really became what I want to continue to do. I would go back in a heartbeat! Back in the States, nurses are tasked with doing everything. We are providing care for patients. We are sounding boards and therapists for families. We are pulled in so many directions. On deployment, you didn't have other responsibilities clouding the mission.

At my stateside hospital, they usually preferred returning nurses to ease back into nursing roles and avoid trauma units for a time. They believed this way, we could acclimate to a nondeployment atmosphere and provide nursing care to patients in a more routine environment. However, this did not prove true for all of us. I thrived in the deployment environment and found stateside care at my hospital boring and not challenging at all.

LIEUTENANT KATE

Kate, a navy nurse, recalled:

Getting reassigned to Guam was a refreshing change of scenery, even though it is an isolated island. I had to start from scratch getting to know a new staff, but it was a welcomed positive change. It was just what I needed after being deployed to a war zone. Afghanistan needed to "move to my rearview mirror," if you know what I mean. I wanted to put the Afghanistan experience behind me, and meet new challenges at a new location. The hospital in Guam was a new beginning.

LIEUTENANT COLONEL TONI

Toni reported how her deployment changed her clinical preference. She recalled:

> On the Reserve side, we don't get much downtime when we re-turn from a deployment. I went back to my job as a trauma ICU nurse, and I just couldn't handle it. I was able to switch to a med-surg ICU at my hospital. I had tried to work in the Level 1 trauma ICU, and we got patients with gunshots, motor vehicle accidents, and I started having flashbacks. You start thinking about that last patient you transported on the helicopter, and you wonder if he made it. Then, you think about the stuff that is still happening over there, and you need to be back there to help them, and you're not. But you know that when you were there you did well, you were helpful, and you know it was rewarding, even though it was a very hard job.
>
> Well, it wasn't very rewarding in the civilian ICU where I worked. It was not the same caring for a drunk driver, or a gang member who shot up some people, or a drug dealer. It was different. The ones I cared for overseas were shot serving their country. The people in my civilian ICU were usually there be-cause of bad circumstances that they brought unto themselves, a lot of criminal activity. I gave it a try, but I just had to get out of the trauma ICU. I transferred to the medical–surgical ICU.

FIRST LIEUTENANT RHETTA

After returning from her wartime deployment, Rhetta wanted to work with posttraumatic stress disorder (PTSD) patients and hoped to get the army to send her for a master's degree in psychiatric nursing. Her desire for a clini-cal change was not because she was burned out.

She recalled:

> I found myself to be a very good listener. Colleagues would come to me with their problems. They said I had a gentle, unassuming way with people. I also related well to my patients and heard their concerns about their future. After serving in Iraq, I am in-terested in the mental aspects of war and I can see myself get-ting a master's in psychiatric nursing to better understand PTSD, compassion fatigue, and burnout. I saw firsthand the toll the war

took on my patients, my peers, and some of the physicians, especially the folks who had done more than two tours of duty. I believe my niche would be as a mental health nurse practitioner or as a clinical nurse specialist in the long run. I definitely want to stay in the army and get advanced education.

LIEUTENANT COMMANDER ZOE

Zoe talked about her work postdeployment and her plan to separate from the active duty navy.

She stated:

Being busy was both good and bad. I love my work and I love patient care and forming relationships with my panel of patients and that's why I love being an NP [nurse practitioner]. There was a benefit to that. But it did take away time from being with my family. Having that 'end date' in sight was very helpful because when I separated from active duty, my plan was to take a year just to be a stay-at-home mom with my girls. We all knew that was the plan. In terms of patient care, I really loved seeing active duty patients. So, when I saw someone who had recently returned from deployment, I would try to engage them by asking, "Where did you deploy? What was your experience with that?" And sometimes I'd say to myself [*laughing*], "Am I that therapist who starts talking about myself?" So, I would say I was there, and often we would end up having a short conversation about where we had deployed to and what our roles had been and how we were doing coming back. I take longer with my patients anyway. I'm always running behind, and they don't mind that. I would be 20 to 30 minutes with a patient. I'd often feel that we were both better off after the short conversation. We had that brief opportunity to share.

LIEUTENANT LAUREN

Lauren is a navy nurse who was deployed to Camp Bastion in Afghanistan. She remarked:

I didn't know what kind of job I was gonna have at Bethesda [Walter Reed National Military Medical Center, Bethesda, Maryland]. My orders were kind of vague. I assumed I was gonna do ICU. I sort of entered the ICU arena in Afghanistan. Then a nursing supervisor said, "We have a different job for you." She wanted me to be the division officer of the medical–surgical floor at the time. I was like, "Oh, dear God." I was the second in command running this 32-bed med–surg unit. So, I didn't go to the ICU and I became a division officer at Bethesda. I was disappointed and didn't have an option, and I was like, "OK, I'll give it a go." You are kind of used to that. It's not a punishment, it's looking at where the needs are. It's like, "We really need you here." So, it ended up being a great learning experience for me. It was very challenging. I was there during the time they integrated Walter Reed Army Medical Center and Bethesda Naval Hospital. At one point we had double the number of nurses because they combined two places, and we renovated different floors and the logistical nightmare was ridiculous. I didn't really like that job in the end, but I think it was really good for me in terms of leadership and seeing the bigger picture and attending meetings about how things operate.

I also think that when they told me that I wasn't going to the ICU, maybe deep inside, I had a little sigh of relief because I knew that all of the guys I had previously taken care of were there. In fact, I had girlfriends who worked in the ICU at Bethesda who were taking care of the guys I had previously taken care of in Afghanistan. I also remember thinking that in Afghanistan, I only had the patients for 72 hours and they would be in the ICU at Bethesda for so long. There they would finally wake up and realize, "Oh my God, I'm missing all my limbs." Then, the infection sets in, and the family is there. That just seemed like a lot at the time for me to continue doing. I think in a way, it was a good thing for me that I wasn't right back in the ICU. It was a good thing. It would have been a lot to have the same guys from Afghanistan. It was so fresh in my mind. That's how it went down.

Lauren talked about her transition back into living in the United States, especially in a large metropolitan area:

Setting routines didn't happen very fast because of having to go back to Japan and pack up my things. I do remember vividly going to a show at a theatre, and we were in line to get a glass of wine and I had to pay in cash and I remember fumbling in my purse to get the right amount of money. I felt like everyone around me was breathing down my neck, like "Hurry up." Everything had to be so fast, and I wanted to just turn around to everybody and scream, "Would you just chill out!" [*Laughing now.*] I was going as fast as I could, and I remember feeling pressured because everything was so fast and busy in DC. Driving for me was a little intense at first again because you're in DC, and everything is too fast.

CAPTAIN CORABETH

Corabeth discussed her nursing career and the decisions she made after doing the detainee care mission in Iraq:

> After November 2008, I got off active duty. I applied for my master's as an NP [nurse practitioner] and graduated from the program in 2011. Now I work for the VA [Veterans Administration] as an FNP [family nurse practitioner]. My deployment experience is very helpful in working with returning vets. I absolutely love my job at the VA. People are supportive, although they don't know my mission was detainee care. Being with veterans, you are surrounded by people who generally understand deployment. Most of the other health care providers I work with are not veterans.

CAPTAIN EARL

Earl is an Air Force Reserve flight nurse who was deployed to Iraq and Afghanistan. Earl described how he felt like he was "pretty much done with nursing." He discussed how he was ready for a clinical change of scenery. He stated:

> So with my new job at the fire department, I got off the medic unit and tried to stay on the fire truck. It helped not having to do patient care. Over time, things improved a bit. You know, time is a great healer for both mental and physical wounds. Over time things got better, and I could re-engage in doing medical things. As time went on, I didn't talk a lot to my peers about being a nurse in the military. We would have continuing education classes for the EMTs [emergency medical technicians] and paramedics, and I would find myself doing more of the teaching. And people would say, "How do you know all of this stuff?" Then I'd tell them that I was a flight nurse in the air force. Over time I felt more comfortable and was able to overcome some of my previous issues."

LIEUTENANT COLONEL DAGMAR

Dagmar had been in the air force and then in the Air National Guard for many years. She worked at a large Veterans Administration Hospital in California for her civilian job. She told of her personal and unique situation surrounding her deployment and her determined plea for a clinical change of scenery.

Dagmar recalled:

> Let me tell you what was going on with me when I went on my first deployment. Back in late February 2003 and into early March 2003 before we actually invaded Iraq, I was home taking care of my terminally ill husband with pancreatic cancer. He died on March 4, and March 19 is when we invaded Iraq. So, I'm home, a grieving widow, and I'm watching all of this on TV. I knew things were building, building, building. I know they were calling people from my unit. They wanted to stage AE [air-evac] out of Turkey. They wanted to stage on the northern front of Iraq to cover that part of the operations. But Turkey would not support it. We were just kind of all held at bay. My squadron knew what was going on with me at the time, and they wanted just to leave me alone. I knew they weren't calling me or trying to pull me in to do anything. But once I saw things on TV, I knew it was just a matter of time before we would be activated or needed overseas. So, I called them up, and said, "If you guys go, I want to go, too. I know you are being kind to me right now, and you are leaving me alone, but if you go, don't leave me home alone. I don't want to stay here by myself; I need to go. I want to go."
>
> Fortunately, I didn't go right away. I don't think that would have been that great. By July, I did go, and that was part of the reason why my deployment was up in November. It was supposed to be for 5 months. But I didn't want to come back home. To come back here and stay alone and face how drastically my life had changed wasn't something I wanted to do yet. Everything was up in the air for me. It was actually easier to be deployed. I was able to dedicate myself to something bigger than myself. I did enjoy it, being deployed. It gave me an outlet that I really needed. It was November, and I didn't want to be home for the holidays. I asked to stay in Afghanistan, but was told I was needed in Iraq. They needed flight crews. There was a lot going on. There were a lot of patients. I just stepped right into a slot in the other war theater. I stayed out, and I was grateful that they

asked me to come along for another deployment. I did not want to be home. I told them I wanted to change my surroundings and be doing something else. I wanted to start another chapter of my life. I knew that was what was going on with me for the first couple of years after my husband died.

It would not have been a good choice for me to come home to an empty house where I didn't want to live and start all over. It was avoidance of that, it definitely was. I know that had a lot to do with why I was doing what I was doing. Then there came a point in those first few years, I was what they call PM, presidentially mobilized, and a bunch of us were. It meant that we weren't mobilized for a specific deployment. They just put you on blanket orders, and you are like on a retainer, and they can use you for whatever they need. You are on continuous orders. I would live in a hotel near the base, and my whole life was just dedicated to the military.

There is an expectation sometimes because I totally volunteered and the PM status is just the status of your orders. You can volunteer or you can be PM'd. When you are PM'd, it is usually for a longer period of time. I thought I was just gonna be on a retainer on orders. I think they can do it for up to 2 years, I believe. You have to be available, but you also perform duty on base at your home station when you are not deployed. If something comes up that the military needs you, you don't have a whole lot of choice of where you are going.

Air-evac tends to send you out on small teams and as individuals, not necessarily the whole unit. When we are "in the bucket" or Air-evac Flight rotation, we are spread all over the place; we fill all the slots. For example, right now it's our turn "in the bucket." I happen to be home this time, but we have people in two different sites stateside that are going; we had some at Ramstein, Kandahar, and Bagram. We are scattered all over the place. Different units, when it is their turn, if they are not able to fulfill all the tasking, there are holes, what we call "short falls." They sometimes need individuals, especially once you go out and have some experience, not just as flight crew, but working in the command center or running operations and some of these other jobs, to support the whole operation. Then, you kind of create a name for yourself, and you may be asked for by name. There are a lot of those opportunities. It was a lot of go, go, go, very involved in the war.

I was living in Fresno at the time my husband died, and I didn't want to stay in Fresno. I didn't want to come back to

Fresno; so, I transferred with the VA to Phoenix. The VA was my civilian job. I just wanted a total change of scenery, but in my mind, I thought of it as a deployment. I thought, I'll just go there for a year, and I'll start a new life. I'll start with all new people. I'll start out fresh.

The military life is like an alter-ego; it is like some hidden shadowy thing that most people aren't even aware of. They don't know what you have been doing or have any clue what are all the things you're involved with. You don't talk about it a whole lot. What I was doing when I was in Phoenix, I'd work five 12-hour shifts in a row; so, I could catch a plane and fly back to California to my unit and do duty there. I worked myself to death to make sure that I could come back and stay attached to the military. It was like my lifeline. Because when you come home, you can feel so disconnected. You know the war is going on over there, but everyone at home seems so oblivious. They have no idea of the nature of injuries, or what kind of conditions you've been living in, or what you have been involved with.

LIEUTENANT SANDRA

Sandra is a navy nurse who served in Afghanistan.
She recalled:

I was dreading going back to work in Guam because the leadership was terrible. They were not very sympathetic, they sent me nothing while I was deployed. There was no way for me to connect with them, since I deployed so soon after arriving in Guam. I didn't have time to get to know people because I was there for "a blink of an eye." By the time we moved into our house and got everything situated and had that time off, I didn't really get to know anyone. I didn't bond with anyone there. I dreaded coming back knowing that the leadership was not that great. It was just as bad as I thought it would be. My schedule was right back to work. I didn't even have time to catch my breath. They were super short on people—that's the way it always is. I didn't really get along with very many people when I first came back, because I really didn't want to talk to people. I didn't like the questions. They weren't glad to see me because they never really met me before. I didn't really fit with the unit. I don't know. I just don't know. I don't think I waited long enough for it to get better,

I requested a transfer. I got out of the ER. Initially, primary care was a very steep learning curve; so, it was stressful. I didn't really get a chance to think about all the things that had happened over the last few months. I was just so busy and stressed.

Once I finally got it after a few months, they made me clinic manager. I ended up really enjoying it. I learned a lot about myself skill-wise and what makes me happy in the workplace. I'm a busybody who likes to know what is going on [*laughs*]. I didn't think the clinic setting would give me that. I was managing the whole overall workings of the clinic. I like having that control; so, I can affect good change. The person before me in the position didn't care. But, I'm internally driven and motivated, and I'm always gonna care. I developed very good management skills [*laughs*]. Now, I'm at the Naval Postgraduate School. I'm furthering my education. I'll go into the administrative side of the hospital. All my jobs with the navy will now be on the administrative side of the house. That comes with rank, and it's especially true in the Nurse Corps. You really don't get power or control until you make 04 or 05 [lieutenant commander or commander]. It takes a while, although I did get picked up early. I made lieutenant in 2010 when I was in Afghanistan, and I just found out last month that I got promoted to lieutenant commander. It's about 3 years early. I have to stay in. It's almost 15 years.

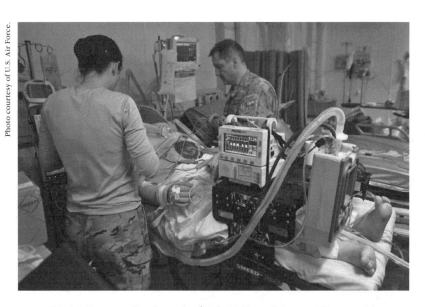

Photo courtesy of U.S. Air Force.

Air force nurse and injured marine at the Combat Support Hospital, Balad Air Base, Iraq.

Photo courtesy of U.S. Air Force.

U.S. Air Force medics from the 455th Air Expeditionary Wing provide care at Bagram Air Base, Afghanistan.

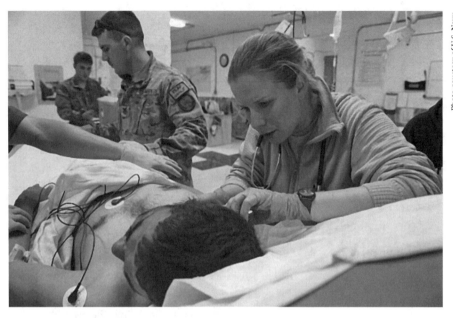

Photo courtesy of U.S. Navy.

U.S. Navy nurse evaluates a patient in Farah, Afghanistan.

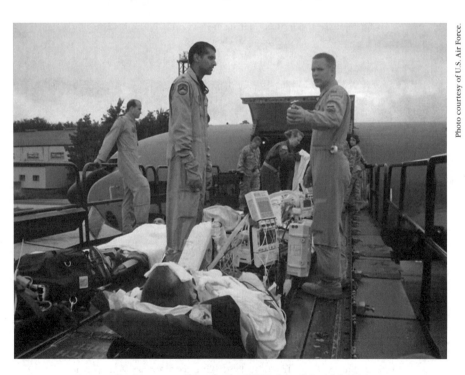

Photo courtesy of U.S. Air Force.

Aeromedical team members load a C-135 aircraft in Afghanistan.

9

Petty Complaints and Trivial Whining: No Tolerance Here

Many nurses reported low tolerance for people's complaints and an impatience on returning home. Some called this "having a shorter fuse" after returning to U.S. soil. After seeing horrendous injuries, they grew weary of trivial whining, people with a sense of entitlement, and those who seem to never be happy or satisfied with anything. Most returning nurses reported having a greater appreciation for life in the United States and the creature comforts of home. Some said other people's dissatisfaction and loud rhetoric about seemingly trivial things rubbed against the fabric of the nurses' appreciation for all that we have in the United States.

We chose the following 10 vignettes that are a reflection of what many of the other 25 participants experienced upon their return home after deployment. In addition to petty complaints and trivial whining, the nurses commented on a general sense of inflexibility and occasional rudeness on the part of others. Examples included being rushed in the grocery checkout line, fast and inconsiderate drivers on the roads, being hurried when paying for a glass of wine at a theatre, and a general lack of consideration for others. One nurse described her fear of parking lots with aggressive people cutting in front of her to get a space. She added that it was not even Christmas time when this occurred. Another nurse told how she was annoyed with the materialism of Americans when many of the children in Afghanistan did not even have shoes. Some of the nurses were concerned about wasteful habits of others such as filling their plates at the hospital cafeteria's salad bar only to throw out more than half of the food taken. Many admitted that the aforementioned behaviors bothered them after returning from war.

LIEUTENANT COLONEL DAGMAR

Dagmar, an Air Force Reserve flight nurse, stated:

> The kind of nursing that you go out and do on a deployment is extreme nursing, like extreme sports. When you come home, it's kind of hard to keep up the momentum because trivial things simply do not hold the same importance. I don't think anything in my nursing career will come close to the "high" that I experienced in Iraq and Afghanistan. I felt tested to my limits. I bent, but I did not break! It was a very tough experience at times, but looking back now, I feel a tremendous sense of accomplishment! On the other hand, I feel that I now have zero tolerance for people back here complaining.
>
> The other night I was at the movies, and a couple ahead of us in line was complaining about the parking, complaining about the price of tickets and popcorn, and complaining about the cost of a babysitter. I wanted to haul off and tell them they are lucky to have a car, to be free to go to a movie, and to know their kids are safe at home. People in the U.S. generally have it so good compared to people in third world or war-torn countries. They need to get a life! They were adult spoiled brats!

CAPTAIN COURTNEY

Courtney, an air force reservist, reported:

> I didn't reintegrate very well back into my civilian job. I just could not tolerate people's whining. I could not listen to it anymore. It wasn't our patients who were whining; it was my coworkers who were whining about their work schedules or time off. I had just come back from war, where soldiers were laying their lives on the line. Then, these other folks are whining about having to work back-to-back call. Some of the staff members were driving me nuts!

LIEUTENANT LORETTA

Loretta, a navy operating room (OR) nurse assigned to the hospital in Kandahar, Afghanistan, remarked:

> I had a lot of anxiety when I came back. There was so much going on at the hospital, and it was not straightforward. It was frustrating because I'd hear about all the trivial things people were

talking about, and it was just not where my mind was. People were talking about who was dating who, and when Macy's was having its next sale, and what surgeon got in trouble for not getting a haircut. I just wasn't into the idle gossip, and I didn't know the people they were talking about anyway. I had just left a war zone where I worked in the OR taking care of young soldiers and marines who got shot or blown up. I helped put little kids back together again after they were innocent victims of a roadside bomb.

LIEUTENANT COLONEL JULIE

Julie, an air force reservist, described how people in her civilian job upset her and angered her.

I was angry because some coworkers seemed to incessantly whine about small stuff or inconveniences, like their schedules, or that so-and-so isn't pulling their weight, or they are complaining about this patient, or that patient, or that they have to pull back-to-back call because someone is sick, or had a serious illness in their family. I just found this very petty and infuriating. I had a very low tolerance for coworkers whining about these little inconveniences. I had just come back from a war zone where young 20-year-old soldiers were laying their life on the line for each other, and they were working 24/7 for the U.S. and all its people, and these other folks back in the States are whining about their schedules! Some coworkers were pushing my buttons!

COMMANDER ROBIN

Robin was a navy nurse who deployed to Afghanistan. Robin shared her feelings:

When I came back I struggled partly because they gave me this huge position for the unit. Fortunately, I had a strong assistant to help me carry it because it was, "Hurry up and do this, hurry up and do that." My immediate leadership did not recognize the fact that I was trying to acclimate after deployment. I would talk to other people, friends and coworkers, who had recently been deployed and coming back. I had primarily employees who wanted to do things like take an hour lunch or were 15 minutes late and

don't want to take leave time or questioned why they had to take
more patients when somebody else only had two and they had
three. I said, "Really?" Then in my mind I was saying to myself,
"Shut the hell up and get back to work! Do you understand that
there are people coming back here with missing arms and legs
who can't go home and hug their children? I don't have time for
your petty bullshit!" But, of course, I just said this in my mind. I
clearly did not actually say that to them. I felt like saying, "You get
to go home to your family, eat your meals, sleep in your bed, and
you are complaining because you don't want to take leave time
for the 15 minutes you were late today." So, for a while, I was like
the Bitch Nurse! I was enforcing rules that had already been established, but that were just not enforced. It was very odd, and I
felt like I had little patience, and that I didn't really have support
from my leadership. It was literally, "just get the job done, and keep
working, just do it." And you just don't have time. It was really hard
to hear people complain about stuff when we came back. You had
to bite your tongue a lot because the people who were complaining had never been deployed. They didn't understand the conditions we had just come from. They had no frame of reference.

LIEUTENANT SANDRA

Sandra, an active duty navy nurse, talked about people not really caring
about your deployment. She said that some went through the motions and
others didn't even bother to do that. She said:

What did they think it was like, a vacation? The living conditions were not very good. You sacrificed a lot, but it was worth
it. Some people asked you "blood and guts" questions. Others
didn't seem to be interested in your experience because they
were too wrapped up in their own lives, like what shifts they
were working, what weekends they were off, the price of things,
etc. What they didn't realize was that everyone's deployment experience is unique. Some people didn't have a bad experience,
but it was not like a walk in the park or a walk on the beach for
anyone. Coworkers were caught up in their own trivial issues
and sometimes seemed oblivious to the concerns of returning deployed personnel. The few that asked me about my deployment
never seemed to ask me about my reintegration, and I was going
through a divorce. My life was certainly leaning in that direction

before I even deployed. I knew that I wasn't coming home to a good situation with my husband.

MAJOR ELIZA

Eliza was an active duty air force nurse who deployed to Afghanistan twice. Eliza mentioned feeling weird when she got home from her two deployments to Afghanistan. She elaborated:

> When I got home, it was kind of weird. I felt like I didn't belong. A coworker told me that she felt the same way. We were used to being in bland, one-color surroundings. It was dry and sandy there. There was not a lot of color. You get home, and you feel overwhelmed with your surroundings. There are crowds and everyone is so busy. It is noisy, and there are all these colors around you. It was easier over there. You just get up and go to work and maybe work out at the gym and just do the same thing the next day. You have everything set up so that things back home are taken care of. Over there, you are only responsible for yourself. You do your job and maintain your health and safety. You get into a routine. Food is provided for you. It is simple. To be honest, it almost felt like a break from my regular, busy life. It felt like a different kind of vacation from the busy world.

Eliza described an air force gathering she attended the summer after returning from her last deployment.

> I got together this past summer with some friends who had also deployed with me. We shared our experiences about working with people who had never deployed. We compared notes about how some people talk about war, having never experienced it first hand, and how some of their comments grate on your nerves. Basically, they just don't get it. What they say can make you irate and bitter. Fortunately, there are enough of us who deployed, and we can talk to each other because there are a great number of people who simply do not understand.
>
> I have never been a person with a temper, but I must say that it has probably gotten a little shorter after having several deployments.

Eliza went further to mention how her collective group of previously deployed colleagues related experiences of having to deal with military personnel who had never deployed. They told of coworkers who belly-ached over weekend and holiday schedules, complained vehemently over patient assignments in the hospital, bitched about their lives in general when it came to household chores, child care, and paying bills. Many turned out to be an unhappy crew in general. Eliza believes that her deployed friends seem to have a greater appreciation for their lives once they settled in and reintegrated.

CAPTAIN AMANDA

Amanda was a captain in the Air Force Reserve, who was deployed to Afghanistan. She reported:

> My biggest hurdle when I got home from Germany was definitely going back to work. I went back to my job at an urban medical center in Boston. It was the new year of 2011 and I worked in the emergency department. It's the busiest Level I trauma center in the area. We are so busy. It is a nightmare [*laughing*]. I went back there, and I started having trouble with the patient population. They were entitled. They were thugs, they were shot for no good reason. They'd come into the trauma room bitching because they were shot with a 22 (caliber handgun) and it was lodged in their fat. It didn't even injure a major organ, and they were crying for their mother and hitting nurses. They were the rudest people you would ever meet in your life. I couldn't stand them. They just didn't seem important. These patients were not important to me, and it was hard.
>
> The staff was appreciative of my service to our country initially. They were happy that I was back. I was on leave for the holidays. I'm sure they were happy to have me back. They were appreciative at the beginning. People always have the weirdest questions. I came back from Afghanistan this year and I got the same weird questions again. Like: "What was the worst thing you saw?" I thought to myself, "You would not want to know." Why would they get into that? I'm back at work, why would I want to talk to you about that. It would be hurtful; it wouldn't be therapeutic at all. People really do ask some very inappropriate questions when you come back. The staff was OK. I went right back on the trauma team, and I was right back in the thick of it. I hated my job. I usually did 12-hour shifts either day or night, and I had to go down to 8 hours because I couldn't stand my job and that was after Germany. It was the patient population. It was not my coworkers. When I was gone, my coworkers sent me CARE (items sent

to show you care) packages and gifts. They didn't forget about me. They were extremely supportive. I am probably the only person that they know from Massachusetts who was deployed. What turned me off was the entitled population who got free medical care and expected you to treat them like a massive trauma when they are not. The patients could be petty, especially the frequent flyers who made regular visits to the ER. They had multiple somatic complaints, which changed from morning to afternoon and usually escalated at night. They often wasted your time with their trivial whining, and I must say that my tolerance for this behavior grew slim after my deployment. I couldn't help but compare my experiences with severely injured soldiers who were more concerned about their injured buddies than themselves and these malingerers who almost occupied a permanent place in the ER.

CAPTAIN EARL

Earl was an Air Force Reserve flight nurse who deployed to Iraq and Afghanistan.

Earl shared:

One of the things that I was acutely aware of when I finally came home was that I had like zero tolerance for people bellyaching about minutiae. I had just come from an exhausting and life-changing experience of serving in war, and people bitching about little inconveniences like traffic jams, or having to stand in a long line at the store, just set me off. I could literally feel my blood pressure rising when I had to listen to this crap. I kept myself from saying anything, and possibly getting in a fistfight, but it was hard to keep my mouth shut.

FIRST LIEUTENANT RHETTA

When Rhetta, an army nurse, returned home from Iraq, she was surprised how oblivious some people seemed to be with what was going on across the world in Iraq and Afghanistan.

She related:

I could sense that people in my rural community wondered why I began my nursing career in the army. It dawned on me that people were so wrapped up in their own little worlds that they could not relate at all to my decision to leave rural Montana. Literally, they thought I belonged on a farm or ranch, not in a war! Things they would say bothered me, always hinting that I should settle down, get married, and have a slew of kids. Some inferred that it was OK for boys to go off to war, but not girls. People were so caught up in small-town politics, the local 4-H club, the county fair and the church supper, who was marrying who, and who was having a baby. I felt that many of my parents' friends simply had their heads buried in the sand. No one seemed to look at the bigger picture of what was going on in the world. This frustrated me to no end. My parents were quietly supportive, but seemed to make excuses for others caught up in local events. I simply could not get excited about the new super-market or the prize-winning apple pie recipe. Basically, I don't think I ever want to live permanently in rural Montana again.

10

Military Unit or Civilian Job: Support Versus Lack of Support

Some nurses were welcomed back with coworkers listening to their stories with empathy, interest, and compassion. A few told how their leadership, both military and civilian, eased them back into the work schedule. A navy nurse remembered how she found solace in talking to people at her base who had also been deployed. She told how they shared their experiences which helped them form a bond. Conversely, some nurses felt ignored by coworkers and abandoned by their leadership. They believed that coworkers expected them to jump right in at work, without needing time to process things and transition back into a stateside work setting. They felt rushed, misunderstood, and pressured to keep up with everyone else. Some vented their frustration and explained that their deployment nursing position was completely different from their stateside one. This was especially true for the nurses who were part of a provincial reconstruction team. It also took the primary health care providers such as nurse-practitioners and nurse-midwives a little time to get back in the groove of seeing patients in a clinic setting after they had done a different mission during deployment.

LIEUTENANT COLONEL TONI

Toni was a Critical Care Air Transport Team (CCATT) nurse who had been deployed to Iraq and Afghanistan. She outlined the predicament of many reservists.

175

She stated:

> For reservists, there are really no resources available for us. When you get home, you are really on your own. The active duty people return to their base, in-process, and are offered mental health counseling. Then, they get 30 days of leave before returning to work. They have resource people who check on them to make sure they are doing OK. On the other hand, reservists have no paid leave; so, most of us return to our civilian jobs a lot sooner than 30 days. We have to hit the ground running because it is like we never left. There are no resources to follow up on a regular basis.

Toni related a vivid example:

> I know a pilot who committed suicide. His wife found him. His friends said he seemed fine, and he looked fine, but he committed suicide. There was no one to follow up with him, and I have to believe that following up can make a difference. He was flying C-17 missions with the back of his plane filled with wounded soldiers. This guy was hurting, and no one knew it. People don't know that having PTSD [posttraumatic stress disorder] is the "new normal" if you served in these wars. It is a normal reaction to an abnormal reality.

Toni described how her civilian colleagues at her hospital were helpful when she returned from deployment:

> My colleagues in the trauma ICU were supportive. They wanted to know what I did, how it went, what I saw, and to hear about the experiences I had. It was helpful to speak of it. I think the more people hear about our experiences over there, the more they can understand why some of us come back with PTSD or compassion fatigue. One thing that bothers me is when people tell me I'm a "hero." I'm not a hero, I did what was important to me and what feels good to me. I'm serving my country in the best way I can. It takes an army of people to save one life. It wasn't just me, it was the pilots that flew the air evacuation plane, the troops working on the flight line to maintain that plane, the medics who carefully load and unload precious human cargo, to the guy refueling the plane, to the communications and admin people reporting the patients who need to be transported. The whole hospital welcomed me back. The new unit I worked on had some wonderful nurses who welcomed me, too.

Toni described her homecoming to her reserve unit:

My colleagues at the base welcomed me back. Many of those folks had deployed before, so they understood. I drill out of an Air Force Base in California. I'm in one of the squadrons there. But, I was asked to start in a new unit there where I didn't know any-one. I felt cheated that I couldn't go back to my old unit. I needed time to recuperate and rejuvenate, and by sending me to a new unit there was no time for that. I thought it would be better to let me return to my old unit and then 4 or 5 months down the road I could get transferred to the new unit. It was too much change too fast. Things worked out OK in the long run, but it would have been better if I had some say in the transition. I felt very respected at my Reserve base. A lot of good reports came back to the wing headquarters about how well our CCATT team did in Afghanistan.

LIEUTENANT COLONEL CHRISTA

Christa, an air force reservist, described her return to work.
    She stated:

I was off for about a month before I went back to work at the hospi-tal. Some people were so happy to see me and they thanked me for my service. Some other people were not very friendly at all, and they took my job away from me, or rather, parts of my job away from me with no real explanation. So, it was pretty tough going back to my civilian job. Then I got my most recent performance evaluation, and they had downgraded my proficiency rating. They put on there that I had been gone for over 6 months from the job, so that is why they downgraded me. I went back in my records, and I saw that they had done the same thing when I deployed the first time. So, it was not a very nice "welcome home" in my civilian job. Now, my friends at the hospital were great, it was just the administrative side that was really bad. Other nurses, the logistics folks, the pharmacy guys, and everyone else, not in nursing administration were great.
    On my first UTA [Unit Training Assembly] back, it was busi-ness as usual. There was nothing special about us having been gone, and there were 60 of us that deployed, which was half of our unit. We didn't have the "yellow ribbon" program back then. That is when the people who were deployed get some time set aside on drill weekends where they can spend time together,

sort of debrief and reflect on what you have just been through. Unfortunately, we didn't have that. We didn't have any time to talk with each other, to just chill out with each other.

Christa went on to explain how she and her deployed colleagues found time to talk. She stated:

One thing that did happen was we got a short field exercise deployment to Kuan-Ju in Korea, and we moved some of our ASTS [Aeromedical Staging Transportation Squadron] equipment over there. We met up with a unit from Luke AFB, Arizona, in Korea. It was an awesome short deployment because we finally had time to chill out, catch up, and debrief each other and just spend time together and rekindle the camaraderie we had. We needed that so much. But it took a year before we could get together as a group.

The leadership from my reserve unit did not deploy to Iraq. I went as the chief nurse and one of our medical services officers (MSCs) was made commander of our unit when we deployed. We both led our unit in Iraq. He was pretty inexperienced and did not always include me in the decision making, even though I had years of administrative experience and he had practically none. However, I found ways to stay informed and work around the fact that he [commander] did not always keep me in the loop. For example, I became very good friends with the chief nurse of the air evac unit and her flight nurses. Her call sign was "Mother Goose." She kept me informed about missions, equipment, and any other things going on. When my commander made up his organizational chart for our deployed unit, he did not even include me [the chief nurse] on the organizational chart. Our Med Group Command above saw what was going on, and they realized that I was the one that should be running the place rather than him [the MSC commander]. It went full circle, because when something needed to be done, the Med Group Command began contacting me instead of him. They respected me and knew I was results oriented.

LIEUTENANT KATE

Kate was a navy nurse who was deployed to Afghanistan.
She reported:

When I came back from Afghanistan my work life at Portsmouth was OK. There was new leadership at the top. I had asked for a couple of things when I returned to work. When I left for Afghanistan I had been the charge nurse of the ER. When I came back, I asked for an orientation and did not want to just jump in and be in charge again. They said that wasn't allowed. So, I had to jump right back into the thick of it. It was difficult for me because my coping skills were not up to what they should be to assume the charge role again. All my staff was new except for the civilian RNs I worked with. It was really hard to go back without an orientation since a lot had changed in a year. I didn't know who any of the military people were, so there was a lot to being in charge again.

I took 30 days of leave when I first got home. That was when my husband and I were having adjustment problems. When I went back to work, the new leadership was pretty poor. They didn't know who I was or what I had done there in the time before I left to deploy. They hadn't had the experience of helping people reintegrate after a deployment to a war zone. So, a lot of things weren't very supportive.

When I compare my homecoming to the way the hospital does things now, it is like night and day. Now, we all go to meet the people coming back from deployment at the airport. The hospital commander or the executive officer, the director of nursing services, the other key leaders make it a point to go to the airport to welcome everyone home. It doesn't matter what time of day or night a flight comes in, they all make it a point to be there to greet all returning hospital personnel. Everyone is so supportive, so caring, and so available. We all pride ourselves on being there and available to meet every single flight. Everyone reaches out to the returning medics and their families, if they have families. We do everything that we can to ensure that they have everything that they need.

It is the opposite of what I experienced when I came home. When I came back the leadership had changed and no one knew who I was or even that I had deployed. I was glad to leave Portsmouth Naval Medical Center to go to Guam because I really didn't feel like I belonged there anymore because I had been there for 3 years before I deployed and I was treated like I didn't count when I came back from Afghanistan. I felt I was "out of sight, out of mind" while I was gone. I think because of the change in leadership, people returning from deployment were lost in the shuffle of the comings and goings of a big medical center.

LIEUTENANT COMMANDER KATHLEEN

Kathleen, a navy nurse, reported:

> It was good coming back to the same unit. They were very sup-
> portive while I was gone. They sent me stuff, and e-mailed me all
> the time, and sent care packages and cards. I really felt appreciated
> and missed. Now, the students look at me differently, I have the
> credibility and respect for having been in a war zone on a com-
> bat hospital tour. All the students were wide-eyed and wanted to
> hear my stories. Through counseling I learned that I have a different
> memory bank now, and at times I have to remind myself that I'm
> not there anymore. I have a picture of every patient we took care of
> on a thumb drive, but I don't even know where the thumb drive is.
> I know it is around somewhere in the house, but I don't feel any ur-
> gency to go look at it. Most of the photos were taken by the trauma
> photographer and was given to us in case we wanted to do research
> or write clinical papers. I haven't looked at it since I got back, and I
> don't even know where it is. It is around somewhere in one of my
> boxes. I even have a picture on there of me with Prince Charles
> when he visited the hospital. Most things are in my head, the memo-
> ries, I don't need to go back through stuff from 3 years ago.

LIEUTENANT LORETTA

Loretta is a navy operating room nurse.
She reported:

> I really didn't know anyone back at the hospital, and I had dif-
> ficulty trusting people. So, I didn't know anyone or what their
> motives were. I had already been in a shutdown mode. I wasn't
> gonna open up to anybody. So, I didn't really have a whole lot
> of friends when I came back. The nature of the military is that
> you always have friends leaving. It was hard. There's definitely
> a difference talking to someone in person as opposed to on the
> phone, even if you are saying the same things. I didn't have much
> of a support system. You have a few days off when you get back
> and then you have to check in to the command. So, even though
> you are staying at the same place, they make you go through this
> process of checking out and checking back in. Then, you don't
> have to be back at work for 2 weeks. All in all, I got roughly
> 2 weeks before I had to be back at work, unless I wanted to take

leave and go on vacation. I was trying to coordinate my schedule with my boyfriend's schedule so, I really didn't take leave until I was back for 2 months. I was pretty much right back at work.

LIEUTENANT COLONEL JULIE

Julie, an air force reserve flight nurse and CCATT nurse, described the lack of support she experienced at her civilian hospital.
She stated:

> I was angry at the facility to begin with, because when I came back I found out that I had been demoted. I was no longer in an assistant nurse manager role. When I returned to work after my deployment, they said they had to move me out of that role because they said they couldn't count on me to be there all the time that I might be deployed again. They were afraid I'd be deployed again. They put me back to being a staff nurse. It was a decrease in pay, and I did not have as much say or control of my schedule as I did as an assistant nurse manager, and I had to pull a whole lot more call.
>
> So I was penalized for being in the air force reserve, and I was in a sense punished for being deployed. This type of situation is not that uncommon for reservists. Some of us come back to our civilian job and are treated this way by our civilian employers. I was just very put off by the lack of support of my medical facility when I returned from Iraq. My friends at work were there for me, but I was just kind of amazed that the leadership was not. I didn't talk about what it was like in Iraq because these people had no frame of reference. They just wouldn't have understood how we had to live and work over there. Truly, I believe only military folks can understand this stuff and empathize, most civilians in my opinion don't have a clue. But my friends were glad to have me home and safe on U.S. soil.

LIEUTENANT COLONEL TAMMY

Tammy, an Air National Guard nurse, described her return to her civilian job after returning from Afghanistan.
She stated:

> I was teaching at a college before I left. I was granted a leave of absence, and I returned to that position when I came home. I was

on active duty orders for a month after returning, and it was mandatory that I didn't work so I had the time to reintegrate with my family. When I returned to work it went OK. I received some honors as well as having some misunderstandings with people I worked with. Some of my peers didn't understand the military at all, and they didn't really understand what I was doing in a mentoring role over there. I did do a presentation for faculty, and that was an eye opener for some of them. I was given some honors for my service to our country. Some of my peers had friends or relatives in the military, and those peers said they were proud of what we did over there. I shared with them pictures of me in military gear and various uniforms, because they only see me on a regular basis when I'm at the college teaching students in my professor attire, or my clinical attire when I'm teaching students in clinical.

Tammy continued to describe some of the misunderstandings and obstacles she encountered in her work environment when she returned from deployment. She reported:

Some of the misunderstandings actually started before I even left. A few other faculty members questioned me about Why would I want to do this? Why would I want to leave? Did I volunteer for this? I responded by saying, I volunteered to be in the military. They just didn't understand why I would want to put myself in harm's way, and why I would want to leave here to go to a war zone. I believe some of them are very connected to what they do at the college, and they don't see the big picture of what is going on in the world. I see the big picture, and have been in the military for 20 years. They thought, Why would someone leave us "short" to go to a war zone? They only saw how it might inconvenience them, not the benefit of serving our country.

Another thing that happened was that the college kept paying me while I was gone. I did not know that because it was direct deposit into my stateside bank account. I wasn't told that I would be paid, but I wasn't told that I wouldn't be paid either. I had heard that some employers continue to pay people while deployed. I didn't know what was going on. My husband handles all the finances, so he didn't know what to expect. When I got home, right away I was asked to pay the money back. They wanted me to pay them back before I returned to work. That was kind of hard to take. I told them I would pay it back, but I couldn't pay it back in a lump sum. Then, I found out I accrued vacation time while I was gone, and I get paid during vacation, so I had to forfeit the vacation time. It would have just been good if all of this was communicated to me ahead of time rather than messing it up and having to straighten it out when I got back. It was irritating, and made my reintegration a little less pleasant. I think the human resources people at the college should have briefed me on the pay and vacation issues before I left.

Tammy described how some people relate to her differently since she returned from deployment. She reported:

I think I get more respect for who I am since I returned. I still feel that some people are envious or jealous, or maybe more competitive. More people seem to want to do foreign travel in terms of humanitarian projects. That's not a bad thing because that will expand their horizons and provide help to others. Some people feel that they have to justify who they are to me by saying things like, "I wish I could have joined the military, but I have three small kids," or "I wish I could join now, but I'm too old, or I have elderly parents." It is interesting to hear what people have to say to me.

I think it is important that nurses experience other cultures when they have the opportunity. I learned a lot about the Afghan culture while I was over there. One important point was not to assume that things mean the same in their culture as they do in our culture. Don't assume that things have the same value. What is nursing there versus here in the U.S.? What are the basic human needs there as opposed to here? Traffic lanes are nonexistent there and they don't have sidewalks. They don't have flush toilets and toilet paper. Feeding yourself and showering is different. People don't frequently shower over there and water is scarce. Drinking water is sometimes hard to come by. Shoes don't fit, clothing is different. The male roles are very dominant. Women are silent. The rules about touching and who you can touch are different. Facial expressions and body gestures are different. How they teach, and how they learn is different. Girls don't go to school over there. If there is a girls' school, it will probably be blown up. The girls are like people who have been starved. Now, they want to learn so much; they want more and more. They are so eager to learn. They can't get enough. They want to hear everything you have to say. They don't have books in their language. To take an individualized exam was a whole new thing for them. They have a different view of cheating; to them it is just helping your brother or sister out.

Tammy admitted that she felt a lack of support from her National Guard unit when she returned from Afghanistan:

> Reintegration into my Air National Guard unit was my major trouble spot. Well, before I left I was the chief nurse of my unit. While I was gone I think there was a whole lot of negativity towards me. I was replaced in my unit by another chief nurse. I would get regular e-mails from the new chief nurse asking me to do this or that. I couldn't do everything they asked because I was in a very austere environment. I was tasked with writing OERs [officer effectiveness reports] on people who used to work for me, and I don't think that was right or fitting to require that of me while I was deployed. I did what I could, but I didn't have the resources available to me to do everything they asked. When I returned we had a new commander. I was basically told I was not needed. I was also questioned on why I had not done a report, and I had proof that I had done it. I have not changed units. I have stood my ground, and I have filed complaints. I'm going to ride it out. Another guy in my unit who had deployed before me said this was not at all uncommon. He was gone for a year, and he basically said they had forgotten about him. I was horrified that people in my unit did this. It took me totally by surprise. The low point of coming home was the way my unit treated me. It was completely unexpected and very, very disheartening.

LIEUTENANT COLONEL REGINA

Regina, an Army Reserve lieutenant colonel who had been deployed to Ramadi, Iraq, as the military senior officer on a Provisional Reconstruction Team (PRT) described how she generally felt supported by the Army Reserve when she returned home from Iraq.

She stated:

> The army transferred me to the reserve brigade headquarters in New York. I had just come back from Iraq, and I really didn't have any peers at the headquarters who had also just come back from Iraq. It was challenging, and it was lonely, but I spent all

that time in Iraq, and I just trusted myself that I would be able to maneuver through this. I had a lot of scary experiences in Iraq, but I tried to see them as challenging rather than scary. I didn't go to Iraq as a young nurse. I went to Iraq as a lieutenant colonel. You are in a world of men, and they are highly competitive, and everyone is trying to do their best, get ahead, and make everyone proud of them at home. If you are scared, you hold that inside, you don't really show that side. I learned a lot in Iraq, and the skills that I learned there I brought home with me. I just tried to be confident, to be positive, and to demonstrate that I was a worthwhile team player, who also just happened to be a woman and a lieutenant colonel. I wanted to get my final promotion to full colonel; so, I worked very hard, and it paid off.

After my promotion to full colonel, I really didn't have a position in the reserves, so I invented one as a war-training consultant for the Army Reserve nurses. Then, I got selected for active duty again. I went to Little Rock, Arkansas, and it was a really good assignment. I had a lot of credibility with our troops there because I was a senior Nurse Corps officer who had spent considerable time in Iraq. I didn't feel alone any more. I had lots of people to teach, and I didn't feel or go through the disengagement that many reservists go through when they come home because I was back on active duty again. We were assigned to training teams because a lot of people were being deployed from there to Iraq and Afghanistan. There was a lot of work to do, and we were inspired to prepare our troops as best we could. It was a soldier readiness processing (SRP) center. We had an SRP team of a physician, a nurse, and a personal affairs officer. The nurse served in a case manager type of position. We served people who were deploying as well as those returning from deployment. It made an amazing difference for these soldiers to talk to someone who had been there. I felt that I made a very valuable contribution on the SRP. I was back on active duty doing this case management job for 2 years. It was very gratifying to make this kind of difference for the troops going over and the troops coming back. I made many referrals and followed up to ensure things were in place for the troops I managed coming home. I was valued for my rank. I was valued for my knowledge. I was valued for my caring and thoroughness. It was a really good experience for me personally as well as professionally. It was a very positive way to end my army career. I felt very supported and valued.

LIEUTENANT COMMANDER CATHERINE

Catherine, a navy family nurse practitioner, had served as a Nurse Corps officer and a member of a provincial reconstruction team.

She talked about returning to work:

When I got back to the hospital, one of the things that was most helpful in terms of workplace reintegration was that other people at the hospital had done the first deployment with me to Fallujah, Iraq. They were from my hospital, so we had gone through some of the same or similar experiences. Having that handful of people around that knew what you knew and had seen what you had seen and who had gone through those experiences was very helpful. It was immensely helpful to have that connection with people. Of course, that wasn't true of everyone who had gone to Fallujah. Some were just one-on-one from a hospital. I can't imagine what it must have been like to go back to their workplaces and try to explain what Fallujah was like. I felt like I had a support system. I'm social when I talk to people, that's how I work things through. I just keep talking about things. I talk about things until I don't need to talk anymore. I think having people around to talk to about my experience was so helpful.

In Afghanistan, I was on a provincial reconstruction team so I was not taking care of patients. So when I went back to work as a family nurse practitioner, there was no way I could see patients at 20-minute intervals as a clinician when I had not cared for patients on diabetic medications or hypertension meds for the last 13 months. It just wasn't my world. So, I knew that it would take me some time to become productive clinically, in terms of clinical output and productivity. I would say that my command was pretty receptive to that. I wasn't gonna let anyone push me around either. I also have been a strong advocate for other people coming back when that hasn't been the case.

Catherine shared her feelings:

I think the expectation as medical personnel, not just nurses, but doctors and corpsmen, too, is to come back and instantly resume their work as if they had never gone anywhere is just ridiculous. It's ridiculous, insensitive, and reflects a complete lack of understanding as to what that deployed person has been through and their readiness to assume their duties. I have been very, very sensitive and a huge vocal advocate and proponent of "let the deployer tell you when they are ready and the pace at which they are ready to resume work." Trust that they know and don't assume anything. You got to have that dialogue and let them set the pace.

It can be hard because you've been gone, you have left a gap, and the work hasn't gone away. So, a lot of times there's this expectation with the hopefulness like as soon as they get back we can put them on the call schedule. You are just another warm body to see the patients and get the work done. You are someone to share the work that maybe other people had to double-up on, but you may not be ready to do the work. It just takes sensitivity, but I can't say we are universally good at that. After 10, 11, 12 years of this, I don't know that we are really good at it. I think a lot of it is leadership-dependent.

There are lots of different variables—tons of them. I don't think there is a one size fits all. I am a factor, my family is a factor, the environment is a factor, and the deployment experience is a factor. There are so many variables that are gonna affect the reintegration experience, what you know, what you expect, what your expectations were. I think for me, resolving some of the issues and by resolving, I mean accepting deployment experiences as part of my life story. You are ever changed by the things you saw and did. You don't forget about these things or your experience. For me, putting it in a place where it makes sense is probably the best way for me to think about my reintegration experience. For me, I'm my own best advocate because I know me and I'm not shy about expressing my own needs. I extend that to advocating for others in my professional and clinical roles as well as in my leadership roles. I'm a director at a medical center. I have a huge directorate with primary health care and the branch health clinics. So, my directorate is 1,500 people and we have people deploying. I talk to them before and after they go. I want to make sure they are whole and well and that they know from the top down that I'm gonna meet their needs. That is something that we just have to be sensitive about.

CAPTAIN SCHUYLER

Schuyler, who separated from the army after being on active duty for 4 years, talked about doing nursing after deployment.

She recalled:

Now, I realize that the nurses I am working with have no idea
what kind of health care I was doing either in Germany or while
I was deployed in Iraq. They don't understand and wouldn't even
be able to fathom it. It was so different; it was on a totally different plane. Sometimes it's frustrating because I do want to talk
about it, but when I do talk about it, it can sometimes come across
as bragging or that I'm trying to outdo someone. This happens
among my nonmilitary nurse friends in civilian health care. I don't
want people to think that all I talk about is my time in the service.
But I also want people to understand what I saw and what I did.
This was even stronger when I got out of the military for the first
couple of months with my first job. I really wanted to tell people.

I would share my experiences if the time was right. Now,
there's more time between my deployment and the present. If I
talk about it a lot now, people will think that I have not moved
on. They'll think, "She's stuck in that time frame" [*laughing*].
But in some ways it feels like only last year. I don't feel like it's
almost 7 years since I was there. It was a very significant time
and a very meaningful time and place because my husband and
I met there and our relationship grew there.

I tell my brother, "I was really glad that I went to war, I
would not have met my husband if I didn't go to Iraq" [*laughing*]. And, it's really weird to say that I'm glad I went to war
[*laughing*]. But I had a really good experience. Not everything
was good. But the majority of my memories are good because of
meeting my husband.

As a nurse, I feel proud of what I did there. It's hard to balance things, and I'm not stuck in that time, and I'm not bragging
about my service either. I don't want people to label me.

LIEUTENANT COMMANDER JUSTIN

Justin, a navy reservist, described his return to his reserve unit.
He stated:

I would say that my unit had no concept of what the hell they
are doing as far as reintegration is concerned. I had some injuries, and I'm still negotiating with the navy to get my injuries
dealt with. They feel absolutely no sense of urgency and have no

concept of timely care when it comes to reservists. I have a fair amount of frustration with my military unit. I still go to reserve drill one weekend a month because I can't do much because I'm in pain 24/7. My civilian health insurance that I get through my civilian job as a CRNA [certified registered nurse anesthetist] says that my injuries were incurred when I was on active duty in the military, so the military has to provide the care I need. I've been to the navy and VA [Veterans Administration] medical facilities, and they can't seem to make a decision as to who is responsible for my postdeployment care.

I think a lot of money has been spent on reintegration of combat troops and rightly so, but I don't think enough money or effort has been spent on the "support" troops like us health care professionals and reservists. I have run into lots of health care professionals who have not successfully reintegrated. We see people at their absolute worst day after day. The trauma comes to us every single day over there. We are much more saturated with the blood and wounds of war than the average combat troop. They may have to live with more danger over there, but we have to live with the burns, traumatic amputations, dead babies, and carnage of the war every single day. I held the hands of Afghan children when they died. I am haunted by their faces. I went as an individual augmentee, so I came home alone. People who deployed with a unit came home with their unit. I had to leave the people I lived and worked with for a year, and get on a plane and go home alone. I felt stripped of my deployment family. I had to go it alone. It was a rude awakening after a year with my brothers and sisters in Kabul, and now we had to head in all different directions and on different flights home. I think the military is failing many of our reservists when they come home. Not much is set up to help them, and they don't live on a base where help activities are in place.

Justin reported that his civilian workplace was helpful in trying to facilitate his reintegration:

My civilian job has actually been pretty good at helping me reintegrate. The chief nurse anesthetist met with me shortly after I got back and wanted to know about my experiences and how I was doing. He basically said we are all here for you and whatever you need just let us know. They have given me days off to go to doctors' appointments and CAT scans. I feel like my civilian employer has given me more than they need to. My family got health care through my employer while I was gone, and they were under no obligation to do that.

LIEUTENANT DARLA

Darla is a navy operating room nurse who was deployed to Kandahar, Afghanistan.

She stated:

My military community was very supportive when I got back. Many people from the hospital met our flight. They had a nice welcome home reception for us. They gave us more than ample time to process back into the base and hospital. We had many leave options available to us. My OR manager was very helpful and supportive, as was the senior management and my peers. After I left active duty, my reserve unit was in charge of the deployment transition program so my OIC [officer in charge] would check up on me all the time. Later, I became the resource officer so I would help people and families get the information they needed before, during, or after a deployment. I tried to keep track of people and their families while they were gone. We tried to provide a lot of the same services and information to reserve families that the active duty facilities provided for active duty families.

All in all, you get roughly 2 weeks before you have to be back at work. I was trying to coordinate my schedule with my boyfriend's schedule. So, I really didn't take leave until I was back for 2 months. I was pretty much right back at work. You feel like you don't have the same purpose with work. You are serving a purpose, but you view your purpose in Afghanistan as more important. You feel like what you were doing before had so much more meaning than what you are doing now. It's harder to be tolerant of all the idiosyncrasies and the trivialities of people. You have to remember that everyone's perceptions are different. The general lack of realization from the general public of what we do and that we are still over there doing it.

I don't know if people are aware enough of what is going on over there. People just don't think about the fact that we have troops over there. But when you come back, it's like, "So what's up?" People know that there is a war going on and that we have troops over there, but they think collectively, not about the individuals. Life continues to be pretty normal for most of the American people, so why shouldn't it be for you when you come back. They just don't realize what you saw and what you did.

CAPTAIN COURTNEY

Courtney is an Air Force Reserve officer.
She stated:

Work was a little different though. My best friend advised me to visit my previous workplace before I was set to work to get my computer passwords, etc. I went in and saw my boss and she told me that I looked like "a deer caught in the headlights." I actually felt like it too. I hadn't done anything but trauma in so long. So what she did was to put me as the "float nurse" who does trauma and helps other nurses in the ER. She did that for about a week and then she'd break up my assignment, giving me 4 hours with patients, 4 hours in triage, and 4 hours on float. She actually broke me in slowly even though I had been there for so long, mostly as triage or charge. I love my boss. I rarely get an assignment anymore. I've been there since 2002 and the burnout in the ER is about 3 years. They don't stay. But there is a group of us who have been there for a long time. The ones who have been there longer than me are ready to retire. I really think I need to do something else because I don't want to end up a 65-year-old ER nurse. I tried to do visiting nurse, and I just don't know.

Everyone at my facility was extremely supportive of what I did with my deployment, especially the female docs saying, "I can't believe what you did, that's awesome. I would never be able to do that." And I tell them, "You'd love it." But the whole separation thing is hard. I loved the clinical part. The army looked at me like I had horns. There's all these guys. I'm a "nursey-nurse"—I like holding hands, telling the patients to look at me, telling them "there's a lot going on right now but we're gonna get through this." I'd talk them through things. Some of the army people had never seen anything like this before and they were stunned. But, that's what we do. I know the army guys are big and strong but when someone just got his leg blown off, he's not feeling so big and strong. You have to be there for that part. I feel like I taught them something, too. They gave me a lot of respect. I had more trauma experience than anyone there. On December 2 when we got attacked, I was running my own trauma table because we had so many wounded. It was really a good experience for me as a nurse.

CAPTAIN EARL

Earl, an air force reservist, talked about his reintegration to the workplace. He reported:

Prior to being mobilized, I was just dabbling with the idea of becoming a fire fighter. I had worked as a nurse in the ER. I was a paramedic nurse educator for my department in the hospital. I got to occasionally ride along with fire fighters. I would teach classes with the paramedics, and I had a really good relationship with the fire department. People would tell me that I'd be the perfect person to work with the fire department and they encouraged me to become a firefighter. So I tried it out with a small town fire department, and I was still working as an agency nurse part time. I started out with that fire department, and it wasn't even a year till I got mobilized.

So when I came back, my last day of practice as a nurse was July 23, 2003. It was my last combat mission. When I came back from deployment, I didn't want anything to do with nursing. I went back to the small town fire dept. It was a bed and breakfast community with white picket fences. We did things like help people get their keys out of locked cars and get cats out of trees. The small town politics was boring. Everyone knew each other. I couldn't get out of there fast enough. Yet, this is another aspect of deployment. I had this need for an adrenaline fix. I interviewed for a job in a neighboring town's fire dept. This is where I work now. It is the biggest fire department in our county and has the most fires. It is the third largest fire department in the state of Washington. It is an aggressive fire department with a lot of action. I work there now, and I must say that going to fires as well as taking care of people who are in car accidents on the freeway fulfills my need for that adrenaline fix. I also do other things that help with the adrenaline need. I went and got my pilot's license for helicopters. But, I also got my commercial rating, instructor rating, and I teach other people how to fly helicopters. At first, I didn't realize that this was tied into my need for adrenaline. I actually fly rescue missions now. That's what I am doing this weekend. I'm "on-call" for the rescue helicopter, Search & Rescue. It's something I do one weekend a month, I volunteer for the county. For me, it's a commitment away from my family. It's reminiscent of military life.

The small town I was working for in the fire department was right next to Fort Lewis, Washington. They bent over backwards to help me. They made sure I had some time off from work before starting back after deployment. They let me adjust my work schedule. I talked to the fire chief, and I admitted that I needed some time to adjust from being back from war. That guy was phenomenal. They were great. When I went to the bigger fire department, I confided in a few people and they became my internal support system in the new job. I kept my mouth shut, too, being a probational employee because they can fire you at any time.

LIEUTENANT COLONEL DAGMAR

Dagmar is an air force reservist with many years of experience, including 13 deployments.
She stated:

I'm in the Air National Guard; so, when I go on active duty I'm in the air force. I live in California, and I'm a flight nurse. I have had many deployments, but some have been very short. My deployments have included Afghanistan, Iraq, Qatar, Kurdistan, and numerous flying assignments out of Ramstein Air Base in Germany. I have been flight medical crew, clinical flight coordinator, chief nurse, Air Evacuation Command Staff, Flight Detachment Commander, and have been in a special operations role at times.

Sometimes I feel like I have two full-time jobs, my civilian job and my air force job. Other times, it's one or the other. I work at the VA in the greater LA area. I worked at the VA Hospital in LA till a year and a few months ago. Now, I work outpatient primary care at a VA outpatient clinic in a different facility across town.

Actually people assume that the VA is very supportive of people like myself who deploy frequently. However, they are one of the worst. I have had a lot of problems. They didn't understand what I was doing and why I was doing it. People asked me why I didn't just quit the military. It kind of becomes a self-perpetuating thing, the more you deploy, the more there are expectations, and they need experienced people. Then when you come home it's hard to settle back and do your regular job. You kind of still want to be back in the war and the opportunity is presented and if somebody is asking me and telling me that we have a short fall and we need someone to go to Bastion and be the detachment commander, I don't hesitate to say yes because we need it. Of course, I'll do it.

When the VA started giving me guff about it, there were times when I was treated pretty poorly, and it was very hurtful. With things that way, it was easier to go. I'm gonna go where I think the higher calling is and where I'm valued and appreciated and when I can contribute to something really important. I don't have any vendetta against the VA, but there were a lot of misunderstandings, and I had to fight for the right to serve in the military and go take care of wounded patients as ironic as that is. There were times that were like that. But to come home and fight after being away in the war, I'll just go. I'll just go away again. I'll go. I can understand their side of it, too, as an employee who is not there for whatever reason. It is still an employee who is not there. But, I tried to position myself. I even joined "the float pool." That's the least impact when I'm gone. I won't be impacting any one department and leaving them short. In the float pool, when I'm here I'll work anywhere in the hospital, I'll help you out. But when I'm gone, no one will really miss me. There were still some problems with that. I got all that straightened out. I'm still with the VA. I've been with the VA for 22 years.

Dagmar mentioned an e-mail she sent, in which she put in quotes, "just a nurse." She laughed when she said this stating:

Because people have images of nurses in safe places, maybe at the rear of the fighting in an air-conditioned hospital, doing pretty much the same things they'd be doing in a community hospital at home. I can't blame them, they had no way to relate to our nurses in combat hospitals, nurses on helicopters, nurses on medevac planes. I found it ironic that I worked for the VA and even those people didn't realize what our nurses were doing, that our nurses were often in harm's way.

People at the VA didn't even view me as a returning veteran. When you are still in the Guard or the Reserves, you don't think of yourself as a veteran because you're still in. I'm still engaged in military service. I may go back to the war. I know I'll still go back. I want to stay active and involved in the war. With the VA, I was never viewed as a returning veteran, I was viewed as an employee. And this is the VA.

I fit in much better with the military than with my civilian job. You just have to take a deep breath and realize that many people don't understand all aspects of it. Eighty-eight percent of air evac is done by Guard and Reservists. There are 30+ guard and reserve air evac units. There are only four that are active duty. As an active duty nurse, you can only do air evac for a few years. Whereas in the Guard and the Reserve, you can do air evac for many years, and those are experienced people. It is also nice to be able to step in and step out of that role. It really is. It's nice to go way and do it. It's nice to be in one place for about 4 months, and then somewhere else for another 4 months. I feel like I've been able to do way more with things this way. I can be less formal with it and play less of the games that sometimes go on, the politics, etc. Wherever we have troops, air evac will follow. There are always mishaps, and we need to move patients. My kinship is with my people in the Air National Guard, the most experienced people, air evac people.

LIEUTENANT COLONEL VIOLA

Viola was a seasoned army nurse, who had served in the Green Zone medical facility in Bagdad, Iraq. Viola shared her reintegration experiences. She recalled:

The first thing when I came back was that I expected to have my old job back because I had orders for Hunter Army Airfield instead of the hospital at Fort Stewart. My orders were specific to the clinic which is near Savannah, Georgia. It's about 45 miles from Fort Stewart. But when I got back, my chief nurse had just put a different person into that position. They had replaced me with someone who was supposed to be there for the duration of my deployment and then when I came back he was supposed to go to another job, and I would resume. I had been the chief nurse at Hunter before I was deployed. When I came back that was not the plan anymore, and they wanted me to be hospital supervisor at Fort Stewart, which was the same job I had been doing in Iraq. It was not something that I was really anxious to do. I wanted to get back to my job at the clinic. I reminded my boss that I had orders specifically assigning me to the Hunter clinic and not the hospital. He still wanted me to work in the position at Fort Stewart. So, I did that from the time that I finished my postdeployment leave until I PCS'd [permanent change of station] the next summer. We lived right in the middle between the Hunter clinic and the hospital at Fort Stewart so it wasn't that I had a longer drive. I actually had suspicions that something like this might happen [*laughing*]. We lived in a little bedroom community right between the two. I think I finished my leave and was ready to start work in February, and we stayed until June. Then I PCS'd to William Beaumont in El Paso, Fort Bliss. I was there for 3 years, and then I went to Germany.

MAJOR ANITA

Anita was an air force critical care nurse who was assigned at the combat support hospital at Bagram, Afghanistan.

She stated:

Going back to work was hard because you compare it all to what you did down range, and down range you really did something incredible. You are taking care of these young guys. I mean these kids. Sometimes they'd be 18 years old. You are saving their lives and getting them back home to their loved ones. Here, at Travis AFB, I'm proud of David Grant Medical Center. We are now the flagship of the air force. We have the largest ICU, we have a cardiovascular ICU, a surgical ICU, and we do some amazing things. We see retired military, we see dependents, and we also see VA patients. Not all military installations see VA patients. There are lots of drug addicts and homeless, especially here in northern California. It is so hard to spend your 13 hours on the floor when you are so busy, and you don't get time to eat or go pee, and then you have a patient who as soon as he is discharged is gonna go right back to snorting cocaine. You get angry about that, you feel like it is a waste of your time. You worry more about them than they worry about themselves; so, sometimes it seems pointless. Those were things I had to deal with early on when I came back.

As I reflect on my anger issues, I must admit that going back to work and taking care of these patients, coming home and dealing with life have been good for me. My life is sheer perfection, and I truly have nothing to complain about. My husband and I have dual incomes, we have no kids, and we have a fabulous house. I have a husband who mops. For heaven sakes, I have it made! I don't even have pets. We like to travel, and we don't even want an animal to tie us down.

Anita continued to talk about going back to work and her anger issues stating:

It's a bit of a touchy subject, and I'm not as angry about it as I was. But when I first got back, no one ever asked me, "You doing OK? Do you feel like you need to kill yourself?" No one asked me anything. Now, I know why. At the time I didn't know why. I kept a log of the days that went by that my leadership failed to ask me how I was. For example, Day 72, no one has asked me how I'm doing. No one said, "Let's do a postdeployment screening on you, let's see if you are suicidal." No one in my air force leadership asked me how I was doing, and I was angry about that. I said, "I'm gonna sit around and wait." I also know that I have to take care of myself, and I can't rely on them. It was just the principle of the matter that no one in my chain of command asked me. I never got a postdeployment physical. Somehow or other, I fell through the cracks.

What concerned me the most was my own leadership. My nurse manager, my flight commander, not once did they ask me if I was doing OK and that's what upset me the most. I think sometimes nurses fall through the cracks because we're nurses. We're expected to do our jobs, we're expected to take care of the injured and ill. We don't get sick at the sight of blood. We clean up poop every day. If you get a little poop on you, you just go and wash it off. We clean up vomit and all kinds of secretions. With that mentality, it's almost like we can't be hurt. We're OK. I think the leadership tends to forget that we are still people. Each nurse is a person. You may have to clean up poop every single day, but there may be that one day where you can't take it anymore. You cannot take anymore poop. It could happen. I think that's why sometimes in our field it gets missed. But the questions should be asked of anyone returning from war. I kept waiting for the question. I have not been suicidal since I came back, maybe a little homicidal at times *[laughing]*. I mean mentally I was OK. I told you I did have some anger issues. It was principal to me that my leadership never once said, "Are you reintegrating OK? How you doing? Is everything at home OK? Not once did they ask."

She summarized her feelings:

I feel very passionate about being emotionless and having emotion because it was literally that black and white for me. Being in

Afghanistan in that environment, you had to have no emotion. There was one time that I let my emotions take over. This is how it works in the ICU when it came to the active duty patients; they get blown up and they are taken to the closest hospital, but they always end up at Bagram because in order to go to Germany, they have to go through Bagram. We were like the hub. When they get to Bagram, they are usually gone on a flight within 12 hours. We don't have them for very long in our ICU.

MAJOR FRED

Fred was a seasoned military nurse with many years in the Air Force Reserve, Air National Guard, and the enlisted forces as well.
He recalled:

When I got home from Iraq, I took my military leave and about 6 weeks off. The kids were back in school. It was not a big deal. I asked my wife what I needed to catch up on. I eased back into things. I took my civilian job leave, too. I went back to work part time. Things had gotten so much worse at the hospital. My wife who has no college education what-so-ever was making three times what I was making. I was working about 3 weeks and I walked into work one morning and they asked me to do something that I didn't think was safe and I voiced my opinion and they said, "You can either do it or you can move on." And I said, "Do you want me to stay and take care of these patients or do you want me to leave immediately?" And I was told to leave immediately. So, I walked right out the door. Later, I called a nurse who I knew at the other hospital nearby who used to work with me and I asked her if they had any openings and she asked me "What are you looking for?" I told her I was looking for a "PRN position." So, I started working at the other hospital after our family vacation. The head nurse at my new job was very accommodating. She knew that I had been a critical care nurse for 20 years. They were well staffed, and they used me appropriately with my skills.

LIEUTENANT SANDRA

Sandra was a navy trauma nurse assigned to the British-run hospital at Camp Bastion, Afghanistan. Sandra shared some details of her reintegration.

She stated:

> I knew I'd be going back to a hospital where I'd be taking care
> of about 60 patients a day in our emergency room. People
> come in with a runny nose and a sore throat compared to
> what I was taking care of in Afghanistan. It made me not
> want to go back to that job. Actually, I ended up switching
> my job 3 months later to primary care, being the clinic man-
> ager. I couldn't handle it anymore. I couldn't handle not being
> in Afghanistan, taking care of people who really needed us
> much, much more.

CAPTAIN AMANDA

Amanda was an air force reservist who primarily worked the aeromedical
staging mission in Afghanistan.

Amanda described what it was like to go back to her civilian job at a
large urban medical center:

> I went straight back to my previous job in the emergency depart-
> ment at a large medical center in Boston. I was sick about it. Sick,
> sick, sick about it. It was the same thing again, but I had such
> dread, but I knew I was moving to Georgia, so it would only be
> for a few months. I knew I had to go in at 11 p.m., and I was so
> sick about it. I cried all day and I was so nervous about going
> back into that place. I would make my husband drive around
> Boston, even out of the way, to avoid going near that place. I just
> didn't want to see that hospital. I really didn't want to go back
> there, and it wasn't easy going back there. We were moving to
> Georgia, and we had already looked at houses there. We were
> going to move to this beautiful new house that we saw when it
> was half built. I knew it was going to be fantastic. I had to work.
> I didn't want to start somewhere else for such a short time; so, I
> sucked it up and went back to work for a few months.

CAPTAIN BRITTANY

Brittany was an army critical care who frequently flew "Dustoff" medevac
missions transporting severely wounded and burned soldiers in Iraq and
Afghanistan.

She told how she was kept from resuming nursing duties because of her mental health issues when she returned from Afghanistan:

Coming back, my workplace was very exclusionary. They isolated me as I told you in an office with paperwork. I am very much a people person. I am an introvert, but I really like small groups. I thrive in that environment. I was pulled away from groups of nurses who were deployed before and at least understand that it's OK to come home feeling different. Instead, I was surrounded by leadership who didn't know what that was like. The chief nurse at my hospital told me that most nurses take 2 months to be able to go back to the floor, and that I've had 6 months so I need to get it together. I said "Yes, Ma'am." It was obvious to me that they didn't know how to take care of someone who knew they were different, who knew they weren't doing well and was actively seeking help. And to not get that help was heartbreaking. I thought about getting out of the army, but I didn't want to do that because it would put me in a world that I didn't understand. I don't understand civilian nursing. I like the military structure, the rank, and the organization of things. Part of me was afraid to get out and the other part of me was so desperate to get away from my current situation. I kept telling myself that I wasn't gonna make any decision for 6–9 months after coming home. I didn't want to make an emotional decision.

MAJOR COLLEEN

Colleen was an army medical–surgical nurse who had been deployed to Afghanistan. She described her workplace issues and experiences.
She stated:

When I got back to the post and the hospital, I kind of got shuffled around a bit because I had decided at that point that I was probably gonna go to Korea and there was some stuff going on in my unit. What ultimately happened was right before I left, our hospital commander was actually relieved of command, and he eventually went to jail and our entire unit was PCS'd [permanent change of station]. He went to jail for 13 counts of sexual assault. He had 3 months of jail, a $30,000 fine and was retired from the military. He was very high ranking and very recognizable. He had other things going on. I was a little overweight when I arrived at that unit and he didn't like me, so he held up my promotion. He would say people were fat, he would say very inappropriate things in formation. He would force people to run 12 miles. He was so crude and said disgusting things in formation. It was just horrible. He was not supposed to stay in that unit. He did not want a NATO [North Atlantic Treaty Organization] mission. Originally, we were supposed to go to Iraq, but he got one last deployment in.

I heard a story about a soldier in Afghanistan. He was having neuro issues and needed to go back to the States to get things taken care of. He was having trouble urinating because of spinal problems, well supposedly this commander told the soldier, "You are fucking pussy, if you come back here I am gonna shoot you myself and kill you." He threatened people with loaded weapons. He was a total loose cannon. He was specialty corps, which is PAs [physician's assistant] and physical therapists and had been our hospital commander.

After I got down range, I actually lost weight because I was having trouble with the food. I lost about 10–15 pounds and he came up to me and told me that I looked great. He said, "You look really good" and looked me up and down. The next day I was in the ICU and walked past the trauma bay. He was in there with one of the other PAs because he had gone for a long run in the morning. He was having trouble with his legs or something, and he called out my name and asked me to come over. He said, "Major ____ is beating up on me, and I want my nurse, I want my nurse. There you are." It has had an effect on me later, the reason I looked good to him was because I had lost some weight [*laughing*].

Colleen talked about her workplace issues and experiences after deployment when she was stationed in Korea:

I went to Korea for a year. I was officially divorced in July 2011. I had decided to go to Korea because one of my mentors was going over there. There is a large hospital in Seoul. I had a lot of friends over there. I decided that after this crazy unit, a deployment, and a divorce that I was gonna have my *Eat, Pray, Love* experience. I wanted to figure out who I was now and hang out in Seoul and have the big city life. And then, I thought, I would be ready to settle down when I got back to the States.

I was out looking at houses and everything. I finally went over to the hospital and asked the assistant chief nurse where my assignment would be. And she said, "Congratulations, you are going to be the head nurse at Camp Casey." I ended up being in a somewhat austere place, and there weren't that many of us there. It's the furthest north post and about 10 kilometers from the North Korean border. I was the head nurse, and I was second in command at my facility, the health clinic. There are very few females up there. There were mostly men with very few officers because it is combat arms. It's kind of a crazy place. Korea is crazy in general, but then you go up north, and it is worse. If you had an emergency walk in, we had to shift them 2-1/2 hours on to Seoul or to Saint Mary's in Oejombu 45 minutes away. It could be a scary place at times. I had gone there the night before, we had an emergency, we had a woman come in, and she was in labor, and I had taken her to the Korean Hospital 45 minutes away. So, I ended up in the ambulance with her while she was contracting, hoping that she wouldn't give birth in the ambulance. I was trying to think back to nursing school [*laughing*]. I don't know how to deliver a baby. I got back at three in the morning and woke up to a phone call at seven o'clock that somebody was "coding" in my clinic. When I got up there, people were crying. It got very busy, people were flying in all day, and generals were coming in trying to calm everyone down. I remember walking into the trauma room where we had coded the patient, and the smell of blood kind of washed over me. I was overtired already, and one of the sergeant majors who had come up with one of the generals said to me, "Oh you know Sergeant Major _____, because he had asked me who I had deployed with." We talked a little bit about that unit which freaked me out a bit, and then I walked into this room where there is blood, and one of my nurses said to me, "You need to go home." [*laugh*] The soldier that coded was maybe 38 years old, and he had a heart attack. The reason there was blood was that he had fallen while he was working out. His jaw was dislocated, and we had a big mess because he had fallen flat on his face. Being up there, we had helicopters for medevac as well.

I remember when I was back maybe 6 months, and there was a helipad right next to my clinic at Camp Casey. Then, down the street maybe 200 yards was the building where I lived. And the first time I was coming up the hill, and a chopper was spinning like it was going to get a patient, and I had to remind myself that I was in Korea at Camp Casey, and that it was different [*laughing*]. One of the things with being up there was that I was 2-1/2 hours from Seoul, and also that we could only have 10% of the unit out of the area at one time. Because I was the head nurse and had only one other military nurse, one of us always had to be there to make sure everything was taken care of. We had medics who were military, but all of our other nurses were civilians. So, I only actually made it out of the country twice which was not my intention. I don't know if you read the book or saw the movie, *Eat, Pray, Love,* but that book made me realize that I was not happy with my marriage.

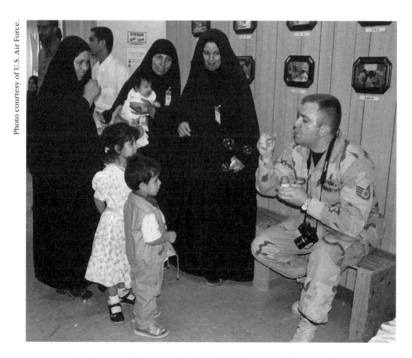

Photo courtesy of U.S. Air Force.

Air force medic entertains Iraqi children and their mothers
at Tallil Air Base, Iraq.

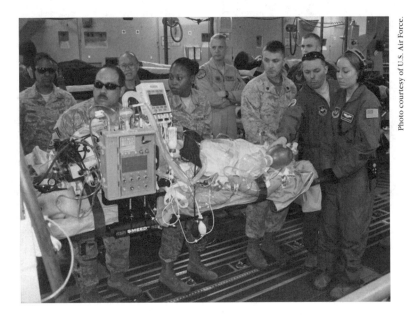

A critically wounded soldier loaded on C-17 medevac aircraft for flight
to Washington, DC.

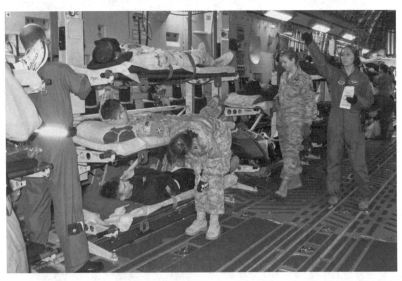

Nurses prepare patients aboard C-17 Globemaster in Germany for flight
to the United States.

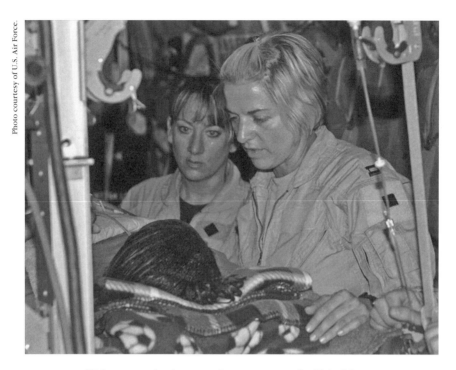

Photo courtesy of U.S. Air Force.

Flight nurses check on a patient en route to the United States.

11

Family and Social Networks: Support Versus Lack of Support

Most nurses received the greatest support from family and friends. Community support was also recognized and appreciated. Some nurses reported a fairly smooth transition with strong support from their families and communities. They wanted people to be patient with them, listen to their stories, and be nonjudgmental. They wanted to be thanked for their service and feel appreciated. On the other hand, nurses who felt a lack of support and connection were devastated. Some nurses struggled in their relationships with family and friends who did not seem to understand that they needed to heal themselves emotionally, psychologically, and spiritually after being deployed. The renegotiation of roles in the family was important, but could be fraught with a myriad of difficulties if the father was tired from childrearing and domestic duties, and if the mother returned fatigued and troubled. Some nurses reported turmoil in their extended families with the sharing of responsibilities for elderly parents. They worried that they would be deployed again when they were needed at home. Some questioned whether they should stay in the military, not knowing what the future would hold for them and their families.

MAJOR FRED

Fred was a critical care nurse who had served many years in the Air National Guard and Air Force Reserve. Fred reported, "I've been gone various times over the last 20 plus years, and my family is always supportive of my military career as well as my civilian nursing career."

LIEUTENANT COLONEL CHRISTA

Christa was an air force reservist who had been deployed to Balad Air Base, Iraq. Her unit performed the Aeromedical Staging mission.

Christa related:

> I remembered one more action that had a huge impact upon me on my return. That action was the regs [regulations] that said we had to stay within driving distance of the base for the first 2 weeks we were back, just in case they wanted to bring us back for something. The impact for me was that I was not able to see my family for almost 3 weeks, and by the time I was able to go, then my leave was almost gone.
>
> For my first deployment to Kuwait in 2004, both my parents were alive, but my brilliant father was dying of COPD [chronic obstructive pulmonary disease]. The lack of oxygen had robbed him of his wonderful mind and spirit. In December while still in Kuwait, I would call home. The first half of the allotted 15 minutes was spent just trying to get connected. The second half was trying to explain to my father (a B-29 pilot in WW II) why I wasn't coming home for Christmas. Christmas was always a very special time for Dad and me. I finally got to see Dad the end of January 2005. He passed away the beginning of March.
>
> Just prior to going to Iraq, I had to put Mom in a nursing home down in Cincinnati where my brother lived. I was sad to have to do this, but glad, because I wasn't going to be able to go home to take care of her. When I returned from Iraq, I just wanted to see her so bad. I was never able to talk to her while I was gone. That first week back from Iraq, I also found out that my brother and his wife had separated, and my family was falling apart. I couldn't go home to be with my brother and my mom because of our travel restrictions. This was very hard to deal with. They were my family, and I just wanted to be with them.

LIEUTENANT KATE

Kate was a navy nurse assigned to a forward resuscitation and shock trauma unit in Afghanistan.

Kate reported:

My reintegration with my husband was pretty difficult. My husband is retired navy and had deployed to Iraq the year before I deployed to Afghanistan. It seemed that every time I tried to talk with him about my deployment, he would cut me off and lead into a story about his deployment. I needed to talk, and he wasn't listening to what I wanted to say. It made me feel awful that he didn't want to hear about my experience, and what I needed to talk about. We both had terrible coping skills. I drank too much after I came home. He drank too much after he came home. This would lead to fights. It was a very negative experience for both of us.

   We lived off-base as did most of our friends. There is no on-base housing at the Navy Hospital complex. We did not have a tight knit community because there were no other military members in our neighborhood. Our neighborhood was a combination of mostly young families and elderly couples. I didn't feel particularly close to anyone in our neighborhood.

Kate talked about her extended family:

When I got back from Afghanistan, it was 2 days before Thanksgiving; so, my husband and I drove from Virginia to New Hampshire where my parents and family were getting together. Everyone in my extended family was supportive. They had lots of questions. They wanted to know what it was like, and everyone sort of had the same questions: Did you see anyone dead? Did you take care of people with their limbs blown off? Did anyone die while you were caring for them? I didn't feel right to be talking about this stuff. I mean, here it is Thanksgiving, and those dead or injured soldiers' families are missing them or missing the way they used to be before getting injured. I was 29 when I deployed, and many of the casualties were a lot younger than I was. Many of those marines were 19 or 20 years old.

   My family was concerned while I was deployed. They knew I was in a hospital, but I never told them about all my helicopter medevac flights outside the wire until I came home. They knew I wasn't out there walking patrols, but they knew that we were all susceptible to bombings. We were shot at when we were flying medevac; I could see the tracer bullets coming up from the ground at night. There were medevac helicopters that crashed over there.

LIEUTENANT COMMANDER KATHLEEN

Kathleen, a navy nurse assigned to the emergency department (ED) at the busy British-run Camp Bastion Hospital in Afghanistan, described her neighborhood:

> I lived in an area near my military base, but it was very densely populated with civilians. There were retired senior citizens, families with kids in elementary school, and young couples. You kind of stuck out when you were in uniform. The community didn't do a homecoming when we came back. I was an "IA" [individual augmentee]; so, it was not like the base deployed a lot of people. We were selected for deployment based on what kind of skills were needed, such as orthopedic surgeon, dentist, or critical care nurse. Only a handful of people from my hospital were needed for deployment.

LIEUTENANT COLONEL JULIE

Julie, an experienced Air Force Reserve flight nurse and Critical Care Air Transport Team (CCATT) nurse, described her difficulties when she returned home from Iraq.

> Coming back from my first deployment from Iraq in 2004 was the hardest for me and my family. My husband was active duty in the air force for 20 years working in Special Operations as a combat controller; so he was gone a lot in that career field. We had always made it work. He retired in early 2001. Then 2003 came around, and I deployed to Iraq. So, he was at home and that was a new role for him, having to manage the kids and do household stuff. He really did a good job in his own way. The kids, twin boys, were 8 years old when I left for Iraq, and our older boy was 14. My husband did quite well overall. I learned over time that it will never be the way you would do it, but your way is not the only right way. Before I left for Iraq, one day my husband said to me, "You know, I haven't gone grocery shopping since I met you, and we started dating." And I laughed and said, "Welcome to my world." On that first deployment to Iraq I was gone for 6 months. I had never really been gone much from my family over the years; so, it took some getting used to for my husband and the kids.

When I came back from that first deployment, I wasn't in the right mindset to step right back into the role of working mother, housekeeper, grocery shopper, child chauffer, and cook. My mind just wasn't there. So, I sort of eased back into it, but he seemed to want me to take over right away, and my mind just wasn't there yet. I think my brain was a little oversaturated with the Iraq war and the trauma patients I had cared for. I'm sure he thought I'd want to jump right in, but I wasn't up to it. I think he was tired, and he wanted a break from childcare stuff. Then 4 months later, I deployed again. I had about a week's notice. I was going to be gone over Christmas; so, I spent that week doing a lot of Christmas shopping before I left. The second deployment was to Ramstein Air Base, Germany, to fly air-evac missions between Iraq and Germany, but we lived in Germany, not Iraq. I was gone that time for 4 months. When I came home, I took some time to go visit my parents.

Julie described her third deployment:

When we did the troop surge, and the casualties went so high, I was deployed again. Because I flew air evac, when casualty counts were high, more air evac crews were deployed because there were more missions that needed to be flown. So, air evac crews didn't have a lot of stability in their lives. By about mid-2008, things seemed to stabilize a bit, and we usually knew how long we would be home, and how long we would be out flying missions. But all these deployments took a toll on the whole family. My husband and I were constantly having role reversals. As the kids got older, they could help their dad more when I was deployed.

Julie described how some people in her community were shocked and surprised to learn that she, a middle-aged woman, had deployed to Iraq. She reported:

One day I was driving home from shopping, and the police were blocking the road because evidently they were blowing up the dam over the river. I stopped and asked, "What are you guys doing here today?" And they said, "Haven't you heard, it has been advertised in the papers and on the radio for months, we are blowing up the dam as an energy conservation project!" I said, "Really, I just got back from deploying to Iraq, so I have no idea." They seemed shocked to hear this response from a middle-aged woman driving a van.

I found that our group of friends would be talking about things in the community as if I was there when these events occurred. Most of the time I had no earthly idea what they were talking about. It might be the high school football games, or an event at the church, or a fire in a downtown store, but they were not consciously aware or mindful that I was gone during those 6 months. Or, someone would say "Did you know that so-and-so and so-and-so are having problems in their marriages and are getting divorced?" I'd say, "No, when did all this happen?" There were huge gaps, although I got e-mails when I was deployed.

Julie described her parents and why she decided to retire from the Air Force Reserve. She stated:

My parents were one of the reasons I decided to retire from the Air Force Reserve. My parents were getting to be elderly, and my dad was a nervous wreck each time I deployed. I had to come home early from my last tour in Iraq because my dad had to have cardiac surgery. He had to have his mitral valve replaced. I only have one sibling, a brother, so my parents depend on me for a lot. Dad had the usual mental fogginess immediately post-op that we see with patients who have been put on bypass during the surgery. When he was waking up, he was talking very loud and saying things like, "Be careful, honey, they are going to blow your plane up." So, somewhere in his psyche, he was thinking about me getting blown up in Iraq.

My parents never told me not to join the reserves, but I think they were always proud and nervous at the same time. They were always supportive when my husband needed help with the kids. They were always wonderfully supportive, but I think they were always scared of what could happen. Even in peacetime as a flight nurse, I still had a relatively dangerous job. Plus, I had other deployments before 9/11 and humanitarian missions, too. I had been to Kosovo, Haiti, and Desert Shield/ Desert Storm. I think all of this took a silent toll on my parents. I think the "in-your-face media coverage of the Iraq and Afghanistan wars" was additionally upsetting for my parents, and a lot of other families as well. Now, you have media folks imbedded with combat units; so, people see the fighting and bombing and blood right in their own living rooms every day. People can have so much more of a connection to the action if they so choose. I think that induced more anxiety in my family.

Whatever they saw in the news, they thought that I must have been there.

FIRST LIEUTENANT ALLISON

Allison is an active duty air force emergency room nurse who was deployed to Afghanistan.

She remarked:

It was great to see my mom and stepdad in person, but the way technology is today, I was able to Skype them and e-mail them fairly often while deployed. We stayed in touch every week while I was gone, even though I was 8,000 miles from home. Finally, being with them was so great and comforting. They were definitely worried about me when I was gone, but I think our frequent contact buffered their worry to a degree. They also knew that I joined the air force to do the kinds of things I was doing, like deploying to war. They knew that I wanted to be where the action was. I was doing exactly what I wanted to be doing, and I think on some level my parents understood. They knew I was happy, motivated, and learning. Being on deployment was one of my goals when I joined the military, and I got to fulfill that goal during my first 3 years on active duty.

Allison believed that she returned to a supportive community of friends. She stated:

I live off-base because I am a single officer and they don't have housing on the base for single officers. It was an easy transition for me. I have friends in the military as well as outside the military in my local community. We all pretty much picked up where we left off.

The only thing that was frustrating for me when I returned from deployment was the types of patients we take care of back in the States. They are mostly older people with chronic cardiac problems. I really miss the deployment environment and the trauma care we provided. It really became what I want to continue to do. I would go back in a heartbeat. I truly loved the deployment environment, and I never really felt threatened, even though we did have periodic rocket

attacks. I lived with the attitude over there that if something
is going to happen to me, it is just going to happen. Coming
back to a stateside medical center was just somewhat difficult for me. It is routine and frustrating. There are always
things in addition to work that you need to take care of, like
PT [physical training], staff meetings, doctors' appointments.
On deployment, you got up, went to work, if you didn't have
patients in the ER, you could take off to do other things, but
you were on call and stayed on the base. You had all the time
in the world to take care of yourself, and do the things you
wanted to do.

LIEUTENANT COLONEL TAMMY

Tammy, an Air National Guard nurse who was deployed to Kabul, Afghanistan, on a mentoring team described the supportive neighborhood:

We have lived in this community for over 10 years. Our neighbors were very supportive. They helped my husband while I was
gone and had us over after I returned. I have been asked to come
to various community forums to talk about my experiences in
Afghanistan. People in our community have been genuinely interested in my story. I've also spoken at nursing forums, such as
the local chapter of Sigma Theta Tau (the International Nursing
Honor Society) and the state nurses' association. I also spoke to
the university group of professors' wives. I never expected so
much local interest and support. I have enjoyed all my speaking
engagements and have met so many people.

LIEUTENANT COLONEL REGINA

Regina, an army reservist, who served on a provincial reconstruction team,
described her trying reintegration after returning from Ramadi, Iraq.
She stated:

My personal reintegration was difficult, challenging, and hard
to explain. I can't seem to be able to talk to civilian people,
mostly relatives, and get them to understand what I'm trying to
communicate. I just don't feel like I have anything in common
with many people anymore, other than military people. Military

people understand how you feel to a great extent, even if they didn't deploy. There is that military bond that is just so special.

I came back to a lot of personal issues because my husband got sick, and my stepson committed suicide. I was trying to deal with those issues, plus the fact that I had just spent almost a year away from loved ones in a war zone. I was so close to completing my 30 years of service and receiving my full retirement benefits. My husband had cancer, so his future was questionable. Deep in my heart, I knew that my husband was probably going to die, and I knew that I'd have to depend on myself for most of my financial support going forward. And, yes, my husband did die. My family, mostly my siblings, wanted me to get out before I reached 30 years of service, but I knew what the benefits were of staying in to reach 30 years. There was a big disconnect between me and most of my relatives, and even some friends. Now, I feel that I just don't have anything in common with them anymore, except for my military friends.

You grieve what your life used to be like, and what your relationships used to be like. My family doesn't value the same things I do, I guess. Sometimes, I think that they see me as deserting the family. It is hard to explain. When my husband and I were serving in the army for all those years, when we were gone from home, it was like we didn't exist. It was not our own children, but our brothers and sisters, who acted this way. I rarely heard from my brothers and sisters when I was in Iraq. Ramadi was an austere area, but I managed to buy trinkets to mail back to all my nieces and nephews. I sent cards for Thanksgiving, Valentine's Day, and birthdays, and I was lucky if I heard from my brothers and sisters once in the year I was in Iraq. When I was overseas, it was out-of-sight, therefore, out-of-mind with my siblings. It was that I chose to go away to war; so, you are out of their life for now. They could have been supportive and helpful, but they chose not to be.

It is kind of interesting and troubling that my siblings turned their backs toward me, while I was very supported by so many of my professional colleagues. I had a very strong and supportive relationship with my local professional nursing organization and its leaders and members. The organization chairperson is a friend, and she has a deep love of military nursing and nursing history. We did a welcome home event at the organization facilities with catered food, a big display of my uniforms and artifacts from Iraq. I put together a power point presentation, and I was able to bring all my friends and my children to this celebration, and show them in one day what my experience was like in Iraq, and to try to fill in the gap for my siblings and friends, so they would better understand what my experience was all about. I had purchased a number of American flags that were flown over my base in Ramadi, Iraq, and I was able to present these flags and their accompanying certificates to my children, brothers and sisters, and organization members as gifts from me representing my service. This meant a lot to me and to my family. My children, my military friends, the organization members and leadership have been really supportive, and this has buffered the rough parts of my reintegration like my husband's cancer and his death, the suicide of my stepson, and estrangement from my own brothers and sisters.

COLONEL SARAH

Sarah, an active duty air force nurse, described a supportive environment when she returned from Iraq.
    She stated:

My husband had been active duty for 13 years, and he deployed numerous times after the first Gulf War. He was flying in a fighter aircraft. I think that reintegration with a spouse might have been a little easier for us because we had experienced separation many times before in our marriage. We had dated for 4 years before we got married. Even then, we had a long-distance relationship because of deployments. We met in Germany where we were both assigned, but he deployed several times during those 4 years. He was gone a total of 11 months during our dating stage. He also deployed several more times after we got married. We learned what to do. We had experienced it before; so, it wasn't something new to us when I deployed.

    I had longevity on my side when I deployed, since I was already a senior officer. I had been a farm girl growing up; so, smells and primitive arrangements weren't anything new to me. Not having all the bells and whistles in my living quarters was not hard for me. I was not too put off by that. Of course, being a senior officer, I had a few luxuries that other people didn't have, such as I had a private sleeping area, and only shared a bathroom with one other woman, as opposed to the gang showers, porta-potties, and group bathroom trailers. I feel like I'm a positive person. I probably excel during adversity. I felt like deploying to Iraq was a very positive experience for me personally. There were a couple of nurses that had to go home on emergency leave. So, not only was I a supervisor of nurses, but I was a clinical nurse as well. I worked the wards to fill in for other nurses or to help when things got very busy. About half of the time, I was a clinical nurse over there, and I worked the wards with everyone else. It was very positive for me. There were certainly horrific things we saw and cared for in terms of injuries, but I think of my experience as very positive.

LIEUTENANT DARLA

Darla is a navy operating room nurse who was deployed to Kandahar, Afghanistan.

She reported:

My family was supportive of me going to Afghanistan. My dad had been in the Marine Corps. He had been deployed to Operation Desert Storm. I talked to my parents two or three times a week while I was deployed. They also mailed me whatever I needed that I could not get in Afghanistan.

However, Darla described the lack of support from her boyfriend when she returned:

Since I came home from Afghanistan, we had not been getting along. He had convinced me our life together would be easier, if I left active duty, so I did. Now, after leaving the active navy, things were not working out. My boyfriend is in the navy, too, and he was good about me being deployed. [*Starts crying and pauses for a long time.*] Before I left, he was very attentive and supportive. He had been deployed to Bagram, Afghanistan, in 2008. I'm a little sensitive about this because he was so supportive while I was gone, and then things fell apart between us, once I got back. That was one of the hardest thing to deal with, he was so supportive while I was gone. He was supportive the whole time I was gone, but our relationship unraveled when I got back. When I got home he was OK for the first 2 weeks, but then he was critical of me, argumentative, and demanding. I wanted out [*crying*]. I had to leave. I couldn't handle the stress of arguing. So before I left, he didn't try to talk me into staying; so, I knew I had to go.

CAPTAIN COURTNEY

Courtney, an Air National Guard member, who was deployed to Afghanistan, shared her biggest disappointment since returning home.
    She stated:

Before I left for Afghanistan, my son was going into high school. I mailed informational packets with a letter to the principal of the high school to give to my son's teachers in September. The letter explained I was going to deploy and that I would not be back until January. Well, none of my son's teachers received the packets. In fact, half of his teachers didn't even know that I was deployed. My son became very depressed while I was deployed. After therapy, my son is doing a lot better now. But I'm very upset that his school dropped the ball and didn't get the information to my son's teachers. When I came back, I noticed that something was not right with him. I took him to his pediatrician, and the doctor said, "I think he has anxiety and let's send him to a therapist."
    At first I took him to a therapist in town who is really unconventional, and my son really never connected with him. Then one day, while I was at work, my sister had taken him to his therapy appointment, and I got a call from the therapist saying that I really needed to take him to Yale (Hospital) because he was suicidal. In the meantime, he had been cutting. I found the cut marks. At Yale, they put him on Wellbutrin. In my opinion, it was the dumbest thing to put him on. He spent a week at Yale, and that's what they put him on. It's not a first line med for depression and anxiety. We found another therapist. They wanted my son to go to this aftercare program, but it started at noon and I told them that he really needed to go to school. The new therapist has been one that my son has really connected with. He sees him once a week, and he's got him on Zoloft. He's up to 50 mg and is doing great. He just slept over at a friend's house last night. He's much more himself.
    It's weird. We always say, that when we are deployed, it's harder for the family than it is for us. The family may worry because we are in harm's way, but you know what to expect to a certain extent. It's almost easier being there, than coming home to bills, the work schedule, and this and that. There, all you have to do is keep yourself alive so you can do your job. You eat three meals a day. You go to the gym. You're on the computer,

and you got to see your family on the computer. You miss your family, but it was almost easier for me being there, than coming home.

You can't beat yourself up about what happens to you and to your family. It is what it is. The teenage years are just tough anyway. Parents almost always feel some guilt, no matter what. We all just do the best we can. I think the teenage years are tougher on kids today, than they were when I was in high school. My son is doing a lot better. But I'm very upset that his school dropped the ball and didn't get the information about me being deployed to my son's teachers. It's not like there are so many deployed parents in my community. It should have been a priority.

Courtney talked about reintegration. She explained:

They have you fill out a questionnaire when you go, and then you fill out the same questionnaire when you come back. After a few months, someone is supposed to call you to check in with you. As I told you before, I didn't get the call when I was supposed to get it. Eventually, I finally got a call, but I was at drill [reserve weekend duty]. They want to make sure you are not suicidal because a lot of people come back, and they kill themselves. I told the woman who finally called that they are not good at bringing you back. The calls are late, and there is no timely follow-up. I had not been sleeping well. I was never suicidal, but I could see how some people could be if they were alone and without a support system. I was maybe sleeping 2 hours at a time; I was tired; I was hearing things; I was scared; I was hyper vigilant; and I was angry that no one called for months to see if I was OK and to see how I was doing. After finally getting a phone call, no one ever called me again. There was no follow-up.

Both the air force and army have had a lot of suicides. I know why, "you are kind of hung out to dry." I get it; I get it; I get it now. Many guys want to deploy again because that's what they know, and it's easier than being here, being home. It's scary; and I'm not the only one. A med tech that I served with wrote on Facebook after her divorce, "I wish I was back in Afghanistan." I wrote back to her, "I get it." The military needs better and more prompt interventions, and I consider myself a very stable person. I recognized that I needed to talk to someone, and I did it with my group of nurses from combat skills training. I'm very close to them. We went through hell together. I'm close to my roommate from combat skills. My group has had our own support system which has been wonderful. I'm hoping everyone is able to find their own support system, but there are no guarantees.

CAPTAIN TENLEY

Tenley was an army nurse and a veteran of two deployments. Tenley emphasized the importance of having someone to talk to who was a good listener. She stated:

> I went from the ER to a clinic. They put me in a plastic surgery clinic. I was stationed in Hawaii. I was single, not married. Going back to Hawaii, I had a friend in Washington state that I would call almost every night while I was unpacking my household goods. Talking to him was probably the most therapeutic thing I could do, because I was just standing there looking at this big pile of crap in front of me. I would have gotten overwhelmed. Having someone to talk to helped so much. He was a good listener.
>
> Work was work. You knew what to do. It was normal because that's what you did for the last year, you worked a lot. I didn't feel overwhelmed with work. It was a mixed group of people in Hawaii. There were some military people, but most were civilians. I made some good friends in the department. They were all good people. Plastic surgery was interesting because there were no boob jobs in the middle of Iraq [*laughing*]. The majority of our work was breast cancer reconstruction. But there was anything from a war injury to whatever. Major war injuries went to Walter Reed Army Medical Center on the east coast or Brooke Army Medical Center in Texas. We see everyone at Tripler Army Medical Center in Hawaii, army, navy, air force, coast guard, and marines. We also get air evacs from Japan and Korea.

CAPTAIN EARL

Earl, an air force reservist, reflected on his return from flying air-evac missions.
He stated:

> The family adjustment was very difficult. My sister and my mom could tell that I was a changed person. It was the elephant in the

room. The civilians in my family, and my friends, pretended like nothing had happened. The military people in my family would acknowledge that I was having a difficult time. My wife saw it, my brother, who is military, would say something to me. They didn't know how to handle it.

 I really didn't get much of a chance to reintegrate with my wife because she volunteered to extend and went back overseas. So, we went for a period of about 3 years not seeing each other. She kept going back on-duty with the military, and I felt like I was pretty much done with nursing. I was pretty burned out. On the civilian side, I trained to become a fire fighter, not realizing at first that I'd have to do the EMS [emergency medical services] stuff. I also had problems with my new job. I had flashbacks of doing patient care. I didn't like the claustrophobic feeling of being in a van/truck/ambulance. It reminded me of being in the airplane. I had been on flight status and was flying missions for over 10 years and was very comfortable. One thing I noticed after being in crowded spaces with lots of people, I was now claustrophobic, and I could not be with large groups of people. That was a real challenge for me, even being in a crowded bar bothered me. I could not stand it. I had lots of anxiety.

Earl described his new job:

So, with my new job at the fire department, I got off the medic unit and tried to stay on the fire truck. It helped not having to do patient care. Over time, things improved a bit. You know, time is a great healer for both mental and physical wounds. Over time, things got better, and I could re-engage in doing medical things. As time went on, I didn't talk a lot to my peers about being a nurse in the military. We would have continuing education classes for the EMTs [emergency medical technicians] and paramedics, and I would find myself doing more of the teaching. And people would say, "How do you know all of this stuff?" Then I'd tell them that I was a flight nurse in the air force. Over time, I felt more comfortable and was able to overcome some of my previous issues.

LIEUTENANT COLONEL DAGMAR

Dagmar was an experienced Air Force Reserve and Air National Guard flight nurse who had served on many deployments over the past 15 years.

Dagmar stated:

My civilian job was with the VA [Veterans Administration].
People at the VA didn't view me as a returning veteran. When
you are still in the Guard or the Reserves, you don't think of
yourself as a veteran because you're still in. I'm still engaged in
military service. I may go back to the war. I know I'll still go
back. I want to stay active and involved in the war. With the VA,
I was never viewed as a returning veteran; I was viewed as an
employee. And this is the VA!

I have no kids, and I'm a widow. That's why it is so easy
for me to deploy. The mother with young kids and the newly-
weds should stay home. It's easier for me to go. I barely even had
houseplants, I could not even manage that for a while because
I was going so often. So, I had no husband, and I had no kids. I
used to write to my mother a lot, almost like a daily diary when
I was gone. She died in 2006. The next time I went out, I really
missed that because I really didn't have anyone else that I really
poured myself out to. I know she appreciated it. You have to be
careful with e-mail; you can't give out that much information or
numbers. I would talk around things, and I'd write an old snail
mail letter that was like a diary for me. I really missed that after
my mother died.

I had my brother and my sister. My sister was always the
one who kept the home fires burning for me. She took care
of my mail and my bills when I was deployed. She was wonderfully supportive. Yes, I'm close to my sister. My sister and
brother are both older. My sister was wonderful about taking
care of the business things for me at home. We didn't live in
the same town. It was a couple of hours drive. My brother was
supportive, too. He was not as involved as my sister. My father was retired military; so, he and I had that connection. He
was pretty much blind; so, he couldn't e-mail me or write to
me, but whenever I came home, we had a very close relationship. I'd talk to him about things, and he'd understand. He just
died on July 6. I just lost him. My mom and dad were always
very interested and supportive of what I was doing, and of the
military. They'd listen to my stories. My mom was a navy wife
for 20+ years and we were navy kids, and we understood the
military.

I had a few close friends from my home town, but most of
my friends are in the military. They are like my family, especially

my Guard unit. They understand and always welcome you back with open arms. They knew what was going on, and what was involved. I didn't feel that disconnect with them that I some-times felt with my civilian job with the VA. I leaned toward my Guard friends and the military more than anything else.

LIEUTENANT SANDRA

Sandra was a navy emergency room trauma nurse at Camp Bastion, Afghanistan. Sandra talked about how hard it was to reintegrate with her family.

She stated:

> You could slice the tension with a knife. The tension was super thick between my husband and me. I didn't even want to be home with him in the first place. I cried a lot for the first 2 to 3 weeks. I didn't know if I was feeling guilty about coming back, leaving my coworkers and the troops that needed me.
>
> I didn't get to talk to my kids very often because the phone connections were terrible. I would have loved to call them every day, but it was probably once every 2 weeks, and it got less frequent near the end. I flew back to Guam by myself. My family was there, and a couple people from the command were there when I arrived. There's a little red rug they rollout, and there were a few people there.

Sandra anticipated parenting issues on returning to her family on Guam. She stated:

> It was difficult with the boys because I am usually the one with the control as far as rearing them. They knew things were gonna be different when I came back. I think Dad had forewarned them. They were just waiting for me to say, "You can't eat that anymore because it's not healthy for you. Mom is a health-nut." It was a little bit rough. It was like an estranged relationship. I think they didn't see my face enough while I was gone because I didn't get to Skype at Bastion. I sent them pictures. They had some nice things to show me that they had done while I was gone. I had given them a bear that they could hug and squeeze while I was gone, and I told them that I would feel it all the way in Afghanistan. They did really believe that. I sent them random

things. I had made them treasure boxes before I left. I had given them things before I left, and I had them put the things in the treasure box. Then, they would add the things that I sent them. I would write letters and cards and send them stuff. They showed everything to me, and that was emotional. We decorated the boxes together before I left; so, they could put stickers on it. They had their own ideas, too.

CAPTAIN AMANDA

Amanda was an air force reservist who served at an aeromedical staging unit in Afghanistan. She was also an experienced ICU nurse.

Amanda stated:

I can't stress enough the support I got when I was deployed, my family and friends back home, my coworkers back home, but also the people who were with me. I didn't know any of the people I was with before. I met some air force people during training; we went to combat skills training before we deployed. The greatest people you ever meet in your life, you meet in war. The bond you form with people who are in a combat zone with you is unlike any other bond you will ever have in your whole entire life. It's just very special, and something I will never get over. I'll never forget the bond that I had when I was there with my friends. They become more critical than your family. They become so important to you.

We left the FOB [forward operating base] on December 26, and I finally flew into Boston on January 7. I was overwhelmingly happy to be home. I was OK leaving my Afghan patients in Afghanistan. I had no guilt about leaving the patients this time. I was so happy to see my fiancé at the time, who is now my husband. We got married this year. I was planning a wedding over in Afghanistan. It was a very last minute deployment. I backfilled, somebody active duty jumped out of a deployment slot, and so I took it. It was my choice. An old commander had come and asked me if I would take this next tasking, and he was at the headquarters here at Robins AFB in Georgia, and he heard there was a last minute need for an ICU nurse. Then, I went to training in 11 days. It was a fantastic deployment. It is a joint expeditionary tasking; so, it's nurses from the air force to go to FOBs and remote outposts. It is the coolest deployment you'll ever get. I'll never be able to replace that experience. It was a great deployment. I felt good about it. I was proud of my behavior; I was proud of my nursing skills; I was proud of how I mentored and taught people. I was proud of getting my troops home and OK. I was just proud of the deployment and happy to come home.

12

Reintegration: Creating a New Normal

The general sentiment among the nurses was that, over time, they came to embrace "a new normal." They felt changed after deploying to war. Their lens for viewing the world was altered as a result of their war experiences. Some found themselves to be more thankful and grateful after what they had seen and done. They appreciated living in the United States with all the opportunities for advancement, comfort, and prosperity. Conversely, others became more impatient and frustrated in dealing with people, in general, once they planted their feet on American soil. It is not that society changed so much while they were deployed; the change came from within, and it posed a very interesting dynamic.

Reintegration needs to be viewed as a process with a beginning, middle, and end. It does not mean that a person going through the reintegration process will eventually be the same person he or she was before deployment. Deployment, as with any significant experience, can be seen as an opportunity for growth as a person, as a nurse. Learning and change are expected on a variety of levels when someone fulfills a mission. Thus, when coming home, all returnees face a new normal. Reintegration is very individual and has no set time frame.

LIEUTENANT KATE

Kate, a navy nurse assigned to a small forward resuscitation and trauma unit in Afghanistan, explained her reintegration to her work setting.

She recalled:

You need time to reintegrate, and the military doesn't always give you enough time. I wanted an orientation to my stateside assignment in the ER, and I didn't get it. They assumed because I was an ER nurse that I'd just jump back into the routine. Well, I wasn't emotionally ready for that. I was mentally and physically tired. I had a real hard time with patients complaining about having to wait to be seen for minor injuries or illnesses when we were busy. I had no patience for them and their whining. The month before I was taking care of soldiers who were dying, how dare they complain about waiting now for a sprained ankle or a stomach ache? I had a hard time doing patient care in a stateside ER. I had an adrenaline high in my Afghanistan ER, which could not be duplicated in a stateside hospital; plus, the soldiers were so grateful for the care we provided over there. It was just so different in the ER once I came home. I had a "short fuse" when I got home in my marriage and at work. It didn't take much to set me off. I was in a bad mood most of the time when I first came home.

LIEUTENANT COLONEL TONI

Toni, a Critical Care Air Transport Team (CCATT) nurse and air force reservist, described things that surprised her when she returned home.
She recounted:

One of the hardest things about coming back was the slow pace of life back home. We were so busy in Afghanistan all the time, and trying to slow down was hard for me. I started taking long walks with my husband, and doing other things that were enjoyable for both of us. We started going to the movies, going out to dinner. My husband made suggestions of things we could do to stay busy, but they were enjoyable things. They were things we could both look forward to. I rediscovered golf and tennis after I came home. We also started playing bridge with some friends.

I would tell the young nurses who have not deployed yet, to know themselves, know their faults, know how they handle stress, and to have outlets besides work. My outlet was getting back into church while I was deployed. I went to church with one of my roommates, and it was very exhilarating to go to a

nondenominational church with coalition forces and government aid workers from about 30 other countries. It was a truly
spiritual experience. But, they need to find that outlet whether
it is going to church, or writing in a journal, or working out, or
playing sports, or taking courses online or by correspondence.
You also have to have someone you can vent to in a deployed
environment. Someone you can go to each week and have a
cup of tea with, and talk about what is on your mind and what
is bothering you.

Toni described some of the differences between active duty nurses
and those in the U.S. reserve force:

For the reserve side, there are really no resources available for
us. When you get home from deployment, you are really on your
own. The active duty returned to their base, and then they in-
process for a few days. They are offered mental health counseling, and they get 30 days of paid leave before they have to return
to work. They have resource people who check on them to make
sure they are doing OK. On the other hand, reservists have no
paid leave; so, most of us have to return to our civilian jobs a lot
sooner than 30 days. We have to hit the ground running because
it is like we never left. There are no resources that follow up
with reservists out here on a regular basis. Most of the reserve
bases, if not all of them, do not have the resources allocated for
post-deployment issues. People don't know that having PTSD is
almost the "new normal" if you served in these wars. It is a normal reaction to an abnormal reality.

LIEUTENANT COMMANDER KATHLEEN

Kathleen served as a navy emergency room trauma nurse at Camp Bastion,
Afghanistan.

Kathleen described her job after deployment:

My husband and I are both doing navy health professions recruiting now. We are not in the same office, but we work for the
same command. I've done everything I've been asked to do in
the navy. Now, this is my selfish choice so my husband and I can
be together. It gives me a break from clinical work, and gives us
some time to start a family. We are both still active duty, and we

plan to stay in the navy as a career. I'm finishing my master's in nursing management, and my husband will be going to school full time with navy sponsorship for a DNP [doctor of nursing practice] after he finishes his recruiting assignment. We are looking forward to our future as career naval officers.

Kathleen described her experience as a woman in a deployment environment, and cautioned what other women coming after her need to know:

They need to know about being a woman deployed with hordes of men from all these countries. No one was real aggressive with me, but you are like a piece of meat on a stick. You are like one percent in a population of 40,000 men. There were like maybe 4,000 women in theater. Anytime you walk anywhere, there are just so many eyes on you. Most of the guys you knew were very helpful and were always giving us women free stuff. But the experience over there was still that you felt like a piece of meat. They weren't physically trying to touch you, but they constantly did things to try to get your attention. You were "a chick in a uniform," and that was kind of difficult for me since I'm an officer. The Afghan men always stared, and they don't respect women. They'd say things like "What is she doing here?" and "How is it that she is an officer?" It was different when the Afghan women came in for care. The men always accompanied them, but the men hung outside the ER with their own group. If you've ever seen a cartoon with a dog salivating over a piece of steak, that is the look the Afghan men gave us female nurses. The Afghan men prisoners who were brought in for care were the worst. The way they looked at us was as if we could be a trophy for them. It was very chilling the way they stared.
      Sometimes, because there were only a few of us navy personnel with this multinational force, we felt forgotten by our administration. We had some of the navy hierarchy visit, and some said they didn't know we were at our base with the other forces. I thought, that is really strange because you folks signed our deployment orders.

Kathleen related that she gained insight about herself while being deployed:

I know for myself, I know more about myself now, than I did before I deployed. I know what my triggers and issues are.

I took care of myself, and I was proactive about going for counseling. It wasn't my command checking up on me, because no one ever asked officially how I was doing. My boyfriend and my other friends asked, but no one in the official chain of command, except my director of nursing service, ever asked. One night my nursing director came by and asked, "Are you doing OK? Whatever you want to do, just let me know. Whatever you need, just let me know." She cared about her nurses. I sometimes worry about the younger corpsmen who might not have their senior officer looking out for them. I was pretty assertive about getting the mental health help I needed, but I don't think some of the younger folks have that insight. They do a post-deployment medical and mental health assessment, but that is usually just with a PA or a senior corpsmen, and people are just checking boxes on a form. There is no real in-depth assessment. No one ever really sat down and made sure I was OK. I went through the "One-Source" system to find a counselor in town, it wasn't through the active military. I think that people assume that because we are nurses, we are used to seeing trauma and blood. However, it is not a normal occurrence for most nurses to see this kind of terrible trauma on a daily basis and to see all the seriously injured and dead children. It does something to you. I feel like we saved a lot of people, but at the same time we saw a lot of people die.

Kathleen described the day during deployment when someone asked her how she was doing and had a special insight:

Only one day on deployment did I break down. The special forces commander came into the ER to see one of his troops who had a back injury, and looked right into my eyes and said to me, "Lieutenant, how are you doing? You have a job where probably no one asks you, and you are so busy asking everyone else. I don't know how you do what you do, because I couldn't do it." And I thought, here's this commander who goes out in harm's way every day, and he thinks our jobs in the hospital are so tough. He was the first person that validated for me that our jobs are so important, and that what we do is so valued by the troops in the field. Some other guys always say that it must be so nice to work in the hospital and to live in a tent with running water and flush toilets. Talking with this commander was a seminal moment for me. It validated a lot for me.

Kathleen believed she picked a good post-deployment job in the navy:

I think going into recruiting was a healthy choice for me. I don't
know what it would have been like for me going right back into
clinical. I don't know whether it would have been OK for me, or
not. It was hard enough for me to be teaching clinical to the new
corpsmen. I don't know what it would have been like for me to
go back to the ER and handle a code right away after returning
from deployment.

LIEUTENANT LORETTA

Loretta, a navy operating room nurse who served in Kandahar, Afghanistan,
described the difference she felt between stateside nursing and her role in
the deployment environment.

She stated:

You feel like you don't have the same purpose with work in the
States. You are serving a purpose back home, but you view your
purpose in Afghanistan as more important. You feel like what
you were doing before had so much more meaning than what
you are doing now. It's harder to be tolerant of all the idiosyncrasies and the trivialities of people. You have to remember that
everyone's perceptions are different. The general lack of realization from the general public of what we do and that we are still
over there doing it, bothered me when I came home. All of a
sudden, you are taking care of a 20-year-old or even an 18-year-
old who 5 minutes ago had all of his limbs and was fine and was
joking with his buddies. And now, he's unconscious and is missing three of his limbs. And another 18-year-old back in the U.S.
would be saying, "Who's having a party tonight?" Or, "Where
am I gonna be going to school after I graduate?" Or, "What color
hair looks better?" We're talking about very different priorities.
And I don't know if people are aware enough of what is going
on over there. People just don't think. Most know that we have
troops over there. But if doesn't affect their personal life, it is
very distant from their consciousness. When you come back,
it's like, "So what's up?" People know that there is a war going
on and that we have troops over there, but they think collectively, not about the individuals. Life continues to be pretty normal for most of the American people, so why shouldn't it be for

you when you come back? They just don't realize what you saw and what you did over there. Now, with time, I've put all this in proper perspective. It took me time to do this. I can't realistically expect everyone to have my perspective because they didn't have my experiences. I'm a wiser and more tolerant person now.

I did some proactive things while I was deployed which I think helped with my reintegration. One of the biggest things to help was to go to school. I was actually in graduate school while I was deployed. I was taking grad school courses while I was in Afghanistan. I continued that while I was over there. So, basically, I did my regular work in the operating room, then I did school work. I kept myself busy and focused. My graduate program was online. It kept me occupied. I'm not like a lot of people and was probably not into networking and socializing as much as some people. I had my few people I could vent to. Others visited different country compounds. I was either at work or doing school work or at the gym. It was nice to have a distraction like school work. I also wanted to plan for the future, and having a graduate degree in nursing administration would certainly help as a Nurse Corps officer. School in a way was therapy for me. It was one more positive step toward my future.

Loretta viewed her deployment to Afghanistan as a positive career move, and something she wanted to do:

I would do it again. No matter how well you know yourself, you are not going to know how you would be in a given situation. I volunteered, and most of us volunteered, but I don't think we really knew what we were in for until we experienced it for the first time. Even if 10 people told me about their experiences, I would still have had that initial shock. That first trauma really does come true. It could be compared to a pregnant woman with 20 people telling her what their labor and delivery experience was like. But the woman would really have to experience it for herself. It's different for everybody.

Loretta described some of the negative emotions she dealt with through her reintegration:

Two emotions I struggled with during my reintegration were irritability and frustration. I wouldn't always know why I was irritated, but I was irritated. It was the silliest thing, I didn't

know what started it or what didn't start it. The littlest thing
could set me off. I remember going to the bank because I had
a safety deposit box, and I wanted to get everything out, and
I had brought the wrong key with me. This was after I came
back, and I couldn't explain why this situation upset me so
much. At the time, my boyfriend was in Afghanistan. He had
been gone for about 3 months. We had an understanding, but
the emotions, it was just hard. He's not medical, but he actually
had a much worse deployment than me. He lost three men from
his unit, and then his training officer committed suicide about
half way through the deployment before Christmas while over
there. I just got so frustrated when my boyfriend was out of
contact with me from Afghanistan, and then he'd come back
from the field and tell me this terrible stuff. There was nothing
I could do but listen, and he'd have to call from a navy phone
which was not very private. So, maybe all this stressed me out
and made me irritable, I just don't know. Needless to say, my
boyfriend is working on his reintegration. He just got back in
June. For the last 22 out of 29 months, one of us has been gone.
He's navy, too. He tries not to show his sadness and stress. I'm
hopeful, and I try not to take things personally. None of us are
the same when we come back.

LIEUTENANT COLONEL JULIE

Julie, a seasoned air force reservist, reported that she got better at reintegration with each successive deployment.
  She stated:

When I first came back in 2003, I think I had not really prepared myself for that type of trauma that I saw in Iraq. Even
though I'm a trauma nurse, I had not prepared myself for all the
burns, traumatic amputations, and the youth of the patients I
had to care for. I felt a real connection to my patients. I have a
son who was only a year or two younger than most of the soldiers I cared for. So, my son was so close in age to these young
troops I was taking care of, and some of them had such terrible
injuries. So, when I first came back in 2003, I had a very hard
time. There was a lot of burnout for me. I was just very angry
about a lot of things.

FIRST LIEUTENANT ALLISON

Allison is an active duty air force triage and emergency room nurse. She remarked:

> My transition back definitely went smooth. I didn't have any issues with that. However, the care we deliver back here in the States is mostly to retired older people with cardiac problems, and you have to deal with the families as well. I just miss the action and challenges that I faced in my wartime environment. I think I found my niche in trauma ICU nursing, and I really miss it now. The active duty patients were so motivated and enthusiastic. They might have just gotten shot or blown up, and they want to get back out there to fight. They are upset that they and their buddies have to be hospitalized. They are just so energetic and motivated. Coming back to the States and my ICU, I'm taking care of these older patients, patients in their 80s who have open heart surgery, and they don't want to get out of bed, and they don't want to walk, and they are just not motivated at all. So, it kind of makes my job more difficult because it is hard to motivate these older folks.
>
> When I was deployed, I found something that I am really passionate about, trauma nursing, and coming back to my stateside ICU I'm finding that I'm clinically frustrated with the pace and the lack of challenge for my ICU skills. On deployment, you just did your job; you fixed them, and you knew you were doing your very best to help these young injured soldiers. We tried to get in touch with unit commanders to let them know how their troops were doing, but once we did, it was up to the unit chain of command to get in touch with their command back in the U.S. who would reach out to the families.
>
> Back here in the States, I feel that the nurses are tasked with doing everything. We are providing care for the patients; we are the "sounding board and therapists" for the families. We are pulled in so many directions. On deployment, you didn't have other responsibilities clouding the mission and your job.

LIEUTENANT COMMANDER ZOE

Zoe, a navy nurse who served in Afghanistan, talked about her reintegration.

She stated:

When you get back from Afghanistan, you are so grateful for everything that you have; your house, your car, being able to take a shower [*laughing*]. We went back to church as a family and started praying nightly together as a family. The prayer that I said to them: I want us each to say three things that we are thankful for and each person would say their three things, and then we'd pray for the rest of our family and friends. Every night we prayed for my friend who was an Afghan midwife, and for her daughters. She was divorced and came to work for the coalition and was in constant danger. We'd pray for her safety, and that she would get a visa. We wanted to get her and her daughters to the U.S.

If my daughters were wasteful, I'd say, "The kids in Afghanistan don't even have shoes." After a couple of months, my oldest daughter said to me, "Mom, I'm really glad that you are back from Afghanistan, and I know that it was a very important experience for you, but I am sorry you deployed because now everything is about being thankful because of what you saw." [*She laughs as she tells me this.*] She was completely blunt and honest. I said, "Honey, I'm not gonna apologize for that and you're gonna keep hearing it, but I understand where you are coming from" [*laughing*]. Being thankful has made a big impact on me and our family. As an individual, I really try not to take things for granted. We connect as a family with the things we are thankful for. Being deployed made me realize how fortunate we are in the U.S. because there are so many in this world who go without the bare necessities. They don't have access to health care, and they don't have running water.

Zoe told how her husband was helpful to her:

My husband, he basically just listened. If I was feeling sad or stressed or anxious or guilty, he would listen. Sometimes he would just hold my hand. He let me talk. He would be open to that. For my first 6 to 8 weeks home, he continued to take the brunt of child care. They were in a routine with school, dinner, and grocery shopping. I was just there. I could take part, but I didn't have to take control. Some of the things I wanted to take control of, and these were some of the functions of the household. I would be a little angry; I would say I want some of this back, and he'd say, "OK, but I don't want to push anything onto you." Then I'd say, "I can handle this," and he'd say, "OK." Now, I think, "What an amazing man! He's a good guy."

I did notice with the pace of life, he continued his active duty job during the whole course of my deployment and had to travel a few times and had to bring my dad in to help out with the kids. He became much more regimented, more serious. I could see his patience was thinner. I gently pointed this out to him. When I was gone, both he and my dad used the Naval Support Center and went for some counseling. The girls had gone for some counseling, too. I guess it was anger focused, but I don't know why. I'll have to ask a little more about that. I remember seeing this thermometer magnet on the refrigerator that was basically to measure mood. My husband and my oldest daughter are very similar in their temperaments, and they would both utilize the thermometer magnet. I would tease them a little about it [*laughing*]. They would go and take 10 seconds to cool off. Also, initially my husband was defensive when I'd try to help. He'd say, "This is how it had to be when you were gone." I'd say, "Yes, I understand." I knew how it was to a certain extent because he had deployed before, and I'd be home alone with the girls. We could communicate about how it was to be the parent at home with the girls. He and I would talk about it. He got to decompress a bit when I got home. I'd remind him that we could share the parenting and the household chores. It wasn't all on his shoulders anymore. We were a team. I'd tell my daughters, too. It made me feel good to be part of it, and it made home feel more relaxed because he realized he had a partner to share things with. I've talked with friends and coworkers who deployed, and we agree that it is hardest when people feel like they have to face the day alone, with no one to share things with.

Zoe described some changes in her life after she returned home.

I got off active duty in July 2011, and I am in the reserves. I struggled when I tried to transition to the active reserves, they didn't have a billet for me, and they still don't. They are overmanned at my rank. I really felt like my identity would be compromised because I've been an active duty nurse and nurse practitioner. I felt like I lost a bit of my identity. When you wear the uniform, you garner that immediate recognition and respect. There is respect that goes with your rank. I actually went back to work last year as a contractor at an air force base clinic in civilian clothes. I wear a lab coat. No one would ever know that I was active duty, and I feel a need to tell them. I try to work it into a conversation. I guess part of it is the need for recognition, but it is also a need for connection. I know the stress of being active duty and being a nurse. Some of my patients are back from deployment. I ask them about their deployment, and I tell them that I was in Ghasni. They are surprised. I want them to realize that I can relate to them because I was active duty, and I was deployed.

I want to tell you about the Afghan midwife. I keep in touch with her to this day. We call each other sisters. I am her American sister, and she is my Afghan sister. I feel like it was important for me to make a connection with a real Afghan. Being there, it was about so much more than combat. It was about real people. She, to me, was the epitome of a real person. She is an Afghan woman who just wants to provide for her children. She just wants food and water for her children. She is currently in Norway. I keep telling myself that we were there for a purpose. I don't know if we'll make any significant changes that will benefit the country. But I think we tried. It can't be a safe haven for the Taliban. We can't allow women and children to be oppressed.

LIEUTENANT COLONEL TAMMY

Tammy, an Air National Guard nurse who performed the mentoring role at an Afghan hospital, described her adjustment and reintegration.

Tammy stated:

It took me a little time to readjust to life in the U.S. One thing I noticed right away is the large numbers of obese people in the U.S. You didn't see any obesity in Afghanistan. I noticed that some people here are really very self-indulgent, spoiled, and have a sense of entitlement. People are into designer-labeled clothes and driving expensive cars, and it was so vivid to me when I came home. Throwing things away bothered me more after I came home. Waste of used household items was apparent to me in the U.S. whereas in Afghanistan people would repurpose items or use items far longer than people do here. I came home much more appreciative of all that I had. I had a family that loved me, a supportive husband, and a happy and secure environment.

LIEUTENANT COMMANDER CATHERINE

Catherine was a navy nurse who served on a provincial reconstruction team during one tour of duty and as an ICU nurse on another tour of duty. She stated:

> I was 44 at the time of my last deployment. Looking at these experiences in my life, reintegration is about trying to share that knowledge and experiences. I help teach and train others and really make a difference in how we manage our own health care assets postdeployment because we've had to learn that as we've gone along. We had to figure it out.

LIEUTENANT LAUREN

Lauren was a navy critical care nurse who served at the British hospital at Camp Bastion, Afghanistan. She reflected on her reintegration.
She stated:

> Decision making in the grocery store was tough. You have too many options. They want you to make a decision from a whole aisle of laundry detergents. I remember thinking, "I just need detergent; I don't care which one." That becomes intense for a while, but then it fades away. It takes a bit of time.

Lauren talked about her boyfriend:

> I remember both of us coming off deployments, and we did a lot of stuff together, and we would talk about things. It was spur of the moment talking, not planned talking. We certainly talked a lot about our experiences and situations, and the things we saw. I kept a journal, an e-mail journal back and forth about things we saw and did, and that was really therapeutic and helpful for me. My boyfriend was in Iraq and Afghanistan. He got home 4 months before I did. We're both in the navy. Reintegration and routines, I remember thinking that life seemed so fast for a while and wanting things to slow down. I feel very fortunate that I didn't have a lot of problems coming back. Some people seem to

think you will. And yes, some people do have significant problems, but I didn't. My boyfriend, who is now my husband, and I did not have a lot of crazy troubles. Yes, anxiety sometimes. It may have been a little more challenging for him. I remember maybe crying with him, but it was pretty normal at the time after our deployments.

I am an energetic kind of person. I learned to cope with anxiety and *breathe*. It was more intense initially. Also, I was coming from Japan and had lived there for almost 2 years. Japan is a totally different way of life. Then, I went to Afghanistan; so, I had been away from the U.S. for a while. It was more like a "coming home" experience. There was a ton of stuff. I was away for more than 2 years; one place was the trauma of a war zone, and the other place was a culture unlike ours, so far from ours. I was 45 miles south of Tokyo.

My husband, who was my boyfriend at the time, got deployed twice when he was stationed in Sicily; once to Iraq and once to Afghanistan. We did manage to see each other over the 2 years. I toured around Italy with him, and it was fantastic. Then, he came to Japan, and we went scuba diving. These were the two times we saw each other during the 2 years. Indirectly, we've been a support system for each other when we got back. Even to this day, he is helpful. He's been deployed five times. We've lost people. He lost a very close buddy when I was living in Japan, and that was really tough. We got married in 2011, and then he deployed one final time to Afghanistan. I was back in the States when he got deployed. During that time, a very close friend of mine who was married to a navy nurse was killed in Afghanistan. I went to the funeral in San Diego when my husband was still in Afghanistan. We've lost some close people. We've been able to work through these things together and talk about them and remember things and honor the people. Those experiences are easier to go through with someone who understands. To this day, we talk about those guys, and we go and visit Bethesda. My husband has a bunch of buddies who have gone through there because they got blown up. We visit them. I have girlfriends who are still in the navy and we talk. My husband and I take part in veterans' things here in Virginia. He is president of the military association here. I am very involved with him in that, just to foster support. We talk a lot about what we saw and did. It is just a common foundation of knowing what deployment has been like.

Lauren talked about a bond between veterans stating:

There's a bond between veterans; it's helpful and it goes without speaking. It's a comfortable group of people to be with. We didn't have trouble incorporating into civilian life. It worked great for us. Our first semester last year in graduate school as civilians went really well, but also seems like a blur [*laughing*]. There was a lot going on. I think we've done pretty well entering a new chapter. We don't expect civilians to know all that we've done. We want to learn from them, and I've been blown away by some of their experiences. It's more like me entering their world. We're really coming back into their world, but we're sharing our world too.

We're using the GI bill for grad school. Our education is paid for, and we get a stipend for living expenses. It's almost too good to be true. It's amazing! All of this has helped us transition quite easily and without a lot of stress. Yes, we're grad students, and we don't make a lot of money right now, but our tuition is paid for. In a year, we'll be looking for jobs. We'll be done in May. My husband had an internship all summer in Boston. He loves what he did in Boston, and hopefully, he'll have a job offer soon.

Lauren spoke of studying to be a nurse practitioner:

With the NP thing, I'd love to go back and work with a veteran population. I might look for work at a VA hospital because I think the VA has a huge amount of guys coming to them. We had to go through our VA experience up in DC as we were leaving the service. We had health assessments. Some VAs are amazing, and others need a lot of help. A lot of them need to get a facelift. Fresh young faces, who are veterans and have had the deployment experience and are health care providers, could certainly offer something positive. I can offer a lot in that arena. I'd love to work for the VA. I'm scoping out some places in Boston. I'd be excited to go up there. That's what we see in our future. And as a country, we are responsible for our wounded veterans now, and for the rest of their lives. They need the best care we can provide.

CAPTAIN SCHUYLER

Schuyler, an army nurse, considered her reintegration easier than that of others because she met her husband in Iraq, fell in love in Iraq, got married in Turkey, and had a promising future to look forward to.

She related:

I feel like my transition was easier and better than most people. I was fortunate to have parents and family members who had experience with combat deployments. Being stationed in Germany, I was surrounded by people who had deployment experiences. So, I was lucky to have a stable support system. We were all in support of the "global war on terrorism" so, we had to wear our combat uniform every day, even though we were in Germany. We had air-evacs coming in every day with traumas that were 1 or 2 days fresh. There was this slow process of dealing with my emotions. I think it was particularly difficult for reservists who go home and have to work at a civilian hospital. Civilians have no idea what returning deployers had just been in 30 days earlier.

I met my husband in Iraq, about 3 weeks into my deployment. We met in the most notorious prison in the world! Actually my husband was working as an interpreter at the prison hospital and I was working in the ER. He worked in a different area of the hospital but I would see him from time to time. I finally figured out how I could talk to him in a respectful encounter that would open the door of opportunity for us to meet. He'll say that I pursued him [*laughing*]. Yeah, he'll say that. That's how we met. He was a civilian contractor. My husband was actually a civilian Iraqi who was an interpreter. He couldn't leave Iraq. He worked with the coalition forces for almost 4 years with various units. So when I left Iraq, he made plans to quit his job and go back with his family and work on our plans to be together. My husband is Kurdish and he's from northern Iraq. All of his family is there. We ended up getting married in Turkey, which is actually one of the easiest places to meet and get married. So, I redeployed to Germany in April 2007. We got married in August 2007.

Then, it was more paperwork to get him to Germany and more paperwork to get him his green card. It's a good story! Turkey became a very special place for us. It is an awesome place to go. It was just me and my husband when we got married. My family and his family were not there. It was probably the best thing for us to get married on our own in Turkey because initially our families were not one hundred percent behind our decision to be together.

Right when I got back to the States on leave, going to the grocery store could be difficult. There was so much going on at the grocery store and so many choices. The options could be overwhelming. I remember talking to my friend, telling her that I started crying in the grocery store when I couldn't find something. I think it was this marmalade that my Mom asked me to pick up. I started crying because I couldn't find it. Finally, a man came up to me and said, "Can I help you?" I said, "I can't find the marmalade." He said, "I'll find it for you" [*laughing*]. Then, he asked me if I was OK. I said, "I'll be OK as soon as I have the marmalade" [*laughing*]. This was probably the most challenging experience for me. It's funny now, but it wasn't at the time.

Then, when I got to Germany after leave, my apartment was really overwhelming. I put everything I needed to live off in one room. I didn't go into any of the other rooms anymore. I had a roommate before I deployed to Iraq, but she had already returned to the U.S. For one person now, it was a huge apartment. You have your housing allowance and what you can afford. So, in Germany, this may end up being a large place, even though you don't need it. I had an 800-square-meter apartment with five bedrooms, a dining room, a kitchen, and three bathrooms. It was huge. Now, here I am with me and a cat. It was just too much after living in a tiny dorm with a roommate when I was deployed. I put all my stuff in my bedroom, and I'd go between there and the bathroom and the kitchen. I closed the rest of the apartment. While in Germany, all my bills were automatically paid. Once I had set them up, it came directly from my paycheck so I didn't have to worry about anything. And with working at the hospital, I'd eat at the hospital most of the time. I didn't make my own food very often. I didn't have a lot of issues.

I met my husband, and at that point I decided to stop drinking alcohol socially. And so, when I redeployed, it was helpful that I made a conscious decision not to drink. For my friends, I think reintegration was more emotional because they were drinking, and sometimes they'd get intoxicated. They'd think about their deployment experiences, and what they saw, and what they did. They did this when they were intoxicated and when they weren't intoxicated. It took an emotional toll on them. For me, not drinking was helpful. The reasoning behind me not drinking was partly because I was starting to think about becoming Muslim. Before I decided to become Muslim, I decided to be a really good Lutheran and not drink [*laughing*]. I guess it was part of my spiritual journey. I didn't think alcohol belonged in that journey whether I was a Lutheran or Muslim or something else. At that point, I just did not think alcohol was good for me. It was a conscious decision not to drink. Technically Muslims are not supposed to drink alcohol. But what I like to joke with my husband about is that most secular nonpracticing Muslims; they will not eat pork, but they'll drink alcohol. A lot of Muslims, especially men, will drink alcohol [*laughing*]. It would be a conscious decision now if I said, "I'm not going to practice my religion right now and I'm going to sit down and have a glass of wine." If my husband and I wanted to have a glass of wine with dinner, we could do that, we could decide to do that. But we don't. It's the degree to which someone wants to observe the basic tenets of their religion. It's the regulation part of the religion.

Drinking and partying are ingrained in the military culture. It was hard for my friends when we got back because they'd want me to go out with them to a bar, and obviously drinking was a big part of a social evening. There would be a lot of peer pressure to participate. After redeployment, I'd suggest things like, "Why don't we just get together for lunch?" [*laughing*]. They'd get frustrated with me. It's this bonding experience, and if you're not drinking, you're not part of the bonding experience. It's this coping mechanism and if you're not drinking with the others, you become this "designated thinker." You're not participating in the activity with the group anymore.

LIEUTENANT DARLA

Darla is a navy nurse.
She remarked:

Deployment was like the straw that broke the camel's back in terms of affecting everything. I think I was in a place in my life where things were going to change anyway. With my boyfriend and I breaking up so soon after I returned from Afghanistan, I'm not sure if being deployed caused that. Maybe us breaking up was inevitable and had nothing to do with deployment. However, I am glad that I deployed, and I am proud of the job we did over there. I'm settled in my new job, in my new apartment, and in a part of the country I never lived in before. I think integration into the reserves was a challenge for me. I sometimes wish I was still on active duty. I might go back, but I'm going to just take it easy for now.

CAPTAIN CORABETH

Corabeth stated:

I think the biggest problem with transitioning back to your family and friends, your workplace, and your community was the lack of understanding of what you saw and did: your experience in caring for detainees in a prison hospital. Nobody knew what you saw and did. That was the biggest problem for most of us that had the detainee care mission. I had 2 weeks back in the U.S. Everyone was glad to see me, and it was "sunshine and roses." But then, I had to go back to Germany. I was home in New Mexico for 2 weeks, and then back to Germany. It was challenging, again, in Germany because no one knew about the experiences you had doing the detainee care mission.

CAPTAIN COURTNEY

Courtney is an Air National Guard nurse.
She related:

Our town has a big 4th of July celebration. At it, our first selectman came over to talk to me. I think everyone in my town knew that I deployed. I'm very low key. People asked me, "How was it?" But they also respected my privacy. I still have the same friends from high school in my town. It was not hard to get back into daily activities. For example, I love cooking and I cooked for everyone in Afghanistan. I loved coming back to my kitchen. But in many ways, it was easier during deployment because you weren't grocery shopping or paying bills or worrying about family schedules. You don't have to do a lot of extra stuff over there. It was easy. You don't realize how easy it is until you come back. It comes back, but it is slow. If you are an impatient person, you may have to seek counseling to deal with all this stuff.

CAPTAIN TENLEY

Tenley is an army nurse.
She recalled:

It appeared fine. We sat through all of the briefings. We figured out, "So, I shouldn't turn to alcohol after all of this." All the things that they told us to watch out for, I think were the stereotypical behaviors of a male soldier, and how he might deal with it. I think being female and not a line person, we didn't see gun shots unless we were flying in a helicopter. We had more emotional trauma. They didn't really teach us about how we might feel when we got home. That was part of the difficulty with reintegrating. They didn't touch on the emotional aspects that females and caregivers might feel upon returning home. So, we got back to our home site and because we were nurses, we only had 3 days together before everyone scattered. All you thought about was going home. Because we only had 3 days, our families were not necessarily there. I got back to Fort Hood, Texas, and my family lives in Washington state. I wasn't gonna make them fly down there just to say, "Hello, I'm home" when 3 days later I'd be flying into Washington state where they were. We got to Texas, and everyone who was from Fort Hood had their family there. The rest of us just wanted to get this over with. It was just irritating to know that others had their families there, but we didn't because we were not from that area. We were the forgotten ones. We kind of banded together, and we all went out to eat. It was the little things after that which made a huge difference. Our perspective on life officially changed because of what we saw, and what we did. For me, a bad day was a day someone died. At the airport, our plane was delayed, and I remember one of the ladies in line complaining that this was, "the worst day ever." I was never an angry person before, but now I could pull the switch and get angry. It was hard for me to hold back because I am a "chatterer," so, I would pretty much verbally, "word vomit" on random strangers because they didn't know what a bad day was. A bad day is when people die, that's where I just came from. I didn't hold my tongue most of the time. Some of the girls and I went to Las Vegas afterwards, and a guy cut in line in front of us. I did not hold my tongue then. I let him have it [*laughing*]. I verbally assaulted him back after he called me the B word. My anger switch was turned on. You don't cut in line. You go to the end of the line where you are supposed to be. I did not hold my tongue.

The little things were huge. For example, in Iraq you could go to the commissary or to this little PX we used to go to, and there would be one choice. "OK, well I need toothpaste, OK, got it." Now, you go into the grocery store at home, and there are ten kinds of toothpaste. Like cereal, in Iraq, there would be maybe four choices of cereal that I could eat. Now, at home, there is a whole aisle of cereal to choose from. It was very overwhelming. Just making a choice was awful. Sometimes, I'd start crying in the grocery store.

Tenley described the beginning of her reintegration stating:

Here I am at home with my mother and my family, and they don't know why I don't feel normal; I don't feel like myself. I was not the type of person who would get overwhelmed in a grocery store. Now, the grocery store overwhelms me to the point of not being able to function in it, and I'd have to leave. I would leave my cart and start crying because I was so overwhelmed. Many different situations would trigger a similar response.

Music is a huge therapy for me. Church was one of those times, and then a situation happened, and I'd go to church. Once in a while, a song would play in church that would speak to me. Then, at home, I'd go to church with my parents, and the same song would be played. I'd feel overwhelmed, and I'd start crying, and I'd have to leave church and go home. All of the Iraq memories would come back to me. It was just awful. This was not me. I was not a crier prior to Iraq. I felt like now I had all these emotions that I couldn't control. I'd start crying in the middle of crazy scenarios. For example, I went to Alaska to visit my sister because I had 30 days of leave. She teaches deaf children, and they put on this play. The play was fine. But afterwards, I could not communicate with anyone other than my sister because I am not fluent in sign language. Again, I'd get overwhelmed, and I'd have to leave. What actually made things better was "calling the girls" or e-mailing them. I'd tell them the scenario that just happened and how I responded. "What is wrong with me?" I'd get overwhelmed, and I'd start to cry, and I could not function. So, we compared notes and stories, and soon I realized that many of us were having the same response to coming home. We agreed that no one ever told us about what we might be feeling and experiencing after coming home. No one spelled out the possible feelings of being overwhelmed or frustrated or angry. This should have been incorporated in classes. Talking to the other nurses, we validated each other's emotions.

So now I realized I was not going crazy and that I was not alone in what I was feeling and experiencing. It was like, "OK, this is normal," and I'll get over it eventually. And, I did. It probably took me over a year before I felt absolutely normal again. Loud noises would startle me. I know this is pretty normal because we were waking up to mortars. Our response was, you hear a sound, wait a minute, you listen for a helicopter, if you hear a helicopter, it meant someone was hurt so you would go to the hospital. Loud noises always meant something to us in Iraq. Being home, the 4th of July almost killed me. I could not handle loud noises. It was awful for me, but you knew it was going to happen because they taught you that you would respond to loud noises the same way at home as you did in Iraq. You knew this would eventually get better. By talking to the girls, I always felt better. Talking through everything was helpful, therapeutic, and made things better. During my 30 days of leave, I told my story over and over again. Each time I did this, things got better.

CAPTAIN MARLEY

Marley is an army nurse.
She stated:

For me, the Afghanistan deployment was different. First of all, it wasn't a year deployment. It was 3 months for training and 6 months of deployment. We worked every single day with trauma, trauma, trauma. We flew out to pick up patients and did stuff for fallen soldiers and their families. A lot of patients died while we were in Afghanistan. Then, when we returned home, there were nine of us together. I had to fly from Afghanistan to Hawaii, which was ridiculous just to turn in my M-9. They made a big deal of this. I actually turned in my M-9 in a hotel on the beach in the parking lot. It made no sense to me why the nine of us had to do this. We stayed in Hawaii for 3 days. We mobilized there, and the FST mission was a week before Christmas. You train in Hawaii and Miami, and then you fly back to Hawaii to Guam to Thailand, and then to Afghanistan. Then you do an amazing mission for 6 months.

I just wanted to go on leave and be by myself. I had a checklist about reintegrating. I had a lot of stuff in my head about surgeries, and some of my medics had been injured and passed away. I just wanted time to myself. I had to go through so many checks to get papers signed to go on leave. It was ridiculous! At one point, I got into an argument with a woman behind the desk. I was very angry. You fly from San Antonio to Albuquerque.

I realized by just driving a few days in San Antonio that I had road rage. So, I told my mom I would rather fly than drive. I was angry and broken down for no real reason. Then when I land there's all these things going on for blue and gold star moms and wives. I just walked through the airport with my mom. No one knew who I was. My mom said, "Well, I'm proud of you," and she started to cry. I was wearing regular clothes. So, I came home to be with Mom and my sisters. I knew from my previous deployment that there were lots of things I couldn't tell her [*starts crying, sobbing*]. It was so hard. I couldn't tell Mom. I said I was fine, but I wasn't. I didn't want her to worry about me. I couldn't tell her what I had seen and done. When I was in Afghanistan, Mom wrote me a letter telling me that she thought it was a good time for me to get out of the military. She said that it was just too hard for her. It was hard for me, too, because I was good at it and some people told me that I'd eventually be a general. Yet, you love and respect your family. I was in for 13 years.

You have to understand, my Mom met me when I was homeless. I was 16 and I had run away from home. I was living on other people's couches. I got a job at 17 or 18. I had graduated from high school. On the way, I had met Mom and she was like, "I'm gonna adopt you." She didn't know that I was living on other people's couches or that I was a drifter. She just took me into her life. She's my adoptive Mom. My biological Mom was a drug addict and had mental health problems. I graduated from high school and joined the army. It was constant feedback and rewards and promotions for doing the right things. I had a lot of mentors. So, when Mom said "I need you home," I wanted to do that. I love my Mom so much. She is an ICU nurse to the core. She influenced me to become a nurse. I was working as a nursing assistant. She told me, "You can do this." I also wanted to be like her. But I found that the ER was for me, more than the ICU. I loved the thrill of the ER.

Marley talked about her deployment:

In Afghanistan, I got to go on patrols through Ghasni. I visited orphanages and places where they had children's services. I did lots of sick calls for soldiers. We had one doctor, and he preferred to play video games; so, I did the sick calls. I got great experience, and that's why I am now a nurse practitioner. I knew that my role would be changed when I came back. I knew I'd be going back to a lesser scope of practice. I took 2 weeks off to be

with my mom and sisters. I got a dog, a puppy. I swear to God
if it wasn't for that dog, I probably would not be doing so well.

CAPTAIN EARL

Earl is an Air Force Reserve flight nurse.
He stated:

When my wife finally came back after her third deployment, we
reintegrated. She now had problems. It was a very unique experience because she was now having some of the same symptoms
that I had had when I came back from deployment, but she was
in complete denial. I went to the flight surgeon pretty quickly. She
refused to go, and I'll never forget this quote she used, "I'm not
one of those people." She was in absolute denial. I said, "OK, fine,
if you don't have problems with what you saw and did that's fine.
But our marriage is having problems; so, we're going to marriage
counseling." And we did that through the active duty military at
Madigan Army Medical Center. We had sessions together, and then
she had individual sessions. It's funny because my wife just came
back recently from 2 weeks of duty in San Diego. This was the
first opportunity to read my book. She's not a book reader. She
doesn't read books at all, whereas I'm reading books all the time.
She thought it was very well written, and she was impressed with
it. But, it opened up a lot of old wounds. She said, "Oh my God,
it recalled so many things that I did over there, and I didn't even
think of them until I read the book. The book brought back so
many memories; memories of fear, memories of flying combat missions. I had just suppressed them." She came home yesterday from
work and was very emotional about this, which is a good thing.

When my wife worked on her master's degree, I helped
edit some of her papers, and she is just not a writer. We eventually got better together. Time helped, and talking about our
experiences and feelings helped. Writing the book helped me,
and reading the book helped her. Also, as my work got out there
and got published, the feedback I got helped, people saying I
read your story, and it really hit home. I had not been able to
explain to my family what I went through, and I was able to
just give them my book and say, "Read this, this is what I went
through, and this is what I did, and this is how I feel." When
Gen. Rank called me and said that she wanted me to do some

work for her, she said that my work tells her that I know what is going on. She wanted me to do some informal research for her, interviewing people returning after war. A lot of them had the exact same symptoms that I had had when I returned. So, there was definitely a common thread. We're all having issues, and we need to talk about it. This motivated me to finish the book. I thought, "I need to get this out there because I think it will help people and get them talking about stuff."

I'd be happy if I could get 4 hours of sleep. That was a good night for me. I have had many nurses, who I have talked to during the informal interviews for Gen. Rank and from the public speaking I do at conferences, come up to me and thank me and say that they are going to go to the VA for help, or to the military for help, or seek private civilian services. I've talked to nurses who have been home for 10 years and still can't sleep. Just recently, one of my friends was over for dinner, and she was showing signs of anxiety. So, I just threw some questions at her: How well did you sleep last night? She looked at me and raised her eyebrows and said, "Why are you asking me this?" I said, "You look a little tired." She added, "I haven't really slept well since we got home from our deployment in 2003." She said, "On a good night, I'm lucky if I get 4 hours of sleep." I have heard this consistently over and over and over again.

Earl shared his own situation stating:

My mental well-being has recovered. Occasionally, there are still some things that occur that will trigger memories. Sleep is my most valued thing when I get 7 hours or so. There was a long period of time when I'd be happy if I could get 4 hours of sleep. That was a good night for me.

Then, Earl talked about reintegration. He said:

I don't think I really completed my reintegration with my family until this last April 2013 when we had a family reunion with all my brothers and sisters. I've got two brothers and two sisters. My mom brought all of us together for a reunion in Snohomish County. So, my brothers and sisters and all the spouses and children got together. I brought a draft of the book from my publishers, and everybody read it during the 4 days that we were there. It forced everyone to talk about what everyone saw in me and my wife and my brother when we came back from war. We actually had an open dialogue as a family about the effect of war on our family. It was a great healing experience. I used the book as a mechanism to get everyone to sit down and talk about things. The book was a perfect vehicle to get communication going. My mom said that all of her uncle's came back from WW II. All of them went into combat. I believe there were six of them, and Mom said that all of them came back as alcoholics. One of my uncles killed himself after WW II. He had a head injury after being on Anzio Beach and could never get over the headaches from his injury and the pain of his memories. Mom remembers being a child during WW II when the veterans came home, and everybody simply did not talk about the war. You just went on with your life, and the only time the memories came out was when your uncles were together at a gathering, and they started drinking. I guess things could get a little crazy.

Ten years after being deployed, I now feel reintegrated with my family. My wife and I have come to terms with our deployments, and what we said and did. We've come to terms in our relationship because there were a lot of open wounds and scars from things that we had said and done to each other. There was verbal fighting; it never got physical. There was a huge disconnect for a long time because her experiences were different from mine. Even now she says, "Oh my God, I would not want to be on a plane with 78 wounded. I don't know what I would have done." And I say to her, "You would have handled it because every time we went on a mission, there were more wounded, and we always somehow made it work."

The true tragedy of combat nursing: Nurses are patient advocates and nurses want to care for patients, but with combat nursing, you are doing an awful lot of triage rather than actually caring for the patient; you employ stopgap measures. You are not really providing the compassionate care you are taught in nursing school; what a nurse is supposed to do. That is very difficult for nurses. There were days when I didn't feel like a nurse; I felt like I was just doing procedures. That makes it difficult when you consider the profession of nursing.

My wife was gone a lot, and there was a lot on my plate. I had to come up with a system. I didn't have anybody to help me with that. I had to map out the entire month between work, my reserve commitment, and my wife being gone. I had to put things on the calendar, such as doing the laundry on this day and grocery shopping on that day. The entire month had to be plotted out, and I didn't have much support. My brother was still mobilized at the time. The support that I did have in the new job was the recruit academy. It was very hard, and it was 16 weeks long, Monday through Friday. I had a military vet friend who had also been through the academy, and he said, "Your wife is gone, your brother is still gone, and your mom can't help you so, every Friday come over to my house for dinner. I'll have a gin and tonic waiting for you. You can just spend time and relax." He did this consistently for 16 weeks, and it was a huge help. He was married, but didn't have any children. His wife was actually deployed with me in the same squadron. He and I deployed to the first Gulf War. We had a strong military connection.

Our military and civilian society needs to accept and embrace the fact that anyone going off to war will return changed. We need to be proactive about this, and educate people prior to the troops being sent overseas, and when they come home. If the civilian population votes our elected officials into office who may ultimately vote to send us to war, they need to accept the responsibility and the burden of the veterans who come back mentally and physically disabled. That is not happening!

I've heard some people say, "Well, you volunteered for the duty." The civilian population agrees to go to war through our elected officials, then you need to accept the responsibility and burden of the veterans who come back with mental and physical problems. The Wounded Warrior Project and many other organizations are doing really wonderful work. Many people are thoroughly engaged. But there are a lot of U.S. citizens who simply pretend it is not a problem, and that it doesn't exist. I had another fire fighter say to me, "Do you think our people (our generation) are just not as tough as the WW II veterans?" He had no military experience. He said, "There's all this stuff on television about PTSD, vets with problems, and vet suicides rates are going through the roof that didn't happen with WW II vets. They came home and went right back to work." I said to him, "Are you kidding me? All my uncles who served in WW II became raging alcoholics. One killed himself. Do you have anything to reference? My great uncle was shot down in WW II, and our grandmother cried every year at his grave site on Memorial Day into her 80s before she died. How can you say that the veterans and society was not affected by WW II?" We have to start training people for the next war we are involved in. Because if we are going to be sending our men and women into war, we have a moral responsibility to take better care of them, and our society needs to put a support system in place for them when they come home.

LIEUTENANT COLONEL DAGMAR

Dagmar is a very seasoned air force reservist.
He recalled:

Every time I returned there's always that initial excitement of coming home, having the luxury of your own bathroom, your own comfortable bed, and getting to do the things you've been dreaming about while you were gone. Then you have to shop and make dinner, and it is an adjustment. I always had a case of the "postdeployment blues." It sets in once you're home and past the initial excitement and jet lag. It's really hard for me to feel left out of the war. You know what's going on, you know who you left behind there. The people who replaced you, maybe you felt that they had less experience or were less qualified. You felt detached. Your whole life was the war. You read *Stars & Stripes*, you watch TV to keep up with the war, and you think about being a good citizen. It's hard to come home and be cut off. My radar would go up if I heard that four soldiers were killed in a helicopter crash or something like that. I would immediately turn on the TV. To me it meant that there were probably 10 others who were injured, and that air-evac was needed to move patients. I knew the implications of that or the report of a suicide bomber. I knew about all the injured kids and civilians. I knew about the horrible injuries of war, and often felt that the American people had no real awareness of any of this. It's hard to be cut off from all of that. You go from living it every single day. On some deployments I worked 12 hour days. The last two deployments were at Bastion; I was the commander and did not take a day off. I would take parts of a day off when it was slow. I never took a whole day off in 4 months. It was hard for me to go from all to nothing. A piece of me always stayed there. I've been to so many places. I've been to so many FOBs, and I can picture all these places, and I know what's there, and what's not there. This was my life. I have very vivid images that everyone around me at the VA was oblivious to. That disconnect is very, very hard.

Each time I came home, I took a little more time off. I said, "I need to walk on the beach, I need to do some yoga, I need to do some 'chilling out' here, I need to decompress." I recognized this. My military friends helped me through the postdeployment blues, and I was able to stay engaged on a limited basis. I needed to do this. Our mission is to stay prepared, and my head still needed to be in the game. I had to form a new life in the process, too, because of losing my husband. I had changed and I had to face it. I realized that I was beating myself up, and questioned why I was going between Phoenix and California with five 12-hour shifts in a row, and then working five more days with the military, and then flying back to Phoenix. So I sort of threw in the towel and quit fighting it. I said, "I am going to live near the base." I realized that this had been no kind of life, and that I needed to make a change. I moved back to California to live near the base because that's what I kept coming home to. That was home for me. I got a condo on the beach, 5 minutes away from the base.

I grew up in Bakersfield, California. My base is the only Air National Guard [ANG] base on the west coast. The next closest ANG bases are in Wyoming and Oklahoma. We cover a huge territory. We are very active, and we have a reputation for being able to do short falls and have experienced people to plug in, and do whatever is needed.

LIEUTENANT COLONEL VIOLA

Viola is an army nurse.
She recalled:

It was not bad getting back into my life. I had the time and the ability because it was so handy to work out while I was gone. Working the evening or night shift as nursing supervisor, I was able to work out in the morning which was nice. The one thing that I did in Iraq which I don't do on a regular basis at home was to eat three large meals. I was going to the dining facility to eat breakfast, lunch, and dinner. I don't usually eat three large meals at home. I gained 10 pounds while I was deployed. I was able to eventually cut back and not gain anymore. I did lose the 10 pounds when I got home. I think it had to do with not cooking yourself, and the selection was good, and there were always large amounts of food available. We not only had our dining facility at the hospital Ipisthina, but we also had access to the dining facility at the palace, which is the headquarters for the Iraqi forces. Our leadership for the U.S. Army was at this palace. It was maybe three-quarters of a mile to a mile from us. We could walk there for meals. Then, there was another dining facility within walking distance too. We had lots of choices. It was fairly safe to walk there, but the Green Zone (the international zone in the city of Baghdad, Iraq) would take indirect fire and could also be a target. A nurse had been killed by indirect fire 6 months or so before we got there. One nurse was wounded, and the other one was killed. They were close to the hospital, too. It wasn't as safe as some people thought the Green Zone would be. Every once in a while there would be minor shrapnel injuries or a tympanic membrane rupture.

I think I had a pretty smooth transition back. My husband was very supportive and understanding. My family was as well. Everything went well. It was my first deployment.

MAJOR ANITA

Anita is an air force nurse.
She recalled:

We live about 40 minutes from Sacramento; so we just hopped in the car and came home. Fortunately, because my husband has deployed before, we know that things are a bit weird that first week when you come home. It's weird between husband and wife. It's hard to put it into words except we've experienced it many times. My husband and I have been together 10 years now, and between the two of us we've had four or five deployments. So, we've had separations, and we know that first week is weird because you want to spend every waking moment with that person. But at the same time, that person needs to get back into the routine of being home. We're big on routines. My husband is very big on routines. But when you are deployed, you do develop a routine. You get up at the same time every day. You pretty much eat at the same place. You don't have to make a decision, you eat what is being served. You don't have to decide where you are going. You don't have to decide what you are going to wear. You don't have to decide what you are going to do either [*laughing*].

All of these things have been taken care of. The only thing you have to decide is what you're going to order from Amazon.com [*laughing*]. But when you come home it's not that way. You kind of miss your routine. You don't miss being deployed. You don't miss Afghanistan. You miss your routine because everything was easy. You even miss your bunk bed [*laughing*]. I called it my little cubby-hole. Let me tell you, I like to fish, I can even bait my own hook but, I'm also a princess. In my little cubby-hole, I had pink sheets, and I had them draped all around. I also hung up sheets from the ceiling, and it looked like a little princess castle [*laughing*]. I had Christmas lights strung up on the inside of my bunk [*laughing*]. It was great, and I literally spent the most time in my cubby-hole. I would read and shop online. It was so nice and cozy.

So, when I came home there were times that I sort of missed my little cubby-hole. My husband would ask me if I missed the cubby-hole, and I said "I kind of do." He'd say, "You're so happy to be home, you love your husband, you're so happy to sleep in the same bed as your husband. But there are times when you miss your life in Afghanistan." You just get so used to it. So, now you have to relearn everything. And I think, honestly, when you first get back, you are ready to go back again. After I was back a month, we had some issues with trying to put people in certain deployment bands, and they approached me, and said we know that you just got back, but we really need you to be in this upcoming deployment band and I said, "Do it, I'm ready." Fortunately, I didn't get tasked to go, and now that I've been home for a while, I really don't want to go back right now. In the beginning, you want to go back because that is what you know. It is kind of strange to people who have not done it. It is strange to my friends back home and my family. My husband gets it. Thank God. I think this may be why we have such a high divorce rate in the military because the other stuff, they just don't know. It is foreign to them. People don't understand why you would want to go back.

MAJOR FRED

Fred is an air force reservist.
He commented:

Reintegration after Afghanistan took some adjustment just because of the isolation. There was just no place to go and nothing to do. Spending so much time alone and in your room can get to you after a while; the movies and reading helped. Within the perimeter of the base, there was just not anything to do. It was a lot different. After 9 months, I can't say I am 100 percent up and running. I think I'm doing pretty well. Oh yeah, I have a wonderful family and a very supportive wife. I have two really good kids. I attempted to go back to school to get my BSN, I lasted all of 2 weeks [*laughing*]. Well, I've been out of school for 20 years. I've been in critical care for 20 years.

Fred shared his personal philosophy relating to his 20+ years as an RN:

Although nursing has been wonderful to me, I am a "patient person." I am definitely patient oriented; I like dealing with my clients. I'm a hands-on person. I was brought up in the military, and I have strong feelings. If someone is not doing their job, I am the one that will tell them so. If you're having a bad hair day, I'm not the one who wants to hear about it [*laughing*]. I am not trying to lie to you, and I'm not trying to hurt you. I'm just telling you to do your job, and do it well.

MAJOR ELIZA

Eliza is an air force nurse with three deployments to Afghanistan and offered her advice to others:

When I came home from my deployments, the key was not trying to do too much too soon. I learned from my multiple deployments. I learned that it was not always good to go right home to family. I found it helpful to take a week to myself in nice surroundings to decompress and have some time alone. It helped to sleep, eat nutritious food, get a massage or a facial, and put things in perspective. It's important not to jump right into a bunch of activities because when you come home everyone wants to see you, and they want you to do this and that. It can be very overwhelming. And when you come home, you are tired, and you have to adjust to a different time zone.

With my 2010 deployment, I was able to take a week to myself, and everyone else was in North Carolina. I had to tie up some loose ends in Alaska; so, I had time to myself. I surprised everyone when I came home to North Carolina, and it was just before Christmas.

With my last deployment, I stayed home a lot during that first week. This was in Texas, and I did my usual routine, but I didn't have to go to work. I kicked back and watched TV and slept when I wanted to sleep. I took it easy. It was calming. Now, I work 8 a.m. to 4 p.m., Monday through Friday, which is really nice. For the 5 years before I was deployed, I worked in the hospital 12-hour shifts, every other weekend, and the holiday rotation. So, this is a nice schedule now. I see my daughter off to school, and I'm home every night. I help her with her homework, and I go to her different events. We do things as a family. She just turned 11 years old.

CAPTAIN AMANDA

Amanda is an air force nurse.
She stated:

Getting back into my life was not problematic after Afghanistan. I remember being at work and saying that it was easier to reintegrate after Afghanistan than it was after Germany. Then— BOOM!—the Boston Marathon bombings happened. I said it out loud, and I hate to think that I actually jinxed it, but it was awful, and I was working that day. I didn't want to be around it either. I had already quit my job, and I asked them for April 12 to be my last day, but they weaseled 2 more weeks out of me. So, I went to work on the 15th, and the bombings happened, and I stayed late to work. Then, we had debriefings over the next few days.

Later that week we were watching a press conference on the TV in the break room, and our chief of trauma surgery, and a social worker, and a nurse practitioner were talking about the marathon bombings, and how America's experience in war has helped the treatment of blast wounds, and how it benefitted that day. And at the end of the interview, they asked if anyone was working that day who had been deployed to Iraq or Afghanistan, and he said "No" [*She starts crying.*]. This doctor had been a retired colonel in the Army Guard, and he had deployed to Iraq a few years back and he said "No" [*crying*]. He didn't know, he doesn't know our staff, he doesn't work in our emergency room [*crying*]. I e-mailed him the next day. I was so upset. I left in tears and never went back. I e-mailed him that there was a doctor in Tent A that day who had Iraq experience, and so did one of our x-ray techs, and I told him that I had just returned from Afghanistan. He answered me and apologized saying that he had no idea, and that was it. I never went back to the medical center. I almost lost it [*crying*]. That was my last day there. I was disappointed and hurt. I had worked there since I graduated from nursing school. That's how it ended.

I lied to my mother about being on an FOB. She thought I was in Bagram the whole time. When I got home, the July 4th fireworks really bothered me. I never realized how much I hate fireworks. It was really overwhelming for me, everything about it, the noise, the smell. I flipped out a little bit; so, now I go to the vet center weekly to talk to someone. The fireworks made me feel hopeless and helpless and very scared; so, talking to someone has helped. In a war zone, you expect loud noises like IEDs every night, but when you get home, you do not expect those noises to continue. You don't expect to be horrified with loud noises. I needed a little bit of help, and now I am good.

LIEUTENANT DOREEN

Doreen is a navy reservist. She talked about her reintegration after Iraq. She recalled:

They flew us out of Iraq to Camp Lejeune and then to New Jersey. My homecoming was OK, the usual, met all my friends at a bar [*laughing*]. I saw my dad, my cousin, and my aunt. My cousin was battling cancer at the time. They were all supportive. I am not married and never have been. I have no kids.

Doreen summarized her reintegration:

I had a lot of ups and downs with my drinking. I also realized that I have often made poor choices with men, and that my behavior has been erratic. Fortunately, I eventually got someone in the VA hospital who helped me get a handle on my problems. My neuropsychiatrist has me doing a battery of tests for TBI [traumatic brain injury]. I am hopeful for my future.

CAPTAIN BRITTANY

Brittany, an army nurse, told about her reintegration after returning from Afghanistan.

She stated:

When I got home from Afghanistan, I moved in with some friends and their teenage daughter. So, I got to ease back into things. I lived with them for about a month and a half, and both the mom and the dad had to go away to army school for a couple of months. So, it was just me and their teenage daughter. It was like living with a little sister, and it was a lot of fun. So, I started cooking again and grocery shopping. I got to reintegrate slowly because I was living with them. They were very gracious and supportive. They had both had deployments in the past, some rougher than others. It was a good fit. They gave me space and time. It was a blessing. In December, I moved into my own place. That was a big shift. It took a while for me to get used to that again. I was super alert to a lot of things, like sounds. That has since decreased. It was different to be back on my own and to be paying bills again. I bought new furniture for the apartment. I have figured out what it is like to take care of myself again. It took a little while, but I feel like things are improving all the time. Most days now are good days for me. I pay my bills on time. I keep enough food in the house. I started volunteering again. I do a lot of things that I liked to do in the past. I love to volunteer, it's a big thing for me. I really enjoy it. I found a small organiza-tion that I really like. I get to go out there and help, but I'm not totally responsible. I don't have to be in charge. It's so nice to be able to help people, but not have the stress of responsibility.

I am still seeing the same therapist, it's been a year now; and it's good. I met with my psychiatrist, and we are gonna start transitioning off some of the meds. Right now, I'm on Wellbutrin and Celexa, which seem to be a good combination for me. When I was in Afghanistan, they gave me Prozac, and it wasn't right for me. I am thankful that things are really looking up for me and that I am enjoying life and work again.

MAJOR COLLEEN

Colleen, an army nurse, talked about her reintegration.
She stated:

The bottom line is that I've been back now for 2-½ years, and I don't know. The whole experience has been difficult. Ultimately,

I think there is a reason all this happened. I guess this is the path that I was supposed to take. It's been difficult. It's sad because I really believe in the army, I love the army. I don't think I belong in the Army Nurse Corps anymore. The experiences I have had over the last few years have been very different from my colleagues. I was around these special forces line-type people, and I really bonded with those people. I was looking to get on a female-engagement team, really any way to get out of here. These teams were just starting when I was over there, and they started attaching females to Special Forces units. They go out to mosque-type environments to speak with the women. I was asked to be on one when I was down range. I have been to 33 foreign countries, and I love dealing with different cultures. I lived in a Muslim country; so, I understand the culture, and I really wanted to go outside the wire and work with people.

I talked to my mentor at length because she had a career in the military and also had a family. I want to do all these cool things, and I have already done some, but I also want to have a family. She talked to me about staying here and dealing with this stuff and not looking to run away, to settle down. So, I decided not to apply for the female-engagement teams. Although every once in a while, I think I should deploy again to do that. This is just not my place anymore. Another thing is that the female-engagement team would only take me out of the Army Nurse Corps for a year. I'd have to come back to this, and I could get stuck again. I guess I'll be in a reserve unit. I wanted to do this so bad. But they told me that I couldn't do it because I'd be gone for 3 weeks at a time, and that with 10 nurses it wouldn't work.

With my deployment and the assignment in Korea, I learned to just push everything away and not deal with life. My first reaction is just to do that. I guess it is something I have to work on, and I am. I also have some difficult stuff left over from college. I was not actually raped or anything, but I have some traumatic experiences left over from college. It's the combination of these things, and the relationships with the men I've been with. I'd say the biggest issue I have, at this point, is relationships with men. In Afghanistan, Korea, and even here in Arizona, there are very few females. And there are very few attractive young females. So, guys are just not good [*laughing*]. I moved around a lot as a child, and I've always had this tendency to "move on." I'd close one book or chapter, and open another one. I've done that my entire life. So, not being able to run away from here has been difficult, but on the other hand, I think it is needed. It doesn't make it any easier, and I hate feeling weak. Other people haven't been through what I have been through. I've moved six times in 7 years.

I've spent a lot of time talking to my family and my friends on Skype. I finally came to the conclusion when I went home on leave in December, that no one is going to fix this for me. I have to fix it for myself. I made a list of things to do for me that would be good for me. They involve the Paleo diet and the rock climbing, and this is where I am now which is a much better place. The final step of that was my decision to go back to school. I'm ready for this now. Although I've had a lot of troubles, I have taken steps to help myself.

Although I have had a difficult couple of years, I would not have changed anything. Because I think that ultimately there is a reason I have dealt with these things. I think that it has shown me more compassion for other people even though in some ways I have less compassion because some people come in with a sore finger. A lot of people have been through worse than me. I think that it has made me grow into wanting even more to help people. It has never changed the fact that I want to help people who have less than me. The whole process that I have been through has trended me more towards the humanitarian thought process. Who knows? I may be working in a foreign country. I don't know. Looking back on everything, I think this was probably not comfortable, but necessary, for me to move on with my life. I have gotten stronger, absolutely.

COMMANDER DARBY

Darby related:

> The horrible experience at this Afghan hospital very much affected my reintegration. I was mad at everybody. I took a year out of my life to go to Afghanistan as a navy nurse, and I thought I would be taking care of our guys. As far as I'm concerned, it was a wasted year away from my family.
>
> Reintegration was very difficult. I am on my own. I had three surgeries on my foot last year. I had surgery for a kidney stone last year. I just had surgery in October on my back. These were not war-related health problems, but nonetheless, they were painful and getting care through the VA was frustrating.
>
> I will never forget what I saw at this hospital. I will always remember the patients that were basically tortured by Afghan

doctors. Surgery without anesthesia is barbaric. Women were beaten unconscious to undergo C-sections without anesthesia. Hemorrhages and infections were rampant. I came home angry, frustrated, and disappointed. I felt let-down, not listened to. I'm a 0–5 [commander] and I have a lot of coping skills. I saved money while deployed. But there were problems with my pay when I got home and also problems with my health care.

I would say that my reintegration has been complicated. It seems like one thing after another, which makes it impossible to reintegrate. I really don't think anybody gets it. [*crying*]. I feel like a train wreck with my foot, my back, and my kidney stone. I'd go back to another place in Afghanistan in a heart-beat if I got to take care of our troops. I'd never go back to that hospital because with that mission nothing mattered. It was a waste of time. It was a horrible experience. I can see why these kids come back from deployments and kill themselves. They are angry; do not feel supported; are frustrated; and do not know where to turn.

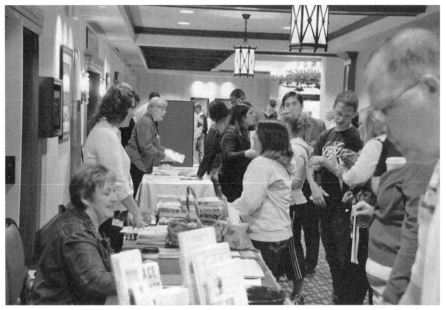

Yellow Ribbon Reintegration event for returning military personnel
and their families, Hershey, Pennsylvania.

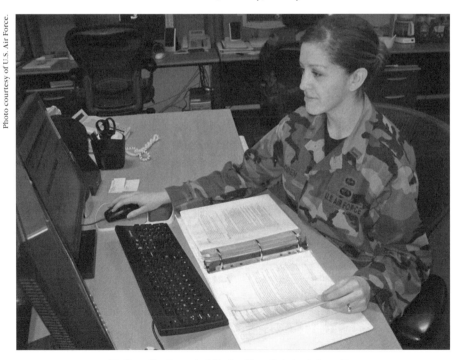

Air force lieutenant visits the SharePoint reintegration
website in Germany.

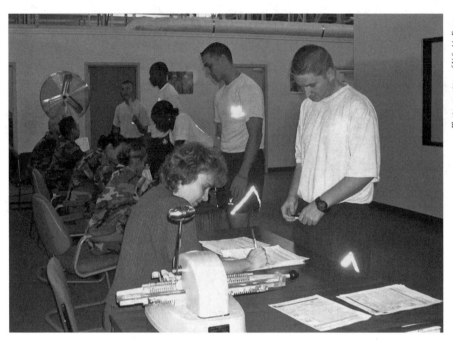

Reintegration processing for airmen at Laughlin Air Force Base, Texas.

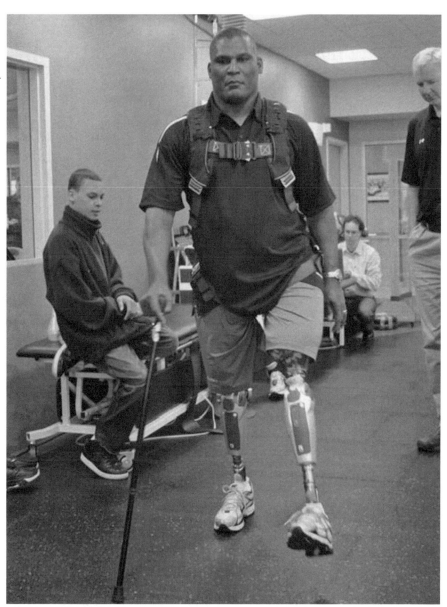

Recovering army officer at Walter Reed National
Military Medical Center.

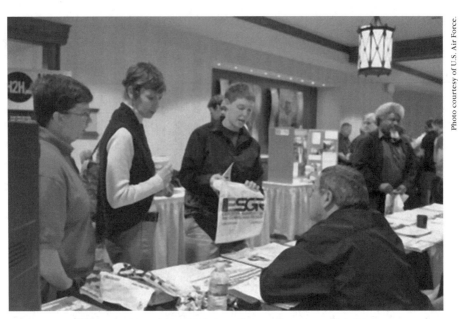

Women veterans attend reintegration conference and job fair.

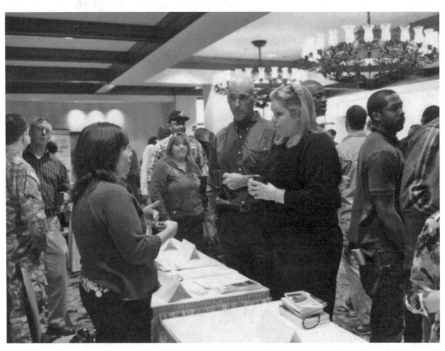

Reintegration seminar for returning service members
and their families.

13

Discussion of Findings

Through the telling of the individual nurses' stories, a readable narrative is constructed that reflects the diversity and eclectic nature of their deployment, homecoming, and reintegration. Their stories reveal a complex reality with regard to their clinical assignments and missions, the patients they cared for, and the military hierarchy in which they practiced. Reintegration for some nurses proved to be complicated as they referenced their social network, workplace, and community. Reactions to coming home were varied; some were met with surprise, guilt, anxiety, and frustration. Others felt surrounded with the love of their families and friends. Some felt appreciated and honored by their social and work networks. Many nurses had difficulty finding their place in society and in nursing because they felt "forever changed." Some assimilated in a more regular fashion, especially when they were graced with a strong support system. Marriages and relationships were tarnished, some ended, others miraculously endured, and still others were strengthened.

When examining the research findings, two distinct elements of reintegration stand out the most. First, reintegration is a very individual process for each returning nurse. Second, there is no specific timetable to complete the reintegration process. As with all processes, there is a beginning, a middle, and an end. Some of the nurses indicated key points in their reintegration and others described when they felt a sense of closure. For example, Captain Earl, who was an air force flight nurse in a reserve unit, exclaimed that he did not feel "reintegrated" until he was home for about 10 years. However, even when nurses recognize closure to the reintegration process, they still readily admit that they are "forever changed" as a result of their deployment experience.

With each theme identified through this research, there were miti-
gating factors that colored each nurse's reintegration. The same could
be said of each nurse's deployment. Just like people could not control
what they did and what they saw, they could not control their homecoming reception or lack thereof. There were positive homecomings
with family, friends, and coworkers greeting returnees with open arms.
Conversely, there were negative homecomings with late night arrivals
and lengthy airport layovers, which led to disappointment and frustration. Yet, many nurses realized that it was relatively easy for the military
to identify aspects of homecoming that could be improved with proper
planning and anticipatory guidance. For example, after a flight back to
the United States, transportation could be provided to deliver returnees
to lodging for the night, which would preclude them having to rent a
vehicle to get them where they needed to go. Military units could make
plans to host a "welcome" reception especially when returnees are traveling in a group.

Although the military cannot dictate what families do to welcome
their loved ones back on U.S. soil, they can encourage military units to see
that their returning members are greeted with gratitude and acknowledgment. The key to all of this is good communication on all levels.

Each chapter introduced a theme that was the thread woven through
the narratives in that chapter. Chapter 1 traced the historical roots of the
wars in Iraq and Afghanistan. Chapter 2 discussed the military medical
assets deployed to each war and the concept of operations and doctrine
underpinning medical unit deployments. Chapter 3 presented the nurses'
narratives regarding positive homecoming experiences. Chapter 4 described disappointments and negative homecoming experiences. Chapter 5
told how the nurses renegotiated roles within their families. Chapter 6 presented the nurses' testimonies of painful memories of trauma associated
with their wartime deployments. Chapter 7 focused on how the nurses
sorted things out and made decisions to seek help. Chapter 8 described
how some nurses sought a clinical change of scenery on returning home,
electing to try a different area of nursing. Chapter 9 told how some nurses
had difficulty tolerating the petty complaints of others after serving in a
war zone. Chapter 10 presented narratives about the nurses' return to work
and the support or lack of support they received. Chapter 11 described the
nurses' families and social networks in terms of support or lack of support.
Chapter 12 focused on the entire reintegration experience and how a "new
normal" was created. Chapter 13 discussed the findings of the research
that led to this book. Chapter 14 presented the clinical implications of the
research. Finally, Chapter 15 presented recommendations for preparing
nurses and their families for wartime deployment, suggested homecoming

and reintegration strategies to foster a smoother transition, and highlighted areas needing further investigation.

This book presented the testimonies of 35 nurses who participated directly in the wars in Iraq (Operation Iraqi Freedom) and Afghanistan (Operation Enduring Freedom). They wanted their stories to be told. Some simply wanted their voices to be heard. Others wanted to awaken the American public about the service they provided as a result of a void in the news about the nurses' mission in these wars. They also wanted people to know that nurses are not immune to posttraumatic stress disorder (PTSD), compassion fatigue, and burnout. These maladies can be a direct result of what nurses see and do. Just like soldiers, sailors, airmen, and marines, nurses are "forever changed" as a result of their wartime deployment.

Reintegration with family and friends, workplace, and community was a challenge for the majority of the nurses. The themes reflected in the chapters depict trials and tribulations, but also victories and triumphs. What came across loud and clear was the individuality and uniqueness of each nurse's reintegration. One size does not fit all.

The nurses' voices are represented in excerpts from verbatim transcriptions of oral testimonies. All names have been changed for privacy reasons, yet their words remain true. The book is replete with vivid descriptions of their clinical experiences in war, which provided the backdrop for their reintegration. Their stories speak of what they saw and did and how these past experiences informed and shaped their reintegration. There is a mention of traumatic amputations, burns, mutilated bodies, and the measures used to treat the injured.

Many nurses talked of what it was like to come home, to return to work, and to resume their previous lives amid much change in themselves. Many wondered if life would ever be the same; others wanted a clinical change of scenery; and some questioned previous decisions. Their stories are full of emotion and convey how deeply these nurses were touched by the human suffering they witnessed. The emotional depth of feelings was clearly evident in their interviews as voices quivered and eyes moistened when the nurses recalled details of their deployment, homecoming, and reintegration.

This book provides a social history told by military nurses, who experienced these wars firsthand. Their accounts detail nursing work set against two major sociopolitical conflicts. It is important to document nursing work in military conflicts because this is definitely a significant piece of nursing history.

The nurses interviewed for this research gave a variety of reasons for joining the military such as to gain clinical expertise, to travel, to seek specialized opportunities, to finance their education, to seek funding for an advanced educational degree, to expand their social network, and an array of other personal reasons. Some came from military families. Others came from rural settings and craved adventure and excitement. All took an oath to support and defend the Constitution of the United States against all enemies foreign and domestic, and to bear true faith and allegiance to the United States. They wore America's uniform proudly and went into harm's way to care for all in need. Sitting and listening to these nurses' stories at their kitchen tables, in their living rooms, or in a booth at their local diner, there was a quiet sense of pride in their military service that clearly emanated from their comments and demeanor. There was no boasting or arrogance about their wartime accomplishments, just a modest acknowledgment that they did their best to provide the highest quality of care possible in the war zone environment.

Nurses join the military in peacetime as well as in wartime. The tragedies of 9/11 sparked the interest of some nurses who had a desire to do something to serve their country. Yet, it is a variety of factors including one's personal and cultural characteristics, coping mechanisms, predeployment preparation and training, military-related experiences during deployment, and postdeployment environment that will shape a person's response to war. Some people enter into a deployment with a past history of traumatic and challenging life events. Therefore, some people already have established a repertoire of coping skills from their life experiences. Others come in with a blank slate and have not mastered stress reduction and management. It is believed that the strength of one's support system is a key factor along with individual coping and resiliency. Just as everyone is unique, so is everyone's story, and so is everyone's response to wartime deployment.

Nurses, as care providers, are always fixated on the physical and emotional pain of others. They try to alleviate or at least reduce this pain. They do so in the spirit of caring and exude a positive presence for their patients. However, in providing an array of therapeutic modalities to lessen the pain, the nurses themselves often suffer emotional trauma. Unresolved and continuous emotional trauma of this nature can lead to compassion fatigue, secondary PTSD, and burnout.

Hochschild (1983) coined the term "emotional labor" to describe the suffering sometimes endured by nurses and other caregivers as they perform their roles. Nursing work can take its toll on the nurse. Empathy is the basis of emotional labor and allows nurses to connect with their patients and show compassion.

Nurses, both in war and after war, deal with stress regularly as they perform their work roles. This stress can be attributed to the complexity of patients, workload, the secondary traumatic stress of witnessing suffering, and the emotional labor embedded in the role. In addition, there may be a lack of appreciation, limited resources, problematic communication, weak leadership, inadequate staffing, and a multitude of other issues. Furthermore, military nurses were not immune to the bombs, bullets, rocket-propelled grenades, and other ordinance of war. They were in harm's ways as they tended to those who needed care at the combat support hospitals, fast forward surgical teams, and in medevac aircraft.

In this study, both active duty and reserve nurses reported an occasional lack of information and education on the part of others in the workplace in understanding the demands of a wartime deployment. Sometimes coworkers simply expected the returning nurse to jump right back into the mix of a busy stateside unit or a large urban medical center. "Happy to be home" did not necessarily translate into workplace readiness and the majority of returning nurses wanted their service to be recognized by coworkers.

It goes without saying that the majority of service members have a variety of reactions after returning from deployment. These feelings and behaviors are normal, especially during the first few weeks at home. Despite the challenges of reintegration, most veterans successfully readjust over time. It is important for them and their families to take advantage of the wealth of resources available to them. Accurate information, coping strategies, and social support will positively influence their reintegration journey.

Although surviving the challenges of war can be rewarding, can foster maturity, and can build character, the impact of war can also be carried by veterans throughout their life spans because of its traumatic and morally devastating nature. Many of the nurses in the research study that lays the groundwork for this book commented on how they were "forever changed." The same holds true for anyone witnessing the ravages of war, civilians and warriors alike.

The chapters on homecoming illustrate the highly individual, personal, and unique accounts of what the nurses experienced in returning home. It was not uncommon for families to go through a honeymoon phase with their returning loved one. This phase was marked by joy, relief, and excitement. However, this phase may soon be followed by a different one in which the veteran feels confused, disappointed, and somewhat lost in trying to renegotiate roles and continue relationships. For example, some nurses who are parents reported feeling displaced by their spouses who had taken over all parenting duties and played a major role in the lives of the children during deployment. In addition, some children exhibited a range of regressive behaviors or had discipline problems, anxiety issues, or depression during the deployment. Parenting can become increasingly complicated when both the children and the returning parent are struggling with psychological concerns.

On a similar note, some of the nurses reported that they were not ready to jump in with household chores, driving carpools to activities, and grocery shopping. They simply needed time to adjust to the colorful world they returned to after being in a basically monochromatic and austere environment for many months. Some complained of physical and mental fatigue. Others felt overwhelmed with the experience of coming home: the long days of travel, having to make decisions, trying to meet the expectations of others, and feeling guilt for leaving colleagues behind in the war zone.

It goes without saying that interpersonal functioning may definitely be impaired as a result of wartime deployment. All people hold a number of roles in society such as husband/wife/partner/son/daughter/sister/brother/ parent and friend. All or any of these roles may be affected by the quality of the relationship predeployment, the level of communication during deployment, and the reality of homecoming and reintegration experiences.

Some nurses reported anger and disappointment with their level of preparedness for taking care of the number and severity of horrific war injuries or dealing with a slew of mass casualty events. Many said the youth of wounded soldiers was hard to fathom. Some nurses had children the same general age as these wounded soldiers. Others expressed concern and dismay with staffing shortfalls or the lack of equipment or supplies. Others complained of austere living conditions, especially if they deployed before 2006. It was evident that feelings of helplessness, unpredictability, and disappointment can give way to anger.

Chapter 6 on memories of trauma clearly outlined the predicament all nurses faced. Going into war, they knew they would be facing injury and death. However, even seasoned trauma nurses from large urban medical centers expressed horror at what they saw and had to do to save lives, ameliorate suffering, and allow death with dignity. Some of the injuries were so severe that the nurses worried about the quality of life that the service members would have if they survived. Moral and ethical dilemmas plagued the nurses as they fought to save lives. In addition, the nurses had to undergo weapon training as part of their preparation to serve in the war theaters of Iraq and Afghanistan. They had to be able to defend themselves and their patients, if necessary. Some reported being fired on, especially if they went out on missions in a helicopter to pick up the wounded from the battlefield or from a forward operating base (FOB). Nurses were definitely exposed to the consequences of combat and took care of war injuries to U.S. and coalition forces, civilians, enemy combatants, children, and homeless refugees. Some nurses saw homes and villages destroyed and were exposed to the sights, sounds, and smells of war. These experiences were intensely vivid, devastating, and demoralizing for some nurses. Also, the memories of the aftermath of war remain etched in their minds and hearts for years to come.

Returning veterans often report feelings of anxiety, panic, and sheer terror in dealing with exposure to the circumstances of war, including a perceived threat to their health and well-being. A plethora of research has documented that, when people perceive that their life has been threatened, their remaining outlook on life may be affected for an indefinite period of time. Thus, their outcome for being able to function comfortably in society is questioned. However, with each passing year, there are more resources available and more supportive services in place for returning veterans. A list of resources and services is provided in Chapter 15.

The nurses' voices in this book mentioned daily stressors, annoying life circumstances, minor irritations, and nagging frustrations. Some of these discomforts occurred during deployments whereas others took on a life of their own during reintegration. During deployment, there may have been a lack of privacy, austere living conditions, lack of food choices, an uncomfortable climate, boredom, and inadequate equipment. After deployment, there may have been a lack of understanding or confusion within one's social network or workplace, an overwhelming variety of choices in all areas of living, a paralytic "mental fog" in terms of making simple decisions, and myriad similar issues. Returning veterans may worry or ruminate about career- and family-related issues. These concerns can tax coping resources and affect performance and functioning. They may accumulate and fester, resulting in a problematic reintegration, or depression, anxiety, and even PTSD.

Some nurses reported unwanted sexual advances or harassment from other unit members, commanding officers, or civilians in a war zone that created a hostile work environment. Any type of harassment, sexual or otherwise, may have occurred while being deployed and may continue to haunt a nurse during reintegration. Such harassment may take the form of threats, constant scrutiny, gossip, and rumors directed toward individuals. In peacetime, these experiences are devastating for victims and create helplessness, powerlessness, anger, and stress. In wartime, they are no less troublesome and may even be worse because of the uncertainty of everything. Similarly, the Department of Veterans Affairs uses the term "military sexual trauma" to refer to sexual assault or repeated threatening acts of sexual harassment that occurred while a veteran was serving on active duty or active duty for training. The term is not specific to women service members. Again, counseling services are listed as a resource later in this book, and are provided at veteran centers in every state.

Although the physical well-being of all returning veterans is of paramount importance, many nurses reported difficulties in the areas of sleep, appetite, energy level, motivation, concentration, and willingness to participate in activities that they enjoyed predeployment. Although these self-reports were not unusual, they caused concern if they continued for long periods of time without improvement and without seeking therapeutic modalities to remedy them. Similarly, many nurses reported impatience with the behavior of others who did not experience deployment. This was particularly evident in the chapter that discussed intolerance to trivial whining and constant complaining about mundane things. The nurses discussed their frustration with others in the workplace who were fixated on their work and vacation schedules, on-call time, workload, lunch and break times, and similar domestic chores. Some were incredulous at the insensitivity of others to the deployment experiences of coworkers and the wars in Iraq and Afghanistan in general. Therefore, many returning nurses expressed anger, impatience, disappointment, and frustration with this behavior.

Chapter 7 on "sorting it out" captured the testimony of nurses as they recalled how they made sense of their experiences and how they decided to get help in the form of mental health counseling. Some stated that they had a sense of guilt retuning home, knowing that colleagues were still in the war zone "doing nursing." Some missed the adrenaline rush and the pride they took in doing meaningful work. Others felt burned out and may have turned to alcohol or self-medicating with drugs to quell or suppress painful memories. Spending money, food binges, and risky behaviors tempted others in an effort to avoid dealing with emotional and psychological trauma they had experienced. Some marriages ended in divorce and some previously promising relationships faltered.

Chapter 12 on reintegration to workplace emphasized the importance of doing nursing in an accepting, supportive environment. Although many nurses found this within the active duty sector and the civilian sector for reservists, others did not. This posed a major disappointment, coupled with extreme hurt. Work-related difficulties had a significant impact on returning nurses. Some felt abandoned, invisible, and unimportant. Others sensed a feeling that they were expected to be immune to being affected by what they saw and what they did because they were nurses. Yet, their self-efficacy, self-worth, sense of identification, and even their financial stability were tied to their chosen profession.

Reservists and National Guard unit members faced even more challenges than active duty military nurses because they returned to the civilian sector. Available resources and services varied depending on location and proximity to veterans' hospitals and centers. Civilian employers differ significantly in the areas of emotional and financial support they offer to returning nurses. In some instances, military deployment may have interrupted career advancement as well. Although Reserve and National Guard bases have enhanced their medical, family, and mental health support facilities over the long duration of these wars, a reservist may live and work a very long distance from these bases. It is not at all uncommon for reservists to even reside in different states from the bases and units where they are assigned.

Although no nurses in our research study decided to leave the profession of nursing, some requested a clinical change of scenery, meaning that they did not want to return to trauma nursing as they resumed clinical work. This was not unusual after what they had seen and done while deployed. Others missed the excitement of the war theater and did not experience the same high in the emergency room of a medical center. Some wanted out of the ICU and others chose to remain there. Similarly, some nurses chose to end their military service after wartime deployment—both reservists and active duty. Issues related to their decisions to separate from the military included a full gamut of responses such as relief, guilt, sadness, and confusion. Some wanted to spend more time with their children and families. Others feared another deployment if they continued a military career. Most of the nurses interviewed for this research expressed a greater appreciation for life in the United States, enhanced devotion and love for their families, and pride in their military careers. Several nurses said they would go back to Iraq or Afghanistan "in a heartbeat."

In summary, this research presents information gleaned from in-depth interviews with 35 nurses who served in Iraq or Afghanistan war theaters. Each nurse has a highly individualized and personal account of what he or she saw and did while deployed. Similarly, each will have a unique set of psychological, social, and readjustment issues. They need to have their voices heard and be understood, validated, and comforted in a way that addresses their service and their uniqueness. They all have their own personal style and it is important to recognize that there is no definitive roadmap or detailed blueprint for addressing a veteran's concerns and needs. The psychological, social, and readjustment toll of war on a veteran can be immediate, acute, and chronic. Time intervals are framed by a variety of individual, contextual, and cultural features.

PTSD is one of the many ways a veteran can manifest postdeployment difficulties. Veterans are also at risk for anxiety, depression, substance abuse, behavioral problems, and a spectrum of severe mental health illnesses precipitated by the stress of war. The absence of immediate signs and symptoms of psychological trauma does not necessarily mean that the veteran is not affected or that he or she will have a satisfactory adjustment to reintegration. Many returning service members are initially so relieved to be home and to have survived a wartime deployment, that they do not realize that they have underlying problems. However, as they settle in and experience life events and circumstances change, the signs and symptoms of distress may become evident to the veteran and his or her family and friends.

Finally, the stories in this book demonstrate that there is no timetable for reintegration. It is a very personal and individual journey filled with positives and negatives, stops and starts, ups and downs. A "new normal" is based on the recognition of change in one's life.

REFERENCE

Hochschild, A. (1983). *The managed heart: Commercialization of human feeling.* Berkeley, CA: University of California Press.

14

Clinical Implications

The majority of previous research on reintegration has focused on combat warriors. Much less is known about reintegration from the vantage point of the nurses who cared for the injured warriors and the innocent civilians who were caught in the horrific chaos of war. Nurses may possess a unique and perceptive insight given the nature of their work and the humanistic and holistic perspectives embedded in their profession.

The findings from our research can be used to encourage meaningful dialogue between military nurses and health care administrators at their various workplaces (military and civilian) to investigate and reflect on how wartime deployment impacts their current and future nursing careers. A lesson can be learned from these veterans because they provide a realistic picture of the reintegration experience. These nurses can be extremely influential in helping other nurses to prepare for deployment to a war zone. The findings in this book inform both military and civilian leadership, as well as families and communities, of the changes that reintegrating nurses have gone through and continue to go through as part of the reintegration process. It is ignorant and unrealistic to assume that nurses will not be changed both personally and professionally as a result of their wartime deployment. The findings presented in this book demonstrate the need for military health care and family advocacy groups to improve outreach services on a regular basis for veterans and their families. Family readiness and outreach services need to make a greater effort and have a more proactive approach to reach all civilian health care facilities that employ nurses who serve in military reserve units. Programs for reservists need to be especially creative and available because reservists often do not reside near a military installation.

Services for all veterans need to include psychological, physical health, social welfare, financial, spiritual, and educational help. A one-size-fits-all approach is inappropriate and problematic in addressing reintegration issues. A more individualized perspective with an open-ended timeline may be key to helping veterans deal with reintegration.

This book expands knowledge about military nursing in war and the sequelae that follow after such service. It elucidates the difficulties encountered upon returning home, such as renegotiating roles, resuming family activities, returning to clinical work, dealing with uncomfortable memories, and addressing possible negative feelings caused by stress, frustration, and disappointment. No one returns to a perfect milieu; even very positive homecomings and seemingly easy reintegrations are not without bumps in the road.

The findings of this current research inform us that it is of paramount importance to have support systems in place to assist military families before, during, and after deployment to address the specific stressors pursuant to each time period. Although the book is concerned with the reintegration process, it goes without saying that reintegration is truly affected by the events that preceded it. It is hoped that future research will build on this foundational work as nurses continue to be deployed to Afghanistan. Some research has led to the development of promising interventions that seem to be beneficial. However, we need to formulate more helpful interventions and specifically address the needs of military nurses to ensure optimal individual and family functioning.

It is important for the American people to hear the stories of these nurses. They not only answered their country's call to serve; they provided high-quality health care for the warriors defending our nation. These nurses served humankind, providing excellent and compassionate care; even for the enemy when needed. They formed a kinship with the oppressed women of Iraq and Afghanistan and never turned their backs on anyone in need. They had a special place in their hearts for the children of Iraq and Afghanistan. Our nurses cared for so many innocent victims in these two war theaters. Their stories inspired us and gave us an appropriate lens to gain a better understanding of the complex reintegration process.

THERAPEUTIC INTERVENTIONS

It goes without saying that all returning veterans need to be "thanked for their service" by everyone coming in contact with them: their families, social network, community, and workplace. Both military and civilian workplaces need to "rally round the flag" and welcome veterans back. Places of worship should acknowledge their service and embrace their homecoming just as the same faith communities prayed for their safe return while they were deployed.

Military personnel and all present in a war zone face an array of multi-faceted stressors on a daily basis. With the constant threat of mass casualty events, nurses had to be on alert 24/7 even if they supposedly had a day off from their regular duty. Thus, nurses were at risk for being injured or being killed even though an attack was less likely to occur at a hospital or clinic. Some nurses volunteered to go "outside the wire" on humanitarian missions specifically directed to help woman and children in nearby villages and towns. The voices of these returning nurses illustrate the need for mandatory mental health screening at homecoming with frequent checkups. Therapeutic modalities and interventions need to be individualized on a case-by-case basis.

Research from the Veterans Administration (VA) and various military services have identified the following factors that increase a service member's chance of developing posttraumatic stress disorder (PTSD). These factors include: a longer deployment time (especially 9–12 months); more severe combat exposure (deployment to "forward" areas closer to the enemy and seeing others wounded or killed); severe physical injury; traumatic brain injury; lower rank; lower level of education; low morale and poor social support within the unit; not being married; family problems; member of the National Guard or Reserves; prior trauma exposure; female gender; and being from an Hispanic ethnic group (National Center for PTSD, 2015).

According to the VA Office of Public Health and Environmental Hazards, more veterans recently returned are seeking care through the VA than ever before. VA data show that from 2002 through 2009, 1 million troops left active duty in Iraq and Afghanistan and became eligible for VA care. Forty-six percent of these troops sought VA services. Of those veterans who used VA care, 48% were diagnosed with a mental health problem. Yet, many veterans with mental health problems have not availed themselves of VA services. Some reasons given for not seeking help include the following concerns: being perceived as "weak"; being treated differently by others; fear that others would lose confidence in them; lack of privacy; a preference to rely on family and friends; lack of confidence in treatment modalities; the possibility of medication side effects; and problems with access to care such as cost and location of treatment facilities (Veterans Administration, 2010).

It is important to note that the National Center for PTSD does not provide direct clinical care, individual referrals, or benefits information. However, they provide a wealth of written and media materials to aid veterans and their families to educate themselves about PTSD and the reintegration experience in general, which will lead to procuring care.

With the greatest majority of nurses in both war theaters being women, the National Center for PTSD in its literature states that women are more than twice as likely to develop PTSD as men (10% for women and 4% for men). In addition, sexual assault is more likely to cause PTSD than many other events. Women with PTSD are more likely to feel depressed and anxious, whereas men with PTSD are more likely to have substance abuse problems (National Center for PTSD, 2015).

Although some caregiver suffering or "emotional labor" may be inherent in the nursing role, some can be reduced by a supportive leadership, understanding coworkers, and a general sense of appreciation (Hochschild, 1983). Also, nurses need to focus on their own mental health and well-being so that they can continue providing quality care and find meaning and satisfaction in their work.

There are several therapeutic interventions mentioned in the literature to aid returning veterans and their families in the reintegration process. Some focus on the returning veteran, others on the couple relationship, and others on family resiliency. There is never a "one size fits all" model.

One therapeutic intervention, about which the authors feel strongly for all nurses preparing for deployment as well as a refresher course for those at the beginning of the reintegration process, is mindfulness training. Mindfulness is the capacity to intentionally bring awareness to present-moment experience with an attitude of acceptance, openness, honesty, and curiosity. It is being awake to the fullness of life at that immediate time as witnessed by the five senses (Kabat-Zinn, 1996, 2001, 2006, 2009).

Mindfulness training can reduce psychological, emotional, and physiological stress. It can also improve empathy, compassion for others, satisfaction with life, and enhance one's overall sense of well-being. Being mindful does not mean altering or stopping one's thinking or purposefully trying to relax. Yet, many people who practice mindfulness on a regular basis report feeling calm, relaxed, and peaceful. Mindfulness meditation can soothe a distracted mind and increase one's sense of feeling grounded.

Many parents, who are juggling a military career as well as child-care responsibilities, describe a feeling of "being on automatic pilot" as they try to reintegrate after deployment. Their bodies operate in a routine manner at work as their minds are somewhere else, often anticipating future events or ruminating over past events. This way of functioning limits how life is experienced both at home and at work, and affects the quality of relationships and one's decision-making abilities. It can also increase feelings of stress and lead to anxiety and depression. Mindfulness practices incorporated into one's daily life can help end negative self-talk, pessimistic thinking, and needless worrying. A conscious shifting of the mind to present-moment experience can interrupt a chain of unhelpful, counterproductive thinking patterns that are detrimental to one's sense of well-being.

Research in the field of neuroscience has indicated that mindfulness practices enhance brain function in the areas responsible for problem solving, while modulating the areas that identify emotions such as fear and anger. Mindfulness practices enhance one's ability to assess situations and circumstances with greater attention and a clearer focus so one can respond appropriately without a quick thoughtless reaction. Although mindfulness practices are relevant for both deploying nurses and reintegrating nurses, their applicability has broad implications for all humans for that matter.

Historically, mindfulness-based stress reduction (MBSR) can be traced to Jon Kabat-Zinn in 1979. His seminal training program was developed to reduce chronic pain in patients. His offered a structured 8-week program which included a variety of stress-reduction exercises geared to increase one's capacity to become more mindful. Its core practices included mentally tuning-in to body sensations, gentle yoga, and breathing awareness. Research examining the effects of MBSR found improvements in the health and well-being of patients who had been suffering from chronic pain.

As a result of the aforementioned training program and the media attention surrounding its success, mindfulness-training programs escalated throughout the United States. In addition, these training programs did not remain just in the clinical sector, but spread to many populations such as athletes, corporate leaders, performers, and educators.

When we consider the nursing profession, mindfulness can foster increased awareness and less distraction in the clinical setting. Mindful practitioners can communicate using better listening skills and speaking abilities. They can deal more effectively with stress because of more efficient coping mechanisms. Mindfulness can also decrease the rate of burnout within the profession.

With military personnel reintegrating after wartime deployment, mindfulness can help them to see things more clearly and with a calmer demeanor. It can help interrupt the cycle of overwhelming thoughts and feelings that often bombard newly returning veterans. Similarly, mindfulness can enhance communication with family, friends, coworkers, and patients. It is a lifelong process that can be developed and cultivated throughout the life span.

Suggestions for practicing mindfulness in daily life include the following steps:

1. For 5 to 10 minutes a day, focus on your breathing. Do not alter it, just tune in to it.
2. When your mind wanders, bring it back to concentrating on your breathing.
3. Awareness of your breathing is a form of meditation and helps to slow your mental activity.

4. Focus on your body sensations to settle your distracted mind.
5. Gentle stretching or walking can also slow down the busy mind.
6. Notice your activities of daily living with greater attention and curiosity about them. Explore them with your five senses (Kabat-Zinn, 1996, 2001, 2006, 2009).

Current research points out that family reintegration can be particularly difficult if there were preexisting family problems before deployment. Preexisting family stresses may include marital issues, financial instability, child behavioral challenges, and mental health problems. These, of course, can become more complicated if combat-related trauma such as physical injuries or PTSD has been added to the mix. Yet, appropriate resources are in place for military families to navigate their difficulties in the short term and in the long term.

Much attention has been focused on couples' therapy in dealing with reintegration issues. Sayers (2010) explored the model of behavioral couples therapy (BCT), which provides a useful framework for intervention with couples, combined with individual treatment and education about the impact of combat deployment. The BCT model can be used to address role transitions, communication, decision making, and general transition-related problem solving. It encourages a team approach for the couple to establish new patterns and adjust to their "new normal."

Another slightly different approach to couples therapy has been described by Greenberg and Goldman (2008). These practitioners argue that, if couples therapy is to produce real transformation, emotion must be activated. As emotion is triggered by conflict, therapists need to help couples get at the primary emotions that power negative interactions and transform these emotions into more functional ones. They discuss the foundations of emotion-focused therapy for couples (EFT-C) and broaden its framework to focus more closely on the development of self and relationships. They explain the major motivational systems central to couples therapy—attachment, identity, and attraction. They illustrate how working with emotions can facilitate change in couples and this can be extended to include all situations in which people may be in conflict with others.

The reintegration period can bring additional challenges to two-parent families in re-establishing a balance in the parenting efforts. There are many programs available to service members and their families to help them navigate reintegration. Many are based on family systems theories and family resiliency theories. One model that has proved particularly helpful for military families is the Parent Management Training-Oregon (PMTO) model, which is undergirded by the Social Interaction Learning model and is a group of empirically supported parenting interventions (Patterson, 2005). The After Deployment Adaptive Parenting Tools (ADAPT) program extended the forementioned PMTO model for military families. All PMTO programs rely on the same core principles and provide information, teaching, practice, and support. The five core principles are designed to reduce coercive tactics and promote positive parenting. These are (a) contingent skill encouragement, (b) limit-setting, (c) positive involvement, (d) monitoring children's activities, and (e) effective family problem solving (Gerwitz, Erbes, Polusny, Forgatch, & DeGarmo, 2011; Patterson, 2005; Reid, Patterson, & Snyder, 2002).

Several family resiliency programs have evolved and escalated as a result of the efforts of the University of California, Los Angeles (UCLA) Nathanson Family Resiliency Center. In 2006, Families Over Coming Under Stress (FOCUS) was founded as a family resiliency program grounded in three well-established interventions. It was founded for families with children and for couples facing adversity and traumatic stress across a variety of situations. FOCUS is a short intervention delivered in six to eight sessions. Some sessions are for parents, some are for children, and others are for the entire family. FOCUS Family Resilience Training helps families to (a) identify and discuss emotions, (b) clarify misunderstandings and respect individual points of view, (c) build on family strengths, (d) feel closer and more supported, and (e) use family-level problem solving and goal setting to empower the entire family. Although FOCUS is structured to ensure that each family learns the program's core skills, it can be tailored to meet the unique needs of each individual family. In 2008, the UCLA Semel Institute for Neuroscience and Human Behavior was funded to implement FOCUS services. Similarly, TeleFOCUS uses a videoconferencing format for families and couples to "meet" with a FOCUS resilience trainer to learn resilience skills. TeleFOCUS is available for families with a wounded warrior (www.focusproject.org).

Operation Mend-FOCUS was established in 2007 as a partnership between UCLA Health System and the U.S. military to help heal the wounds of war by offering the most advanced medical care available. Operation Mend services are offered free of charge to all service members seeking medical treatment for specialty injuries sustained while serving in Operation Iraqi Freedom (OIF)/Operation Enduring Freedom (OEF) while on active duty. Current services provided through Operation Mend include treatment and consultation for a multitude of injuries including the invisible wounds of war—mental health services for PTSD and traumatic brain injury (TBI). It should be noted that, with treatment at UCLA, all transportation and housing for each patient and family are arranged and paid for by Operation Mend (http://operationmend.ucla.edu).

A novel endeavor was launched in 2009 in conjunction with the FOCUS program. It was called the National Military Family Association Operation Purple Camps and Healing. These outdoor adventures are designed to bring families together for 4 days in a national park setting. The camps give families the opportunity to participate in fun, family-centered activities to allow them to renew and strengthen relationships while exploring and enjoying the environment. The Operation Purple Family Retreat program helps families to reintegrate following deployment. Activities are designed to promote parents' understanding of the effects of deployment on children and rekindle a sense of family bonding. The retreat fosters communication, teamwork, and reconnection (www.militaryfamily.org/our-programs/operation:purple).

The UCLA Welcome Back Veterans Family Resilience Center is supported by the McCormick Foundation and Major League Baseball. The Center works to adapt, evaluate, and disseminate innovative programs that decrease the negative effects of deployment for OEF/OIF service members and their families. The Center articulates two missions. The Research Core mission seeks to develop and evaluate promising interventions to improve the lives of returning service members and their families. The Services/Educational Core mission seeks to develop and enhance a community-level continuum of health care for veterans and their families in the Los Angeles area that can be adapted and implemented nationally (www.nfrc.ucla.edu).

It should also be noted that the UCLA Nathanson Family Resilience Center has recently expanded its services to better reach female veterans in LA County. With support from Newman's Own Foundation, there is a Female Veterans Initiative. FOCUS Family Resilience Training allows female veterans and their families to learn resilience skills and build strengths.

The Combat Operational Stress Control (COSC) program provides decision-making tools for service members and their families. They are taught to build resilience, identify stress responses, and mitigate problem stressors. The end-state goal of the program mirrors the COSC goal of creating mission-ready service members, families, and commands. In this program, peer counseling has been proved to be an effective strategy to normalize access to mental health services (www.dcoe.health.mil).

The Coming Home Project began in 2006 as a nonprofit organization devoted to providing compassionate care, support, education, and stress management tools for Iraq and Afghanistan veterans and their families. The program addresses the psychological, emotional, spiritual, and relationship challenges experienced during reintegration. It utilizes peer support and offers offsite retreats to reinforce concepts learned in the program (www.dcoe.health.mil).

The Joint Family Support Assistance Program (JFSAP) augments existing family programs to provide a continuum of support and services. The primary focus of support is families who are geographically far from a military installation. Coordination with state and local agencies and communities is essential (www.dcoe.health.mil).

Operation BRAVE Families (OBF) refers to Building Resilience and Valuing Empowered Families. This family-centered program focuses on the children of service members while supporting parents. OBF specifically serves the children and other family members of injured service members. Engaging family members in reintegration services is of paramount importance in this program (www.dcoe.health.mil).

The Red Cross Coming Home Series is a series of learning modules geared for returning service members and their families. A key insight or lesson learned in this program has been that the offering of mental health services to returning service members through a third-party organization may reduce the stigma associated with accessing those resources (www.dcoe.health.mil).

The Returning Warrior Workshop is a 2-day weekend event that helps promote successful reintegration and continued growth as a person. It emphasizes thankfulness and appreciation for serving one's country. It is most enjoyed by service members if it is held at an upscale offsite venue (www.dcoe.health.mil).

Warrior Mind Training (WMT) is based on mind-focusing techniques that warriors have used for thousands of years to maintain focus in battle and to reintegrate back into their community after war. Key insights and lessons learned tell us that psychological and emotional inoculation are important components of preventing combat-related stress (www.dcoe.health.mil).

The Yellow Ribbon Reintegration Program (YRRP) is sponsored by the Department of Defense in partnership with federal organizations including the VA and the Department of Labor to help National Guard and Reserve service members and their families connect with local resources before, during, and after deployments. The reintegration phase is the most critical and programs need to be held in several regions of the country (www.dcoe.health.mil).

Many strategies used to deal with reintegration vulnerabilities are based on a strengths-based, resilience-building approach, rather than a treatment of psychopathology approach in working with military families. However, these strategies are not a substitute for the treatment of returning veterans who are experiencing severe individual distress. Many individuals need individual therapy for PTSD, depression, and substance abuse and dependence. Yet, the aforementioned strategies may be important adjuncts to a variety of treatment approaches.

REFERENCES

Combat Operational Stress Control Program (COSC). (2015). Retrieved from http://www.dcoe.health.mil
Coming Home Project. (2015). Retrieved from http://www.dcoe.health.mil

Gerwitz, A. H., Erbes, C. R., Polusny, M. A., Forgatch, M. S., & DeGarmo, D. S. (2011). Helping military families through the deployment process: Strategies to support parenting. *Professional Research Practice, 42*(1), 56–62.

Greenberg, L. S., & Goldman, R. N. (2008). *Emotion-focused couples therapy: The dynamics of emotion, love, and power.* Washington, DC: American Psychological Association.

Hochschild, A. (1983). *The managed heart: Commercialization of human feeling.* Berkeley, CA: The University of California Press.

Joint Family Support Assistance Program (JFSAP). (2015). Retrieved from http://www.dcoe.health.mil

Kabat-Zinn, J. (1996). *Full catastrophe living: How to cope with stress, pain, and illness with mindfulness meditation.* London, UK: Piatkus Books.

Kabat-Zinn, J. (2001). *Mindfulness meditation for everyday life.* London, UK: Piatkus Books.

Kabat-Zinn, J. (2006). *Coming to our senses: Healing ourselves and the world through mindfulness meditation.* New York, NY: Hyperion Books.

Kabat-Zinn, J. (2009). *Letting everything become your teacher: Lessons in mindfulness.* New York, NY: Dell Publishing.

National Center for PTSD, United States Veterans Administration. (2015). Retrieved from www.ncptsd.va.gov/ncmain/veterans

National Military Family Association Operation Purple Camps and Healing. (2015). Retrieved from http://www.militaryfamily.org/our-programs/operation:purple.

Operation BRAVE Families (OBF). (2015). Retrieved from http://www.dcoe.health.mil

Operation Mend. (2015). Retrieved from http://operationmend.ucla.edu

Patterson, G. R. (2005). The next generation of PMTO models. *The Behavior Therapist, 28,* 27–33.

Red Cross Coming Home Series. (2015). Retrieved from http://www.dcoe.health.mil

Reid, J. B., Patterson, G. R., & Snyder, J. (2002). *Antisocial behavior in children and adolescents: A developmental analysis and model for intervention.* Washington, DC: American Psychological Association.

Sayers, S. L. (2010). Family reintegration difficulties and couples therapy for military veterans and their spouses. *Cognitive and Behavioral Practice, 18,* 108–119.

UCLA Nathanson Family Resiliency Center. (2015). *Families OverComing Under Stress (FOCUS) Program.* Retrieved from http://www.focusproject.org

UCLA Nathanson Family Resilience Center. (2015). *Welcome back veterans.* Retrieved from http://www.nfrc.ucla.edu

Veterans Administration Office of Public Health and Environmental Hazards. (2010). *An analysis of VA health care utilization among Operation Enduring Freedom (OEF) and Operation Iraqi Freedom (OIF) veterans.* Washington, DC: Author.

Warrior Mind Training (WMT). (2015). Retrieved from http://www.dcoe.health.mil

Yellow Ribbon Reintegration Program (YRRP). (2015). Retrieved from http://www.dcoe.health.mil

15

Recommendations

Existing knowledge of reintegration experiences is largely dependent on using clinical samples focusing on those who have documented post-traumatic stress disorder (PTSD) and its impact on family life. However, to study reintegration broadly and deeply, further research is needed with nonclinical samples because the majority of returning veterans do not have PTSD. The research study that culminated in this book was an attempt to capture the reintegration experience with such a sample. A qualitative, phenomenological approach allowed the 35 nurses participating in this study to tell their stories. This method yielded personal, anecdotal, and meaningful information about their reintegration journey, which is far different from checking boxes on a survey. In addition, there needs to be a balance between strength-based and resiliency approaches and those emphasizing psychopathology (Marek et al., 2012).

Family-focused, longitudinal studies would add greatly to knowledge development about the reintegration process and could lead to the formulation, implementation, and evaluation of effective support programs, resources, and services. Collaboration between military and civilian communities would be needed to put forth a research agenda of this nature. Yet, the mission of helping military families to build resiliency during reintegration is of immense importance (Marek et al., 2012).

Family and friends of active duty and reserve nurses could benefit from family-readiness training to help the reintegration process. This training is usually military-service-branch specific, base specific, and unit specific for active duty families. It frequently consists of biweekly meetings for families of deployed personnel. Attendance is voluntary. The meeting agenda is usually developed by the base family support center in concert with mental health services, financial services, and family advocacy and readiness services. Attendees normally have input for the following meetings so their concerns can be addressed. Sometimes reserve component units try to hold similar meetings, but geographical distance from the base can impair attendance.

All returning veterans need a comprehensive assessment to check their level of functioning and to formulate a treatment plan if necessary. Areas to evaluate include: work functioning, interpersonal functioning, recreation and self-care, physical functioning, psychological signs and symptoms, past stress-reduction activities and coping mechanisms, a history of previous traumatic events, and deployment-related experiences.

The assessment process should commence by focusing on current psychosocial functioning and the immediate needs of the veteran. Trauma exposure should take place later in the assessment process, if possible. It is of utmost importance that reintegrating veterans feel safe, secure, comfortable, and accepted. Reintegration has no specific time frame or map. It is a very individual process for each returning veteran.

Vet Centers provide counseling services for various problems affecting reintegration. All veterans can utilize the resources and services at a Vet Center. A Vet Center is a place where veterans can come for professional help with combat-related trauma, harassment, employment, bereavement, benefits, and educational services. Families of deceased service members are welcome as well. Currently, there are 232 community-based Vet Centers located in all 50 states, as well as Washington, DC, Guam, Puerto Rico, and the U.S. Virgin Islands.

Although Vet Centers were originally set up to help returning Vietnam veterans, they are now available to counsel all combat veterans from all military conflicts, including World War II, Korea, Lebanon, Grenada, Panama, the Persian Gulf, Somalia, and Kosovo/Bosnia. Most veterans being seen at Vet Centers today are veterans of Operation Enduring Freedom (OEF), Operation Iraqi Freedom (OIF), and subsequent operations within the Global War on Terrorism (GWOT).

There is also a national center for PTSD. This center provides written materials for families of returning military personnel. The mission is to help the service member and his or her family understand what to expect when returning from a war zone and how to help the returning veteran adapt to life back home.

CONCLUSION

In writing this book, we followed an enlightening and insightful path to get at the heart of the reintegration experience by capturing the words, phrases, and narratives of nurses who had served the United States in the Iraq and Afghanistan wars. Our travels took us from Maine to North Carolina. Our telephone interviews spanned to Hawaii, Alaska, and Guam. We interviewed nurses who served as early as 2003 and as late as 2014. Numerous books have been published describing the experiences of reintegration for returning soldiers, sailors, marines, and airmen serving in these wars. Yet, very little has been written about the reintegration experiences of military nurses. Therefore, the mission of this book is to do just that—to identify, describe, explore, and document the reintegration experiences of nurses who served in Iraq (OIF) and Afghanistan (OEF). A rather lengthy and in-depth research study was conducted by the authors in an effort to tell the nurses' stories, which has culminated in this book.

As nurses ourselves, we feel a kinship to the nurses in this study. Their words resonated with us, staying in our minds and hearts. Occasionally after an interview, we had difficulty sleeping because of what they told us. Sometimes, they made us laugh with their anecdotes. Other times, their stories caused our eyes to well up with tears and get a sinking feeling in our stomachs. Their narratives were never boring and we often got the feeling that the nurses experienced a kind of catharsis as a result of telling their stories. We listened intently and were never judgmental. We marveled at their sense of duty, patriotism, selflessness, kindness, and compassion. Repeatedly, they told us how much they loved America and how much they appreciate the freedoms and way of life they enjoy at home. No matter how much they struggle with reintegration issues, a sense of home was important to them. They saw up close and personal the devastation and carnage resulting from the wars. They saw maimed, burned, and slaughtered children. They witnessed firsthand the lack of regard for women in both countries, in terms of education and social status. They learned how precious and fragile human life could be and how easily it could be gone in an instant. Many stated that they never felt truly safe while deployed and that they are having issues with fear, safety, and uncertainty here at home as well.

Most nurses doubt that any human experience will exceed their wartime deployment in terms of stress, horror, and vulnerability while at the same time they feel that they benefitted with the growth of their professional nursing expertise, decision making, and leadership. Yet, the majority of the nurses feel like they took the war home with them. They think about their patients and colleagues, the elderly villagers, and the women and children. They wonder how the amputees are getting along or if the traumatic brain injury (TBI) patients are making progress. By the nature of their work, nurses tend to live with trauma almost every day when deployed. They learn to anticipate and prepare for mass casualty events. However, many of the nurses were not prepared for what they would be dealing with on U.S. soil when they came home.

The voices of reintegrating nurses were heard loud and clear in this book. They tried to make sense of their experiences within the framework of reintegration. The ones who had positive experiences had less difficulty adjusting, such as the nurse who met her future husband in a prison hospital when he was serving as an interpreter or some of the air force nurses who had shorter deployments. Long deployments seemed to be the most difficult, and reintegration for reservists who did not live near a military installation could be problematic. It could also be quite troublesome when reservists had to return to their civilian nursing positions before they felt ready but needed to do so for economic reasons. A plethora of variables could impact the reintegration process.

Although military units can plan "welcome home" events on a regular basis, it could be a crapshoot with families. Some families went all out to make their loved ones feel loved and appreciated whereas others did nothing or the bare minimum. The same held true for military units, with some hosting a welcome home event and others not doing anything to recognize returning service members. Probably the most neglectful thing was not providing transportation to lodging or having individual augmentees arrive home without anyone to greet them. If people had preexisting marital strife or estrangement from family members, homecoming was not necessarily a positive experience. Yet, returnees were essentially out of harm's way, which was somewhat of a consolation.

Returning to nursing work could be a blessing or a curse depending on the individual nurse, the position, the leadership, the facility, and the clinical unit. Some nurses reported that they were welcomed back with open arms; people wanted to hear their stories, digest their lessons learned, and thank them for their service. Others felt ignored and pressured to catch up as fast as possible to the heartbeat of their clinical unit. People wanted them to resume a full workload immediately and did not give them time to catch their breath. Any warm RN body would have been welcomed! Conversely and thankfully, this was not the case for many nurses who were thoroughly appreciated.

Some nurses wanted to transition to a new clinical area, not wanting to return to the ER, ICU, or operating room (OR). Nurse practitioners welcomed a clinic schedule, replete with well-women gynecology visits, college physical examinations, hypertension and diabetic management. Others changed to the recovery room, day surgical unit, and the birthing center. Yet, there were the adrenaline junkies who chose to stay in the thick of it with trauma cases from motor vehicle accidents, gunshot wounds from gang fights and domestic violence, and serious burns from house fires.

Nurses are not immune to PTSD and the sequelae that go along with it. Many could not escape fearful thoughts, hypervigilant actions, horrific nightmares, roller-coaster emotions, and the physical sensations that accompany this disorder. They brought the war home with them; it dwelled in their bodies and souls. They were forever changed as a result of their experiences. How can one ever forget being ankle-deep in blood, holding brain tissue in your hands, seeing burns so severe that you do not know if the victim was male or female, or holding an innocent child in your arms as she takes her last breath? Memories like this are hard to let go of, even though the nurses wanted to forget them.

Personal relationships ebbed and flowed like the tides. Most intact marriages and close relationships survived and troubled ones crumbled. The chances were that, if the foundation was shaky to begin with, a wartime deployment was not going to improve it. One nurse in the study commented that her boyfriend was extremely supportive before and during the deployment, but that her relationship with him crashed and burned during reintegration. Another nurse reported that she did not have a supportive, healthy relationship with her husband prior to deployment but that she needed him to take care of their two young sons while she was gone. Although the children were fine when she came home, she stated that the tension between herself and her husband was palpably thick. They are now divorced.

The nurses in the study were quick to point out their anger and frustration with coworkers back in the States who were lazy, complaining, and self-centered. They had no tolerance for trivial whining about their lot in life, work schedule, patient load, and anything that resembled needless gossip. After what the deployed nurses had seen and done in the war zone, they had no patience for the whining of coworkers. Besides the injuries of war, they had seen children without shoes, without food, and without parents. As a result of their war experiences, everything their coworkers bitched about paled in comparison to the ravages of war.

The nurses in the study emphasized the individual nature of reintegration. There is not a one-size-fits-all model. Also, the timetable of the reintegration process is unique and specific to the individual nurse. It should not be rushed; it should be allowed to flow freely at its own rate. Support, guidance, and nurturance are important, whereas control and rigidity have no place. It is fortunate that the military services and the Veterans Administration (VA) have made significant strides in the past few years to screen all returning service members for PTSD. This screening is performed incrementally because PTSD often has delayed symptoms. This initiative is of paramount importance and is long overdue. We applaud the military services and VA for its continued efforts to improve mental health services for all veterans.

Nurses going through the reintegration process should be encouraged to talk freely about their experiences within a supportive and accepting environment. They are in a strategic position to inform and prepare other nurses who will soon be deployed. These seasoned nurses have the experience, credibility, and insight to provide anticipatory guidance, which will be of great benefit to others.

We will never forget the 35 nurses who were willingly interviewed for the research study, which led to this book. They believed in our work and wanted the world to have a lens into the reintegration period. They hoped that others would benefit by reading their narratives and understanding the meaning and feelings behind their words. The nurses wanted to debunk the myth that implies that nurses have any kind of immunity from PTSD, compassion fatigue, or burnout. Nurses are susceptible; it is just that they embrace a healing mission.

After interviewing these 35 nurses, transcribing their audio-recorded interviews, and listening to the tapes frequently, we believe we learned a great deal about the reintegration process. We gained a thorough understanding of the totality of the reintegration experience as much as possible without having been actually deployed to these two war zones. The nurses and their stories had a profound and substantial effect on our lives. We gained increased respect, admiration, and appreciation for military nurses and for the entire nursing profession.

The purpose of this book was to describe and document the reintegration experiences of U.S. military nurses who served in the Iraq and Afghanistan wars, 2003 to 2014. We wanted to inform our readers of the reintegration process and the challenges faced by these compassionate and brave nurses as they transition home after wartime deployments. Mission accomplished!

RESOURCES

It is recommended that returnees from the wars in Iraq and Afghanistan peruse the following programs in gaining help during the reintegration process.

Family Support Programs
  Family Assistance Centers (FAC) are located at armories throughout the Unites States. Originally, they were created by the National Guard, but are available to all service members and their families in all branches of the military: www.jointservicessupport.org
  Family Readiness Groups (FRG): Army units have groups of volunteers to help with communication to families of deployed troops. They can be located through the service member's unit.
  Families at Ease: 1-888-823-7458
    Air Force: U.S. Air Force Service Agency: www.usafservices.com/default.aspx
    Army OneSource Family Programs and Services: 1-800-342-9647: www.militaryonesource.mil
    Army Reserve Family Programs: 1-866-345-8248.

Army: U.S. Army MWR (Family and Morale, Welfare, and Recreation Programs): usarmy.jbsa.imcom-hq.mbx.army-mwr-webmaster@mail .mil (2016 MWR.com).

Marine Corps Community Services (MCCS): www.usmc-mccs.org

Military Homefront: Official U.S. Department of Defense website for service members and families, which features online government resources and links: www.militaryhomefront.dod.mil

National Military Family Association (NMFA): www.militaryfamily.org

Navy Fleet and Family Support Services: www.cnic.navy.mil

Navy One Source: 1-800-540-4123.

Veterans Affairs: www.va.gov. 1-800-827-1000

America Legion: www.legion.org

Homeless Veterans: www.va.gov/homeless/index.asp

National Veterans Foundation: 1-888-777-4443: www.nvf.org

Nurses Organization of Veterans Affairs (NOVA): 202-296-0888, 1726 M Street NW, Suite 1101, Washington, DC, 20036.

Strategic Outreach for Families of All Reservists (SOFAR): 888-278-0041 or 617-266-2611, PO Box 380766, Cambridge, Massachusetts, 02236.

Veterans Crisis Line: 1-800-273-8255 (press 1) or 1-877-927-8387.

VA National Suicide Prevention Hotline: 1-800-273-TALK.

VA Center for Women Veterans (1-800-827-1000): www1.va.gov/womenvet

Vet Centers: 1-800-905-4675 (Eastern); 1-866-496-8838 (Pacific): www .vetcenter.va.gov

Women Veterans: Center for Women Veterans: 1-855-829-6636.

Women Veterans Health Care in the VA: www.publichealth.va.gov/ womenshealth/index.asp

Other Federal, State and Community Resources

Defense Centers of Excellence for Psychological Health and Traumatic Brain Injury (DCoE): 866-966-1020: www.dcoe.health.mil

National Alliance on Mental Health (NAMI): 703-524-7600, 2107 Wilson Blvd, Suite 300, Arlington, Virginia, 22201-3042.

National Association of Veterans Advocates, Inc. (NOVA): 877-483-8238, 1425 K Street, Suite 350, Washington, DC 20005.

National Center for Post Traumatic Stress Disorder (PTSD): 1-800-296-6300: www.ncptsd.va.gov/ncmain/veterans

National Suicide Prevention Hotline: 1-800-273-8255.

Real Warriors Campaign: www.realwarriors.net

U.S. Department of Defense Sexual Assault Prevention and Response: 1-800-342-9647.

USO Services: 888-484-3876.

Other Resources

American Red Cross: www.redcross.org

Care for the Caregivers: 407-805-8566, 1035 Greenwood Blvd, Suite 205, Lake Mary, Florida, 32746.

The Coming Home Project: 415-353-5363, 1801 Bush Street, San Francisco, California 94109.

Disabled American Veterans: PO Box 14301, Cincinnati, Ohio, 45250-0301; 877-426-2838 or 859-441-7300.

Gift from Within: 207-236-8858, 16 Cobb Hill Road, Camden, Maine, 04843.

Give an Hour: PO Box 5918, Bethesda, Maryland, 20824-5918.

Hearts Toward Home International: 360-714-1525, 1050 Larrabee Avenue, Suite 104, Bellingham, Washington 98225-7367.

Iraq and Afghanistan Veterans of America: 770 Broadway, 2nd floor, New York, 10003: 212-982-9699.

The Mission Continues: www.missioncontinues.org

ONE Freedom, Inc: 303-444-1221, PO Box 7418, Boulder, Colorado 80306.

Operation Comfort: 210-826-0500, 4900 Broadway, Suite 400, San Antonio, Texas 78209.

Operation First Response: 888-289-0280, 20037 Dove Hill Road, Culpepper, Virginia 22701.

Operation Homefront: 210-659-7756 or 800-722-6098, 8930 Fourwinds Drive, Suite 340, San Antonio, Texas 78239.

Rand Corporation: www.rand.org

Returning Veterans Project: 503-933-4996, 907 NE Thompson Street, Portland, Oregon 97212.

Soldier's Heart: 518-274-0501, 500 Federal Street, Suite 303, Try, New York 12180.

The Soldiers Project: 818-761-7438 or 877-576-5343.

UCLA Nathanson Family Resilience Center, Semel Institute for Neuroscience and Human Behavior at the University of California, 760 Westwood Plaza, Room A8-153. Los Angeles, California 90095: (855) 231-9500: info@nfcr.ucla.edu

Veteran Love: 305-673-2856, 930 Washington Avenue, Suite 206, Miami Beach, Florida 33139.

Veterans for America: 202-483-9222, 1025 Vermont Avenue NW, 3rd floor, Washington, DC 20005.

Vets4Vets: 520-319-5500.

REFERENCE

Marek, L. I., Hollingsworth, W. G., D'Aniello, C., O'Rourke, K., Brock, D. J., Moore, L, . . . Wiles, B. (2012). Returning home: What we know about the reintegration of deployed service members into their families and communities. *National Council on Family Relations Report (spring)*, *52*, 16-18.

Afterword

I was delighted to learn earlier this year that Dr. Elizabeth Scannell-Desch and Dr. Mary Ellen Doherty were going to be writing a second book addressing the results of their fourth joint research study involving deployed nurses to Iraq and Afghanistan. I felt honored to be asked once again to support this endeavor by providing feedback on chapters during the writing stage and by authoring the Afterword for their latest book, which addresses the challenges of reintegration for nurses after deployment. I applaud their willingness to address the critical issues associated with nurses reintegrating back into their families, work settings, and communities.

Their first book, *Nurses in War: Voices From Iraq and Afghanistan*, was a very important addition to the nursing literature, addressing the impact of these two wars on the largest personnel category of combat medics, the nurses. The lived experiences of the participating nurses made combat nursing "come to life" for readers, just as the stories of this fourth cohort of 35 nurses make the multitude of reintegration issues "very real" for any reader of their latest book. I have a much greater appreciation for how significantly a nurse's life can be changed as a result of serving in a war zone.

Their second book, *Nurses After War: The Reintegration Experience of Nurses Returning From Iraq and Afghanistan*, I believe may well be an even more important contribution to the nursing literature. There are several important factors that set this book apart from other publications on the topic of reintegration. First, this book addresses the specific population of nurses and their homecoming and reintegration experiences; there is very little material currently in the health care literature on this issue. Because of the research methodology used by Beth and Mary Ellen, their research results have a much more powerful impact on readers. I will remember these compelling stories for many years to come because they have made a lasting impression on me. Some of the larger research studies conducted with combat veterans resonate less because they lack the personal element. This book can be a catalyst for a raised consciousness level across the entire health care industry, military and civilian settings, about how we can better support our returning combat veterans. We can not only make their homecoming and reintegration more positive experiences for them, as well as for their families and communities, but also provide a more supportive and sustained environment for them.

I personally want to thank the 35 nurses who voluntarily shared their very personal and moving stories in the hope that lessons learned from their experiences could be used to more dramatically impact future military deployments, as well as help with the reintegration of current and past combat veterans. Each nurse's story reinforces for the reader the complexity and multifaceted nature of reintegration. It is a personal journey that varies greatly from individual to individual. This book makes it exceedingly clear there should not be a "cookie-cutter" approach or a belief that a "one-size-fits-all" strategy can be used to best support our returning combat veterans.

Scannell-Desch and Doherty are to be commended for the time and effort they put into researching the many different resources that are available to veterans of the Iraq and Afghanistan wars, their families, and their communities. This level of support is so different from the Vietnam War and the two world wars of the past. There needs to be an increased awareness generally in society about the resources available to veterans to facilitate their homecoming and transition after deployment.

Scannell-Desch and Doherty have indicated that they do not plan to do any further research studies involving deployed nurses to the wars in Iraq and Afghanistan. Personally, I hope they will consider additional studies with the four different cohorts of nurses they have studied. I believe there could be considerable value in a longitudinal study with these 35 nurses that examines how they have continued to reintegrate over time, as well as any long-term impact that may be associated with their deployments to war zones.

Regardless of whether there are future studies and/or books regarding nurses in or after war in Iraq and Afghanistan, I want to express my gratitude to both Scannell-Desch and Doherty for their commitment to studying and sharing the research results on this important subject with the health care community and society. They can and should take pride in their legacy and the contribution they have made to all veterans for a more positive homecoming and successful reintegration as they resume their stateside lives with their families, coworkers, and communities. Their research efforts will make a difference in the lives of combat veterans because these authors and the nurse participants have made combat nursing, and its impact on the nurse, as real as possible, short of experiencing it personally.

In closing, I find this book to be the more profound of the two books by Scannell-Desch and Doherty because it portrays how health care providers themselves are adversely impacted as a result of providing combat casualty care in a hostile environment in order to save lives and limbs. The authors plus the nurse participants have captured so articulately and comprehensively the complexities of the entire deployment experience, especially the postdeployment impact. One of the major ironies of war is that countries and individuals become involved in conflicts with an ultimate goal of trying to make the world a safer and better place for all. Yet, in the process, combat medics themselves return home with emotional and mental health scars from their deployment. *Nurses After War* documents these phenomena in an unforgettable manner.

Linda J. Stierle, Brigadier General (Retired)
United States Air Force, Nurse Corps

Index

aeromedical evacuation,
13, 14, 15-16
Afghan National Army (ANA)
Hospitals, 14-15
Afghan war (2001-present), 5-6
After Deployment Adaptive
Parenting Tools Program
(ADAPT), 284-285
Air Expeditionary Force (AEF),
10-11, 13
Air Force C-18, 21, 23
Air Force C-132, 23
Air Force Theater Hospital, 11
Air Force: U.S. Air Force Service
Agency, 294
Air National Guard, 10-11
Al-Qaeda, 5
America Legion, 295
American Red Cross, 296
Army Medical Service, 9
Army OneSource Family Programs
and Services, 294
Army Reserve Family
Programs, 294
Army: U.S. Army MWR, 295

Base Realignment and Closure
(BRAC) commission, 10
Behavioral Couples Therapy
(BCT), 284
Bin Laden, Osama, 5
Building Resilience and Valuing
Empowered Families, 287
Bush, George H. W., 1, 3, 4

Camp Bastion, 14
Care for the Caregivers, 296
clinical change of scenery,
need for, 277
Allison, First Lieutenant, 156
Corabeth, Captain, 160
Dagmar, Lieutenant
Colonel, 161-163
Earl, Captain, 160
Julie, Lieutenant Colonel, 155-156
Kate, Lieutenant, 156
Lauren, Lieutenant, 158-160
Rhetta, First Lieutenant, 157-158
Sandra, Lieutenant, 163-164
Toni, Lieutenant Colonel, 157
Zoe, Lieutenant Commander, 158

clinical implications, 279–287
  therapeutic interventions, 280–287
combat exposures, of nurses, 274
Combat Operational Stress Control
    program (COSC), 286
combat support hospital (CSH), 12, 13
Coming Home Project, 286, 296
coping, 290
couples therapy, 284
coworkers' workplace readiness, 273
Critical Care Air Transport Team
    (CCATT), 15–17

Defense Centers of Excellence
    for Psychological Health and
    Traumatic Brain Injury
    (DCoE), 295
deployable medical facilities, 9–18
Disabled American Veterans, 296

emotion-focused therapy
    (EFT-C), 284
emotional labor, 272, 282
emotional trauma, 272

Families at Ease, 294
Families Over Coming Under Stress
    (FOCUS), 285
family and social networks, support
    versus lack of support, 293
  Allison, First Lieutenant, 213–214
  Amanda, Captain, 224–225
  Christa, Lieutenant Colonel, 208
  Courtney, Captain, 218–220
  Dagmar, Lieutenant Colonel, 221–223
  Darla, Lieutenant, 217
  Earl, Captain, 220–221
  Fred, Major, 207–208
  Julie, Lieutenant Colonel, 210–213
  Kate, Lieutenant, 208–209
  Kathleen, Lieutenant
    Commander, 210
  Regina, Lieutenant Colonel, 214–216
  Sandra, Lieutenant, 223–224
  Sarah, Colonel, 216–217

  Tammy, Lieutenant Colonel, 214
  Tenley, Captain, 220
Family Assistance Centers (FAC), 294
family readiness, 279
Family Readiness Groups (FRG), 294
family-readiness training, 289–290
family resiliency programs, 285
family support programs, 294–295
Female Veterans Initiative, 286
FOCUS Family Resilience Training,
    285, 286
Forward Resuscitative Surgery System
    (FRSS), 12
forward surgical teams (FSTs), 10,
    11–12

Gift from Within, 296
Give an Hour, 296

harassment, 275
Hearts Toward Home International, 296
Heathe N. Craig Joint Theater
    Hospital, 14
help-seeking, 276
  Amanda, Captain, 142–143
  Anita, Major, 135–138
  Brittany, Captain, 144–148
  Catherine, Lieutenant Commander,
    121–123
  Colleen, Major, 148–152
  Corabeth, Captain, 125–127
  Courtney, Captain, 127–128
  Darla, Lieutenant, 124–125
  Doreen, Lieutenant, 143–144
  Earl, Captain, 116–118
  Eliza, Major, 140–142
  Fred, Major, 138–139
  Julie, Lieutenant Colonel, 119
  Justin, Lieutenant Commander, 124
  Kate, Lieutenant, 118
  Kathleen, Lieutenant
    Commander, 116
  Marley, Captain, 130–132
  Natasha, Lieutenant Colonel,
    123–124

Rhetta, First Lieutenant, 153
Robin, Commander, 132-135
Sandra, Lieutenant, 139
Tenley, Captain, 128-130
Toni, Lieutenant Colonel, 118-119
Zoe, Lieutenant Commander,
    120-121
homecoming, disappointment, 270,
    273-274
    Catherine, Lieutenant Commander,
        68-69
    Christa, Lieutenant Colonel, 61-62
    Darby, Commander, 79-82
    Doreen, Lieutenant, 75-79
    Fred, Major, 73-74
    Justin, Lieutenant Commander,
        70-72
    Kate, Lieutenant, 62-63
    Kathleen, Lieutenant Commander,
        63-66
    Loretta, Lieutenant, 67
    Marley, Captain, 72-73
    Natasha, Lieutenant Colonel, 69-70
    Sandra, Lieutenant, 74-75
homecoming, positive reception, 270,
    273-274
    Allison, First Lieutenant, 34-38
    Amanda, Captain, 40-42
    Anita, Major, 29-30
    Brittany, Captain, 49-50
    Catherine, Lieutenant Commander,
        27-28
    Christa, Lieutenant Colonel, 44-46
    Colleen, Major, 50-53
    Darla, Lieutenant, 53-55
    Fred, Major, 48
    Lauren, Lieutenant, 32-33
    Natasha, Lieutenant Colonel, 49
    Regina, Lieutenant Colonel, 26-27
    Robin, Commander, 43-44
    Sarah, Colonel, 46-47
    Schuyler, Captain, 33-34
    Tammy, Lieutenant Colonel, 28-29
    Tenley, Captain, 47-48
    Toni, Lieutenant Colonel, 38-40

Viola, Lieutenant Colonel, 42-43
Zoe, Lieutenant Commander, 30-32
Homeless Veterans, 295
humanitarian missions, 281
Hussein, Saddam, 1, 2, 4

individual therapy, 287
individualized perspective, and
    reintegration, 280
interpersonal functioning, 274, 290
interventions for optimal individual
    and family functioning, need
    for, 280
Iraq and Afghanistan Veterans of
    America, 296
Iraqi war (2003-2011), 3-5

Joint Base Balad Air Force Theater
    Hospital, 13
Joint Family Support Assistance
    Program (JFSAP), 286
Joint Military NATO (North American
    Treaty Organization) Hospital, 14
Joint Services Military Medical
    Center, 13

Kabat-Zinn, Jon, 283
Kandahar Air Base hospital, 14

Marine Corps Community Services
    (MCCS), 295
medevac aircraft, 12, 14-15, 273
Medical Force 2000, 10
Military Homefront, 295
military medical doctrine, 10
    echelons of care, 12-13
military sexual trauma, 275
military unit or civilian job, support
    versus lack of support, 292
    Amanda, Captain, 199
    Anita, Major, 196-198
    Brittany, Captain, 199-200
    Catherine, Lieutenant Commander,
        186-187
    Christa, Lieutenant Colonel, 177-178

military unit or civilian job, support
    versus lack of support (*cont.*)
    Colleen, Major, 200–203
    Courtney, Captain, 191–192
    Dagmar, Lieutenant Colonel, 193–195
    Darla, Lieutenant, 190–191
    Earl, Captain, 192–193
    Fred, Major, 198
    Julie, Lieutenant Colonel, 181
    Justin, Lieutenant Commander,
        188–190
    Kate, Lieutenant, 178–179
    Kathleen, Lieutenant
        Commander, 180
    Loretta, Lieutenant, 180–181
    Regina, Lieutenant Colonel, 184–185
    Sandra, Lieutenant, 198–199
    Schuyler, Captain, 187–188
    Tammy, Lieutenant Colonel, 181–184
    Toni, Lieutenant Colonel, 175–177
    Viola, Lieutenant Colonel, 195–196
mindfulness-based stress reduction
    (MBSR), 283
mindfulness meditation, 282–284
The Mission Continues, 296
Mobile Army Surgical Hospital
    (MASH), 9
moral and ethical dilemmas, 274
multifaceted stressors, 281
MUST (Medical Unit Self-Contained
    Transportable), 9

National Alliance on Mental Health
    (NAMI), 295
National Association of Veterans
    Advocates, Inc. (NOVA), 295
National Center for PTSD, 281–282,
    290, 295
National Military Family Association
    (NMFA), 295
National Military Family Association
    Operation Purple Camps and
    Healing, 285–286
National Suicide Prevention
    Hotline, 295

National Veterans Foundation, 295
Navy Fleet and Family Support
    Services, 295
Navy One Source, 295
"new normal," 278
Newman's Own Foundation, 286
Nurses Organization of Veterans Affairs
    (NOVA), 295

Obama, Barack, 4, 6
ONE Freedom, Inc, 296
Operation BRAVE Families
    (OBF), 287
Operation Comfort, 296
Operation First Response, 296
Operation Homefront, 296
Operation Mend-FOCUS, 285
Operation Purple Family Retreat
    program, 286
outreach services, 279

Parent Management Training-Oregon
    Model (PTMO), 284–285
parenting complications, 273, 282,
    284–285
Persian Gulf War (1990–1991), 1–3
personal relationships, 293
petty complaints and trivial whining,
    276, 293
    Amanda, Captain, 172–173
    Courtney, Captain, 168
    Dagmar, Lieutenant Colonel, 168
    Earl, Captain, 173
    Eliza, Major, 171–172
    Julie, Lieutenant Colonel, 169
    Loretta, Lieutenant, 168–169
    Rhetta, First Lieutenant, 173–174
    Robin, Commander, 169–170
    Sandra, Lieutenant, 170–171
physical functioning, 290
physical well-being, 275–276
posttraumatic stress disorder (PTSD),
    271, 277, 289, 292–293
    risk factors, 281
preexisting family problems, 284

Provincial Reconstruction Team
(PRT), 17-18
psychological signs and symptoms, 290
psychological trauma, 277
psychosocial functioning, 290

Rand Corporation, 296
Real Warriors Campaign, 295
reasons for joining military, 271-272
recreation and self-care, 290
Red Cross Coming Home Series, 287
reintegration, 276, 290-294
    Allison, First Lieutenant, 239
    Amanda, Captain, 259-260
    Anita, Major, 256-257
    Brittany, Captain, 260-261
    Catherine, Lieutenant
        Commander, 239
    Colleen, Major, 261-263
    Corabeth, Captain, 245
    Courtney, Captain, 245
    Dagmar, Lieutenant Colonel,
        254-255
    Darby, Commander, 263-264
    Darla, Lieutenant, 244
    Doreen, Lieutenant, 260
    Earl, Captain, 250-254
    Eliza, Major, 258-259
    findings, 269
    Fred, Major, 257-258
    Julie, Lieutenant Colonel, 234
    Kate, Lieutenant, 227-228
    Kathleen, Lieutenant Commander,
        229-232
    Lauren, Lieutenant, 239-241
    Loretta, Lieutenant, 232-234
    Marley, Captain, 248-250
    Schuyler, Captain, 241-244
    Tammy, Lieutenant Colonel, 238-239
    Tenley, Captain, 245-248
    Toni, Lieutenant Colonel, 228-229
    Viola, Lieutenant Colonel, 255-256
    Zoe, Lieutenant Commander,
        235-238
renegotiating family roles
    Anita, Major, 87-88
    Eliza, Major, 89-90
    Fred, Major, 88
    Julie, Lieutenant Colonel, 83-84
    Kate, Lieutenant, 85-86
    Sandra, Lieutenant, 88-89
    Tammy, Lieutenant Colonel, 87
    Toni, Lieutenant Colonel, 84-85
    Zoe, Lieutenant Commander, 86-87
Reservists and National Guard, 276
resiliency during reintegration, 289
Returning Veterans Project, 296
Returning Warrior Workshop, 287

September 12, 2001 attack, 5
sexual harassment, 275
shock-trauma platoon (STP), 12
Soldier's Heart, 296
The Soldiers Project, 296
stigma
    defined, 115
    getting help for (*See* help-seeking)
Strategic Outreach for Families of All
    Reservists (SOFAR), 295
stress management, 272-273, 290
support system, and coping and
    resilience, 272, 275
support systems, 280

Task Force Med, 13-14
TeleFOCUS, 285
therapeutic interventions, 280-287
trauma, painful memories of, 273,
        274-275, 290
    Allison, First Lieutenant, 98-99
    Amanda, Captain, 102-103
    Anita, Major, 99-101
    Brittany, Captain, 105-106
    Catherine, Lieutenant Commander,
        95-96
    Courtney, Captain, 97-98
    Darby, Commander, 106-111
    Darla, Lieutenant, 97
    Doreen, Lieutenant, 103-105
    Julie, Lieutenant Colonel, 93-94

trauma, painful memories of (*cont.*)
  Justin, Lieutenant Commander, 96–97
  Loretta, Lieutenant, 91–92
  Rhetta, First Lieutenant, 92–93
  Robin, Commander, 99
  Sandra, Lieutenant, 101
  Zoe, Lieutenant Commander, 94–95

UCLA Health System, 285
UCLA Nathanson Family Resilience
  Center, 285–286, 296
UCLA Welcome Back Veterans Family
  Resilience Center, 286
USCENTCOM (United States Central
  Command), 11
U.S. Department of Defense Sexual
  Assault Prevention and
  Response, 295
USN Mercy, 21
USO Services, 295

VA Center for Women Veterans, 295

VA National Suicide Prevention
  Hotline, 295
Vet Centers, 290, 295
Veteran Love, 296
Veterans for America, 296
Veterans' Administration (VA), 281, 293
Veterans Affairs (VA) Services, 295
Veterans Crisis Line, 295
Vets4Vets, 296

Warrior Mind Training (WMT), 287
welcome home event, 292
Women Veterans Health Care in the
  VA, 295
Women Veterans: Center for Women
  Veterans, 295
work functioning, 290
worries and concerns of returning
  veterans, 275

Yellow Ribbon Reintegration Program
  (YRRP), 287